BACKPACKING CALIFORNIA

Mountain, Foothill, Coastal, & Desert Adventures in the Golden State

From the Expert Authors of **WILDERNESS PRESS**

 WILDERNESS PRESS ... *on the trail since 1967*

BERKELEY, CA

Backpacking California:
Mountain, Foothill, Coastal, & Desert Adventures in the Golden State

1st EDITION May 2001
2nd EDITION July 2008
  2nd printing 2010

Front cover photos copyright © 2008 by (clockwise from top) Bill Stevenson c/o Mira, Michael McKay, Mathew Grimm, and John Elk
Section opener photos by the following: David Money Harris, pp. 9 and 37; Matt Heid, p. 70; Mike White, pp. xiv, 160, 254, 438, and 459; Elizabeth Wenk, p. 209; and Jeffrey P. Schaffer, p. 343
Interior photos: All photographs placed in a particular trip are by that trip's author, except the following: Tim Oren, p. 114; Tom Winnett, p. 378; and Laura Shauger, pp. 95, 98, and 120.
Maps: Bart Wright, Lohnes + Wright
Cover and book design: Larry B. Van Dyke
Book editors: Laura Shauger, Roslyn Bullas, and Eva Dienel

ISBN: 978-0-89997-446-0
Manufactured in China

Published by: **Wilderness Press**
           1345 8th Street
           Berkeley, CA 94710
           (800) 443-7227; FAX (510) 558-1696
           info@wildernesspress.com
           www.wildernesspress.com

Visit our website for a complete listing of our books and for ordering information.
Distributed by Publishers Group West

Cover photos (clockwise from top): Hiking near dawn at Truckee; Marble Canyon, Death Valley National Park (Trip 35); Coast Trail, Point Reyes National Seashore (Trip 23); and Garnet Lake in Ansel Adams Wilderness (Trip 49)

*Wilderness Press dedicates this book to
California's wild places and their defenders—
past, present, and future.*

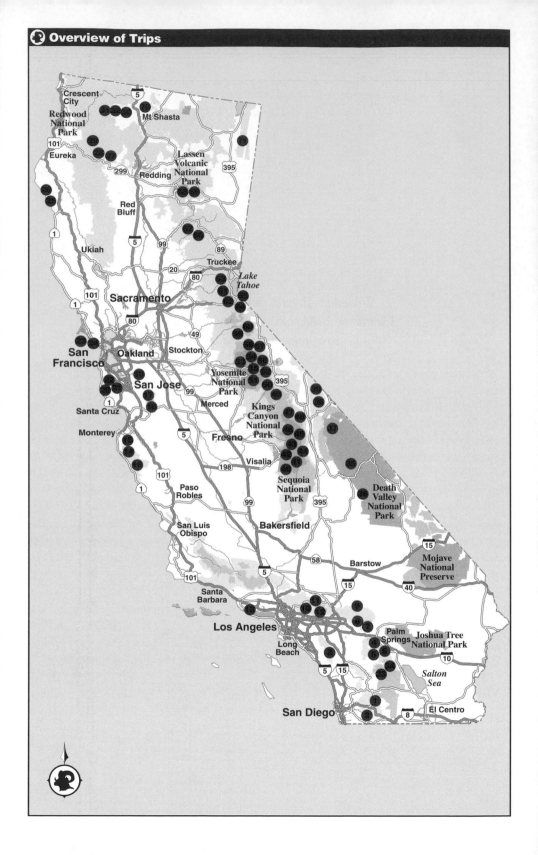

CONTENTS

WESTERN CALIFORNIA

FOREWORD *by Eric Blehm*

I grew up on Sunny Mountain Ranch, which wasn't a working ranch but rather 34 acres on the west side of North Lake Wohlford Road, in a rural town called Valley Center in east San Diego County. I learned "directions" at a young age, and scoured every inch of our property in search of blue-bellied lizards, veins of gold (the fool's variety), and a certain tree, rock, or brush pile that would become the foundations of my next fort.

Our property butted up against the Mountain, as we called it, the geographic feature that both consumed the bulk of the acreage and was the inspiration for the name of our home. Most of my young life was spent between the boundaries of the road and the property line that was drawn (north to south) along the top of the Mountain, not far above a huge granite slab we named Zebra Rock because of its striping.

The Mountain, which may as well have been Everest, was around a thousand vertical feet from our driveway to the top and densely vegetated by chaparral, manzanita, and sagebrush. It was shaded generously by giant oaks spilling down into a pasture that was my parents' garden, and, for a time, our Christmas tree farm. As a kid, I was never satisfied until I reached the top of every climbing tree, so when it came to exploring I always gravitated up onto the Mountain—higher and higher as my parents played out more and more leash, trusting, even by age six or seven, that I probably knew the ranch better than they did.

But it was easy to get lost up there on the Mountain, both figuratively and literally, especially when my eyes were fixated on the immediate surroundings—alert to rattlesnakes, red ant piles, poison oak, and the source of the wild howls we heard every night. It was the Mountain that introduced me to the idea of wilderness and how little is needed to escape. It was also a constant reminder to never forsake what's in our own backyard.

Like most outdoor-minded kids in Southern California, I was initiated to overnight hiking and "real" mountains with the High Sierra. The Range of Light brought perspective to things I had once considered big, tall, and vast. I was fourteen at the time of my first backpacking experience and Cottonwood Pass, my doorway to the high country, still evokes nostalgia twenty-six years later. Once my father and I made camp and counterbalanced our food bags, I stalked golden trout in a narrow stream that crossed a lush green meadow. The creek gurgles through my memory. The Shakespeare Rod and Garcia reel my oldest brother gave me is still vivid: the feel of the cork grip, the red-handled needle-nosed pliers I used to bend down the barbs on Eagle Claw hooks that I drifted weightless with salmon eggs for bait into likely pools and undercut banks.

I found romance in the beckoning narrow line of the trail cutting across the meadow and disappearing into the distant treeline. Imagine the excitement when the ranger checking our permits told us that our trail was a day's hike to a lake whose name I can't remember, but what he called a "sure thing."

I woke the next morning before the sun—if I slept at all. The meadow had a mist hugging its contours, and the thick slabs of Spam my dad fried up for breakfast atop slices of hearty wheat bread were wrapped in tin foil that was hot to the touch when I tucked it inside my jacket pocket. We stirred the mist with our legs as we followed the trail. I felt like the man in Jack London's "To Build a Fire" when I pulled out the still-warm Spam sandwich from my jacket pocket an hour later. The man had noted the same comforting warmth of his biscuits—cut in half and soaked in the grease from the slab of bacon he'd fried for breakfast that morning—when he lunched on them.

After our meal, we climbed out of our Yukon to a clear blue, tropical reef–like lake that proved to be loaded with trout. When I left the group to circumnavigate its shores alone, I was Robinson Crusoe angling for my lunch. There's magic in wild places, and there's not a spot I've ever visited that doesn't call me back.

I'm often drawn back to my earliest jaunts into the wilds of my childhood, before my sojourns into the Sierra, Dolomites, Alps, Alborz, and Himalayas, to when I was eight or nine, chugging a warm canteen of Kool-Aid in the shade of an oak tree at the upper elevations of Sunny Mountain Ranch. By that point I knew, or had blazed myself, every trail on the Mountain and had been recruited more than once to guide "old people" up its face. My older brother's Harley-riding friends dubbed me Eric the Red because I was always exploring, always finding new ways up the Mountain.

That's what this book is all about: finding new ways up the mountain whether it's in our own backyard or over yonder. California's wilderness areas are like Never Never Land. Just tighten up your laces, pick a trailhead, and keep on hiking straight 'til midnight.

Eric Blehm is the author of *The Last Season*, the true story of the life and mysterious disappearance of legendary backcountry ranger Randy Morgenson in the high country of Sequoia and Kings Canyon National Parks. Learn more at www.thelastseason.com. Blehm won the prestigious 2006 Barnes & Noble Discover Award, naming him the best new author of the year in the category of nonfiction. He lives in Southern California with his wife and two young children and is currently working on his next nonfiction book, which is set in Afghanistan.

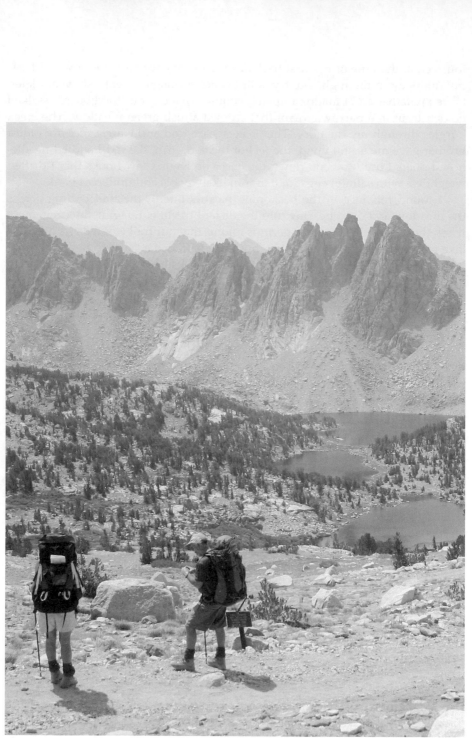

View of Kearsarge Lakes, Trip 43

INTRODUCTION

First and foremost, this book offers you some of the best and most diverse California backpacking trips, as selected by Wilderness Press editors and documented by 16 of our experienced authors. Some authors have described their favorite trips elsewhere; others are presenting them here in print for the first time. Taken together, these 71 trips cover the major bio-regions of California, including the mountains, foothills, coast, and desert. The book divides the state into eastern and western sections; within those sections, the trips are organized south to north. This second edition features expanded coverage in Big Sur, Anza-Borrego, Death Valley, and the White Mountains.

For Wilderness Press, California is home turf, where our founder Tom Winnett coauthored a new kind of guidebook geared toward the serious backpacker. Tom launched Wilderness Press with *Sierra North* in 1967 and followed it with other titles for and by keen hikers, which soon became the core of our extensive list. Those men and women who approached Tom with their first manuscripts have grown older, but, in so doing they have covered thousands of trail miles and gained a wealth of backpacking experience. And since then, many younger Wilderness Press authors have joined their ranks, compiling meticulous trip descriptions and highly detailed maps. Short of hiring a Wilderness Press author as your guide, this book offers you the most complete repository of what these expert authors have learned and the wonders they've seen.

While ensuring the overall high standards of this book, we didn't crimp our proven authors' styles, for style is a direct reflection of personality. A response to the glorious, majestic places of the earth is a person's own. When we enter the wilderness—whether savoring a pristine cirque below sawtooth pinnacles, camping high above crashing waves in the coastal range, or trekking remote desert canyons—we come away with an expanded sense of freedom borne out in the rich variety of life everywhere apparent. Delve deeply, enjoy, and pass it on.

HOW TO USE THIS BOOK

This book's 71 trips are divided into geographic regions within two main sections: western and eastern California. Within those sections, the trips are organized roughly south to north. The western portion is subdivided into the following sections: the Peninsular Ranges, Transverse Ranges, Coast Ranges, and Klamath Mountains. The eastern portion is subdivided into desert, the southern Sierra Nevada, northern Sierra Nevada, Cascade Range, and Warner Mountains. Referring to the table of contents and corresponding locator map, as well as the appendix of trips-at-a-glance, you should be able to easily identify the trips that most interest you.

Each of these geographic subregions begins with a short introduction to the area, with very brief background information on geology, geography, history, and managing agencies, for instance. The introductions are each written by that region's contributors, Wilderness Press's best guides to the region.

Because this book assumes you have basic knowledge of and experience backpacking, there are not introductory chapters covering basic techniques and gear. If you are looking for that sort of information, consult more general how-to books like *Joy of Backpacking* also published by Wilderness Press. Sprinkled throughout this book are sidebars focused on side trips for a given route and tips from the contributors, sometimes specific to a given trip or region and other times more general.

THE TRIPS

Each trip includes a simple trail map showing the starting and ending points, as well as all the trip's major locations. Each trip is divided into the following sections: summary information, permits, take this trip, challenges, how to get there, a trip description, and build-up and wind-down tips.

SUMMARY INFORMATION ·

Each trip begins with a block of summary information, with the following categories of information: miles, recommended days, elevation gain/loss, type of trip, difficulty, solitude, location, maps, and best season.

> **MILES:** Each trip's distance is listed in miles to the nearest tenth.

> **RECOMMENDED DAYS:** Each trip lists the number of days (if it's a short trip) or a range in which the average backpacker can complete it.

> **ELEVATION GAIN/LOSS:** Each trip includes elevation figures. Separate loss and gain figures are provided where they're available. If those are not available, the elevation fluctuation of the trip is provided.

TYPE OF TRIP: Each trip falls into one of four types: point-to-point, out-and-back, semiloop, or loop.

DIFFICULTY: Each trip is assigned a difficulty rating, based on what backpackers they're most appropriate for:

> **Easy:** Suitable for beginners
>
> **Moderate:** Suitable for physically fit hikers
>
> **Moderately strenuous:** Suitable for experienced hikers in extremely good physical condition
>
> **Strenuous:** Has one or more of the following characteristics: high mileage, substantial elevation gain/loss, cross-country travel, or navigation challenges

SOLITUDE: Each trip is assigned a solitude rating, based on its popularity:

> **Crowded:** You'll see many other hikers or backpackers for most of the trip.
>
> **Moderately populated:** You'll definitely see other hikers or backpackers, but they'll likely be spread out.
>
> **Moderate solitude:** You'll see others only occasionally.
>
> **Solitude:** You're virtually guaranteed to see few, if any, other people for most of the trip.

LOCATION: This section lists the location of the given route, whether it be a local park, state park, wilderness area, national forest, or national park.

MAPS: This section lists the applicable 7.5-minute U.S. Geological Survey topographical map or other commercial map available for the area and appropriate for backpacking.

BEST SEASON: This section lists the seasons the trip is accessible and most enjoyable.

PERMITS

This section mentions any permits necessary for a particular trip and provides details about how to obtain them.

TAKE THIS TRIP

This section conveys the highlights of a given trip and explains why it's worthwhile.

CHALLENGES

This section explains the main challenges of a given trip beyond those involved generally when backpacking in the wilderness. Any unusually challenging sections or special problems that the average backpacker would need to prepare for are covered.

HOW TO GET THERE

This section provides directions to the trailhead(s) from the nearest major interstate or highway.

TRIP DESCRIPTION

In this section, the author provides a detailed description of every segment of the trail, with mention of the available campsites, water sources, vegetation you'll see, any wildlife you might expect to see, where to turn at each junction, possible side trips, and much more.

BUILD-UP AND WIND-DOWN TIPS

This section features places or experiences in the vicinity of the trip that backpackers can enjoy right before or after a trip, such as a restaurant, nearby hot springs or swimming hole, frontcountry campground, and more.

Map Legend

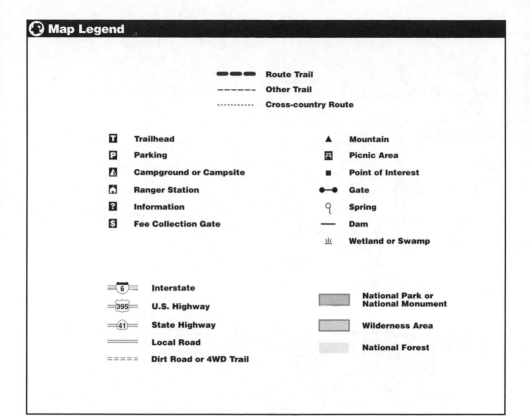

▬ ▬ ▬	Route Trail		
- - - - - -	Other Trail		
....	Cross-country Route		

T	Trailhead	▲	Mountain
P	Parking		Picnic Area
	Campground or Campsite	■	Point of Interest
	Ranger Station	●—●	Gate
?	Information	♀	Spring
S	Fee Collection Gate	—	Dam
		ⅶ	Wetland or Swamp

⑤	Interstate		National Park or National Monument
395	U.S. Highway		Wilderness Area
㊶	State Highway		National Forest
	Local Road		
=====	Dirt Road or 4WD Trail		

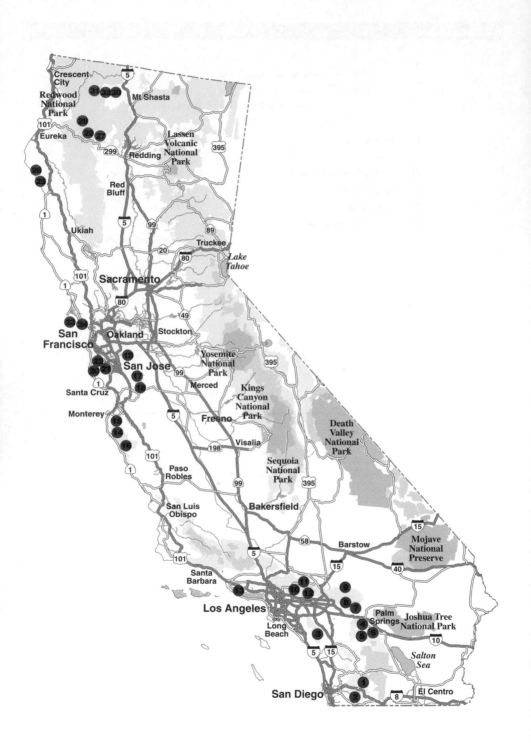

WESTERN CALIFORNIA

THE PENINSULAR RANGES

The Peninsular Ranges in the southernmost part of California belong to a series of mountains stretching some 1000 miles south—all the way down the Baja California peninsula. These ranges are generally parallel to one another, and they trend northwest-southeast, which is typical of the "grain" of almost all the major mountain ranges in California. As in the Sierra Nevada range (the backbone of the northern two-thirds of California) the Peninsular Ranges tend to have dramatically steep eastern slopes and more gradually inclined western slopes.

The northernmost and highest peak in the Peninsular Ranges is San Jacinto Peak, elevation 10,804 feet, in Riverside County. South from there the range slopes down to somewhat lesser elevations in the Palomar, Cuyamaca, and Laguna mountains of San Diego County. A bit lower still are the Santa Ana Mountains, which form the eastern border of Orange County.

Because the Peninsular Ranges stretch from near the coast to the desert, and rise (sometimes abruptly) from elevations of near sea level, there is a startling diversity of climate and vegetation. Nearly every major climate zone and major type of plant community found in the whole state of California can be found here. For example, desert scrub vegetation endures summertime temperatures as high as 120°F at the foot of San Jacinto Peak, while the top of the peak, only a few miles away, barely pokes into the arctic-alpine climate zone, where even the hardiest evergreen trees cannot survive. In between are belts of chaparral and various zones of oak and coniferous forest.

Since no part of Peninsular Ranges territory lies very far away from paved highways and dirt roads, dayhiking is more popular than overnight backpacking. Most wilderness-oriented backpacking trips are of the weekend variety. Multiday trips along the Pacific Crest Trail are possible, but these excursions tend to cross roads fairly frequently.

9

LAGUNA MOUNTAINS

East of the Cuyamaca Mountains—the first great moisture-wringing barrier to Pacific storms within central San Diego County—lies a slightly lower and drier range, the Laguna Mountains. Here, storm clouds yield enough precipitation to support a patchwork forest of Jeffrey pines and black oaks. Farther east still, the land falls away abruptly. Below this sheer escarpment lies the desert.

The Laguna Mountains lie mostly within the jurisdiction of Cleveland National Forest, though some private lands on the mountain have recently been purchased for inclusion in Anza-Borrego Desert State Park, which sprawls east over a space of about 1000 square miles. About 70 miles of hiking trails lace through Laguna mountain territory, including a roughly 25-mile stretch of the Pacific Crest Trail, and a 10-mile stretch of the Noble Canyon National Recreation Trail. For several miles the PCT edges close to the spectacular eastern escarpment (the "sunrise" side) of the Lagunas. Nowhere else in San Diego County can you so dramatically experience the interface between mountain and desert. Much of this stretch, however, closely parallels the scenic Sunrise Highway, and is suited best for casual dayhiking. Somewhat more remote areas on the mountain can be explored on the Noble Canyon Trail.

PINE CREEK WILDERNESS

The Cleveland National Forest's Pine Creek Wilderness, created in 1984, encompasses more than 13,000 acres of chaparral-covered slopes and riparian woodland south and west of the Laguna Mountains. A 15-mile stretch of Pine Valley Creek (or "Pine Creek" as it is often referred to) meanders through the heart of the wilderness, flanked by sloping walls up to 1000 feet high.

Since elevations in Pine Creek Wilderness are generally quite low (typically 2000 to 4000 feet), and the area lies close to San Diego, this is a good place for a quick getaway during the cooler, wetter, greener months of the year—typically February through April. The logical destination for backpackers is Pine Creek itself, which may carry anywhere from a trickle to a torrent of water, depending on the amount of recent rainfall.

SAN MATEO CANYON WILDERNESS

Deep within the Santa Ana Mountains, east of the Orange County metropolis and near the spreading suburbs of southern Riverside County, San Mateo Canyon Wilderness covers 62 square miles of Cleveland National Forest territory. Some 5 million people live within 30 miles of the wilderness, yet this proximity does not guarantee easy access. Some formerly unpaved access roads have recently turned into marginally paved ones; still, they may be closed during periods of bad weather. Other, former fire roads have been abandoned for motorized use and turned into trails.

Exploring the inner sanctum of the wilderness, which is basically the bottomlands of San Mateo Canyon and its several tributaries, can be both physically taxing and mentally stimulating. Trails sometimes melt into the scenery, making it easy to lose track of your position. If you're willing to put up with these difficulties, though, this is your paradise! Just be sure to choose a time of year (winter and spring) when the landscape is green with new growth and the canyon bottoms whisper with the sounds of cascading water.

THE SAN JACINTO MOUNTAINS

Of the Peninsular Ranges, only the San Jacintos and the Sierra San Pedro Martir in Baja California rise above 10,000 feet. San Jacinto Peak is the loftiest summit in the entire mountain province. The summit country of the San Jacintos, well above the highways and byways that penetrate the lower slopes, is a sky island of delectable alpine wilderness, unsurpassed in Southern California. Under white granite summits and boulder-stacked ridges lie little hanging valleys and tapered benches lush with forest and meadow. A multitude of bubbling springs nourish icy-cold streams that tumble and cascade down the mountain.

San Bernardino National Forest (which mostly covers the San Bernardino Mountains to the north) has primary jurisdiction over the San Jacintos, though the topmost elevations of the mountains are administered as a wilderness area by the California state parks department. A multitude of trails radiates across San Jacinto territory, primarily from trailheads near the resort community of Idyllwild on the west slope, and from the upper (mountain) station of the Palm Springs Aerial Tramway. Backpacking opportunities range from easy overnight (mostly on the tramway side) to multiday loops or traverses across the north-south length or the east-west width of the mountain range.

The San Jacinto Mountains are popular, not only because of their alpine beauty, but also because they are conveniently accessible to a population of some 20 million. In certain seasons camping or wilderness permits are hard to come by, so advance planning is wise.

THE SANTA ROSA MOUNTAINS

The Santa Rosa and San Jacinto Mountains National Monument was established by the U.S. Congress in 2000 to protect these outstanding natural and cultural resources. Encompassing 272,000 acres, the land is administered by a wide variety of governmental agencies, the Agua Caliente Band of Cahuilla Indians, and many private landowners. In general, the U.S. Forest Service is responsible for the higher mountains, the Bureau of Land Management is responsible for the desert regions, and the Agua Caliente Band is responsible for Palm Canyon. The national monument contains three notable wilderness areas, including the 64,000-acre Santa Rosa Mountains Wilderness.

The Santa Rosa Mountains are one of the few remaining homes for the endangered Peninsular bighorn sheep. An estimated 350 of the majestic but shy animals roam the rocky desert slopes. Count yourself fortunate if you catch a fleeting glimpse of them during a winter of hiking in these mountains. Their numbers have been steadily declining as human development encroaches on their habitat.

The Coachella Valley and Santa Rosa Mountains are among of the hottest and driest parts of the U.S. When much of the Los Angeles basin shivers under winter rain clouds, the Santa Rosas are usually sunny and mild, perfect for hiking. Nevertheless, be ready for anything—the desert is known for rapid changes of weather and for rare but intense showers that will chill the unprepared hiker and unleash flash floods down the canyons.

Santa Rosa is a popular name in California. Be careful not to confuse the Santa Rosa Mountains with the Santa Rosa Plateau Ecological Preserve (near Murrieta) or the seat of Sonoma County.

Numerous trails crisscross the cactus-clad wilderness, but few are shown on U.S. Geological Survey maps. A new map of the area depicting these trails should be available from the Santa Rosa Monument Visitor Center by the time you are reading this. Plan carefully because reliable water sources are scarce. Adventurous backpackers will relish exploring the ancient Indian paths that lace the hills and canyons, including Palm Canyon, the Guadalupe Trail, and the Cactus Spring Trail.

NOBLE CANYON TRAIL

JERRY SCHAD

MILES: 10.0 total; 5.0 to wilderness campsites
RECOMMENDED DAYS: 2
ELEVATION GAIN/LOSS: 650´/2400´
TYPE OF TRIP: Point-to-point
DIFFICULTY: Moderate
SOLITUDE: Moderately populated
LOCATION: Laguna Mountain Recreation Area,
    Cleveland National Forest
MAPS: USGS 7.5-min. *Monument Peak*, *Mount Laguna*, and *Descanso*
BEST SEASONS: Fall, winter, and spring

PERMITS

A remote camping permit is required for overnight stays. Campfires are prohibited; stove use is permitted when fire-hazard conditions are not severe. Cars parked at the trailheads must display a National Forest Adventure Pass. Contact Descanso Ranger District, Cleveland National Forest at 619-445-6235 or visit www.fs.fed.us/r5/cleveland.

Photo: Lower Noble Canyon panorama

TAKE THIS TRIP

Freeway-close to San Diego residents, Noble Canyon in the Laguna Mountains offers a look at the way rural Southern California used to be a century ago. It's nice to explore an area where the wind sweeps through pine needles, raptors soar overhead, and a crystal-clear brook sings as it tumbles over stone—all with barely a hint of modern civilization. Botanically, this one-way downhill trip takes you from a zone of conifers and oaks into fragrant chaparral.

CHALLENGES

The route, officially known as the Noble Canyon National Recreation Trail, is designed for multiple uses, including mountain biking. Naturally the bikers prefer the downhill direction, and some are likely to be moving excessively fast.

Snow visits the canyon on several occasions during winter, but it usually melts within a day or two. By late summer or early fall, the brook in Noble Canyon could dry up.

HOW TO GET THERE

North End: Exit Interstate 8 at Sunrise Highway, just east of Pine Valley. Drive north, uphill, on Sunrise Highway, observing the mile markers, which increase from approximately mile 13.5 at the I-8/Sunrise Highway interchange. Drive to the Penny Pines Trailhead, mile 27.3, where parking space is plentiful along the highway shoulder.

South End: From the town of Pine Valley, drive west 1 mile on Old Highway 80 to Pine Creek Road, next to a bridge over Pine Valley Creek. Turn right and proceed 1.6 miles to the Noble Canyon Trailhead on the right.

TRIP DESCRIPTION

From the Penny Pines Trailhead, head west along the marked Noble Canyon Trail. After passing through a parklike setting of Jeffrey pines, you rise a bit along the north slope of a steep hill. From there, the tree-framed view extends to the distant summits of San Jacinto Peak and San Gorgonio Mountain. Next, you descend to cross dirt roads three times and then climb and circle around the chaparral-clad north end of a north-south trending ridge. Three varieties of blooming ceanothus brighten the view in springtime.

Next, you descend into the upper reaches of Noble Canyon, where the grassy hillsides show off springtime blooms of blue-purple beard tongue, scarlet bugler, woolly blue curls,

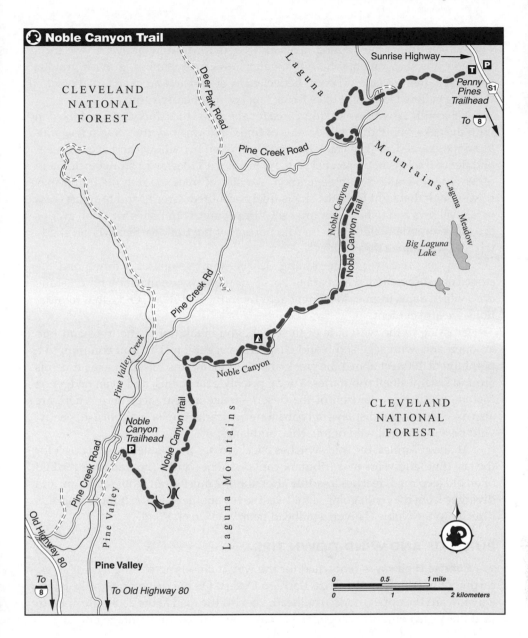

Noble Canyon Trail

yellow monkeyflower, Indian paintbrush, wallflower, white forget-me-not, wild hyacinth, yellow violet, phacelia, golden yarrow, checker, lupine, and blue flax.

The trail sidles up to the creek at about 3.0 miles, and stays beside it for the next 4 miles. Past a canopy of live oaks, black oaks, and Jeffrey pines, you emerge into a steep, sunlit section of canyon. The trail cuts through thick brush on the east wall, while on the west wall only a few hardy, drought-tolerant plants cling to outcrops of schist rock.

Back in the shade of oaks again, you soon cross a tributary creek from the east, which drains the Laguna lakes and Laguna Meadow above. Pause for a while in this shady glen, where the water flows over somber, grayish granitic rock and gathers in languid pools bedecked by sword and bracken fern. Look for nodding yellow Humboldt lilies in the late spring or early summer.

You continue within a riparian area for some distance downstream. Mixed in with the oaks, you'll discover dozens of fine California bay trees and a few scattered incense cedars. The creek lies mostly hidden by willows and sycamores—and dense thickets of poison oak, squaw bush, wild rose, wild strawberries, and other types of water-loving vegetation. The line of trees shading the trail is narrow enough that light from the sky is freely admitted. Greens and browns—and in fall, yellows and reds—glow intensely. Impromptu campsites for small groups are fairly abundant along this middle portion of the trail, particularly on shady terraces well above the creek.

You may discover some mining debris—the remains of a flume and the stones of a disassembled arrastra (a horse- or mule-drawn machine for crushing ore), which dates from gold-mining activity in the late 1800s. Old cabin foundations are also evident.

Crossing to the west side of the creek, you break out of the trees and into an open area with sage scrub and chaparral vegetation. The trail contours to a point about 100 feet above the creek and then maintains this course as it bends around several small tributaries. Yucca, prickly pear cactus, and even hedgehog cactus—normally a denizen of the desert—make appearances here. There are also excellent vernal displays of beard tongue, scarlet bugler, paintbrush, peony, wild pea, milkweed, wild onion, chia, and larkspur.

At about 7 miles, the trail switches back, crosses the Noble Canyon creek for the last time, and veers up a tributary canyon to the south. The trail joins the bed of an old jeep road, reaches a saddle after about 2 miles from Noble Canyon, and diverges from the road, going right (west) over another saddle. It then descends directly to the Noble Canyon Trailhead near Pine Creek Road.

BUILD-UP AND WIND-DOWN TIPS ·

Sunrise Highway is renowned for the way it chisels across the face of an escarpment overlooking the Anza-Borrego Desert. On the drive up Sunrise Highway toward the upper (north) trailhead, veer off the road at the 23.8-mile mark to visit the Vista Point near Stephenson Peak, one of the better vantage points.

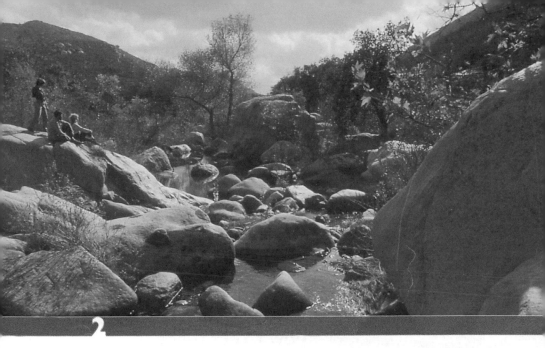

HORSETHIEF CANYON

Jerry Schad

MILES: 2.8 round-trip (easily extended with dayhikes)
RECOMMENDED DAYS: 2
ELEVATION GAIN/LOSS: 500´/500´
TYPE OF TRIP: Out-and-back
DIFFICULTY: Moderate
SOLITUDE: Moderate solitude
LOCATION: Pine Creek Wilderness, Cleveland National Forest
MAPS: USGS 7.5-min. *Barrett Lake* and *Viejas Mountain*
BEST SEASONS: Winter and spring

PERMITS

A wilderness permit is required for overnight stays. Campfires are prohibited; stove use is permitted when fire-hazard conditions are not severe. Cars parked at the trailhead must display a National Forest Adventure Pass. Contact Descanso Ranger District, Cleveland National Forest at 619-445-6235 or visit www.fs.fed.us/r5/cleveland.

Photo: Pine Valley Creek near Espinosa Trail

CHALLENGES

You may encounter groups of undocumented immigrants traveling north from Mexico on foot. It's safer to hike in groups in any area close to the border. You should also hide your camping gear when you are away from camp.

Large portions of the Pine Creek Wilderness have burned repeatedly. The Horse Fire of July 2006 consumed chaparral in the southern one-third of the wilderness area, including the area covered in this trip. Although the trails have reopened, it may take several years before the oak-woodland and chaparral landscape fully recovers.

HOW TO GET THERE

Exit Interstate 8 at Tavern Road in Alpine, 25 miles east of San Diego. Go south on Tavern, which after about 3 miles becomes Japatul Road. After a total of 9.5 miles from I-8, turn right on Lyons Valley Road. Go 1.5 miles south to the Pine Creek Wilderness trailhead on the left.

TRIP DESCRIPTION

Since this trip is so short, plan to start hiking in the afternoon, and make use of the next morning, when the air is fresh, for dayhikes. From the trailhead parking lot, walk north along a gated dirt road for about 300 yards. Then veer right on the Espinosa Trail, which quickly enters Pine Creek Wilderness. After a fast, 400-foot elevation loss, Espinosa Trail bends right (east) to follow live-oak- and sycamore-lined Horsethief Canyon. True to its name, this corral-like canyon was used in the late 1800s by horse thieves to stash stolen horses in preparation for their passage across the international border. The canyon bottom is dry about half the year, but always agreeably shaded.

After another mile and not much more descent, you cross over to the left side of

TAKE THIS TRIP

The croak of a soaring raven cracks the morning stillness as you saunter down from your campsite to the placidly flowing creek. A groggy dragonfly flits through a beam of sunlight. Cool air, slinking down the night-chilled slopes, caresses your face and sets aflutter the papery sycamore leaves overhead. You cup the clear, cold water in the palms of your hands and splash it across your head. Ahhh! If you want this kind of escape from the city—and you want it relatively quickly—Horsethief Canyon and Pine Valley Creek, just east of San Diego, is one good place to find it.

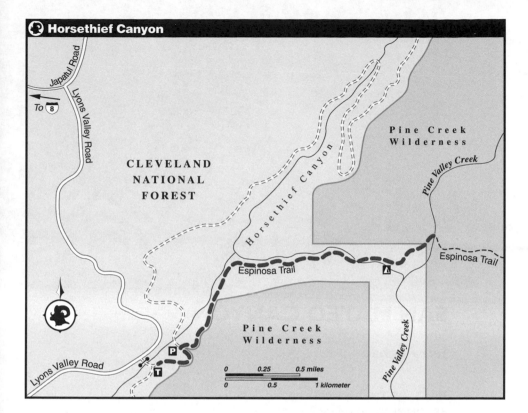

Horsethief Canyon's little creek, a couple of minutes short of its confluence with the much wetter Pine Valley Creek. Look to your right (south) to spot a broad, grassy bench, densely shaded by coast live oaks. This is one possible wilderness camping spot in the immediate area.

In the morning you can try heading a mile or two downstream (south) along the bank of Pine Valley Creek. This involves easy walking and is fine for wildflower watching in the spring season. More adventurously, you can head upstream into the Pine Valley Creek gorge. Beyond a large pool immediately upstream from the Espinosa Trail crossing is a picturesque jumble of car-sized boulders and several mini-waterfalls. Watch your step on the slippery rock, and watch out for poison oak and rattlesnakes. If the water level is too high, don't do this. Beyond the narrowest constriction, the rock-bound canyon widens somewhat and remains scenic for miles ahead.

BUILD-UP AND WIND-DOWN TIPS ·

Food cravings can be satisfied at the **Bread Basket** restaurant in the Alpine Creek shopping area, on the east side of Tavern Road, 0.2 mile south of Interstate 8. The restaurant features a large, shaded patio area for outdoor dining.

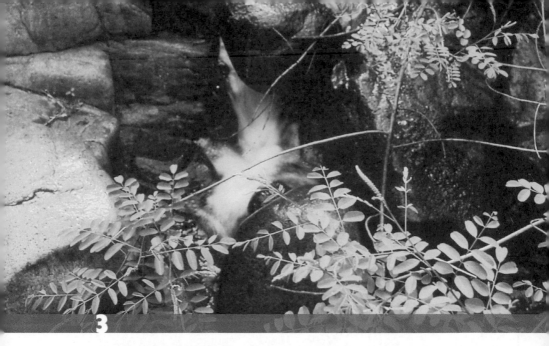

3

SAN MATEO CANYON

Jerry Schad

MILES: 7.4 (easily extended with dayhikes)
RECOMMENDED DAYS: 2
ELEVATION GAIN/LOSS: 1300´/1300´
TYPE OF TRIP: Out-and-back
DIFFICULTY: Moderate
SOLITUDE: Moderate solitude
LOCATION: San Mateo Canyon Wilderness, Cleveland National Forest
MAPS: USGS 7.5-min. *Wildomar* and *Sitton Peak*
BEST SEASONS: Winter and spring

PERMITS ·

A wilderness permit is required for overnight stays. Campfires are prohibited; stove use is permitted when fire-hazard conditions are not severe. Cars parked at the trailhead must display a National Forest Adventure Pass. Contact Trabuco Ranger District, Cleveland National Forest at 951-736-1811 or visit www.fs.fed.us/r5/cleveland.

Photo: *Mini-cascade in San Mateo Canyon*

CHALLENGES

The San Mateo Canyon Wilderness is hot and dry much of the year, and exceedingly parched in the month or two before the first substantial rainfall—which may not come until December or January. The area also harbors plenty of rattlesnakes, which are mostly out and about during the onset of warm weather in April and May. If it's very warm, bring plenty of water for the hike back out, which is almost entirely uphill.

HOW TO GET THERE

Exit Interstate 15 at Clinton Keith Road in Murrieta. Proceed 5 miles south on Clinton Keith Road (passing into the Santa Rosa Plateau Ecological Reserve), and curve sharply right where the road becomes Tenaja Road. After 1.7 miles more make a right turn to remain on Tenaja Road. Continue west on Tenaja Road for another 4.2 miles, and then go right on the one-lane, paved Cleveland Forest Road. Proceed another mile to the Tenaja Canyon Trailhead.

TRIP DESCRIPTION

From the Tenaja Trailhead, start downhill on the trail going west. A few minutes' descent takes you to the shady bowels of V-shaped Tenaja Canyon, where huge coast live oaks and pale-barked sycamores frame a limpid, rock-dimpled stream. Mostly the trail ahead meanders alongside the stream, but for the canyon's middle stretch it carves its way across the chaparral-blanketed south wall, 200 to 400 feet above the canyon bottom. As you descend, notice Tenaja Canyon's obviously linear alignment. You're following a northwest-trending rift called the Tenaja Fault.

After 3.7 miles of general descent, you reach Fishermans Camp, a former drive-in campground once accessible by many miles of bad road. Today the site, distinguished by its parklike setting amid a live oak grove, serves

TAKE THIS TRIP

Amid a chorus of droning bees, you hear the soft melody of water sliding over polished rock and your own crackling footsteps on brittle leaves. A fat gopher snake lounging by the creek stiffens at your approach. Tiny fish dart about in the stream eddies, while a pond turtle launches itself from a rock shelf, deftly slicing through the surface of a crystalline pool. You're in the San Mateo Canyon Wilderness—a roadless area almost completely surrounded by the Southern California megalopolis. This is a perfect destination for a cool-season weekend escape, no more than a two-hour drive away from any part of greater Los Angeles or San Diego.

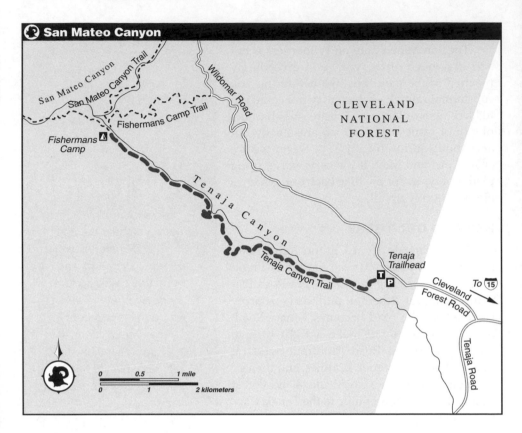

as a fine, uncrowded wilderness campsite. On quiet winter nights cold air drains off the nearby slopes, and you may wake up to morning frost.

The campsite's name hints of the fishing opportunities afforded by the near-by creek—in the rainy season, at least—in the bottom of San Mateo Canyon. Keep an eye out for steelhead trout swimming up the creek to spawn. Sightings suggest the revival of a southern subspecies of steelhead formerly thought to be extinct.

From Fishermans Camp, you could dayhike in three distinct directions. First, you could travel uphill on the Fishermans Camp Trail—the remains of the old road to the camp—going east toward Wildomar Road. Hiking partway up this route nets you a comprehensive view of San Mateo Canyon and it tributaries.

Second, you could follow the narrow and sketchy San Mateo Canyon Trail upstream (northwest) alongside San Mateo Canyon's stream and reach the Tena-ja Falls Trailhead along Wildomar Road. From there you can venture just 0.7 mile farther north to visit Tenaja Falls, which is a series of cascades dropping a total of 150 feet.

Third, you could head west and eventually southwest, downstream, through a superbly scenic section of San Mateo Canyon. The canyonside trail becomes in-creasingly indistinct the farther you go. Several miles away lies the boundary of the Camp Pendleton marine base, where hikers are not welcome.

SUMMER IN SOUTHERN CALIFORNIA

"Summer equals hiking" in much of California and the U.S.—but it ain't necessarily so in Southern California. The summer months may be too hot and dry for pleasant backpacking in Southern California's mountain ranges, and downright lethal in the lower desert areas. Think of the other three seasons instead—except for high elevations where snow lingers through winter and into spring.

BUILD-UP AND WIND-DOWN TIPS

Either on your drive in or on your way back home, don't miss stopping at least briefly at the 8000-acre **Santa Rosa Plateau Ecological Reserve**. The reserve's main entrance and nature center lie on the east side of Clinton Keith Road, 4 miles south of Interstate 15. A 39-acre vernal pool on the reserve property is one of California's largest. Springtime displays of wildflowers throughout the entire area can be eye-popping.

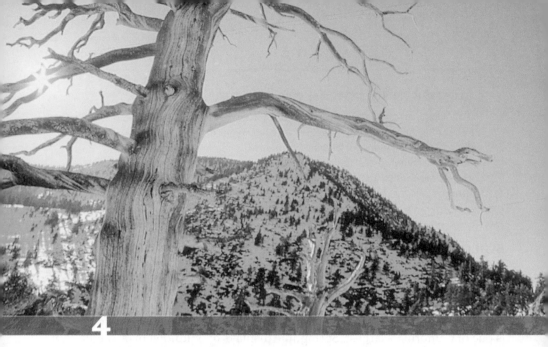

4

SAN JACINTO PEAK

Jerry Schad

MILES: 4.0 round-trip to campsites in Round Valley,
       11.0 round-trip to summit of San Jacinto Peak
RECOMMENDED DAYS: 2
ELEVATION GAIN/LOSS: 2600´/2600´ to peak and back
TYPE OF TRIP: Out-and-back
DIFFICULTY: Moderate
SOLITUDE: Moderately populated
LOCATION: Mount San Jacinto State Wilderness,
       San Bernardino National Forest
MAP: USGS 7.5-min. *San Jacinto Peak*
BEST SEASONS: Late spring, summer, and fall

PERMITS

A wilderness permit is required for all travel into the Mount San Jacinto State Wilderness. For information call the Mount San Jacinto State Wilderness ranger office, 951-659-2607. National forest lands surround the state wilderness, and overnight camping outside the immediate San Jacinto Peak area requires a national-forest wilderness permit. Visit www.fs.fed.us/r5/sanbernardino for more information.

Photo: Pine snag below San Jacinto Peak

CHALLENGES

You ascend to the mountain station of the tramway (elevation 8500 feet) in almost no time at all, and there's no time to adjust to the thin air. To condition yourself to higher altitude, consider hiking at some mid-elevation site (5000–8000 feet) a few days prior to your San Jacinto trip. Also, be aware that the tramway may be closed in August for maintenance, and that high winds or snow may result in temporarily suspension of service. Call the Palm Springs Aerial Tramway, (760) 325-1391, for current information.

HOW TO GET THERE

From Highway 111 just north of Palm Springs, turn west on Tramway Road and continue to the valley station of the Palm Springs Aerial Tramway. Purchase a round-trip ticket there and ride the tram to the mountain station, which includes a restaurant and a gift shop. Start your hike on a paved pathway leading 0.2 mile downhill from the mountain station to the San Jacinto State Wilderness ranger hut in Long Valley, which normally has a ranger on duty and present. There you must obtain a wilderness permit for travel beyond Long Valley.

TRIP DESCRIPTION

From the Long Valley ranger hut, follow the wide trail leading toward Round Valley (about 2 miles), where the primary trail camping sites are located. Additional sites can be found at Tamarack Valley, 0.5 mile north of Round Valley. During these first 2 miles, you'll ascend through one of the better examples of mixed coniferous (cone-bearing) forest in Southern California, with mature Jeffrey pines, sugar pines, and white firs offering abundant shade.

On your dayhike to the peak, you climb steeply through mostly lodgepole-pine forest to Wellman Divide, where you get your first

TAKE THIS TRIP

The north face of San Jacinto Peak, at one point soaring 9000 feet up in 4 horizontal miles, is one of the most imposing escarpments in the U.S. Upon witnessing sunrise on the peak a century ago, John Muir exclaimed, "The view from San Jacinto is the most sublime spectacle to be found anywhere on this earth!" Perhaps Muir was exaggerating–especially after seeing so many high places in California–but the emotion and exhilaration behind his statement is easily understood. Today, there's no great hardship involved in reaching the 10,804-foot summit. You simply take the Palm Springs Aerial Tramway all the way to the main trailhead, which lies only 2300 vertical feet below the peak.

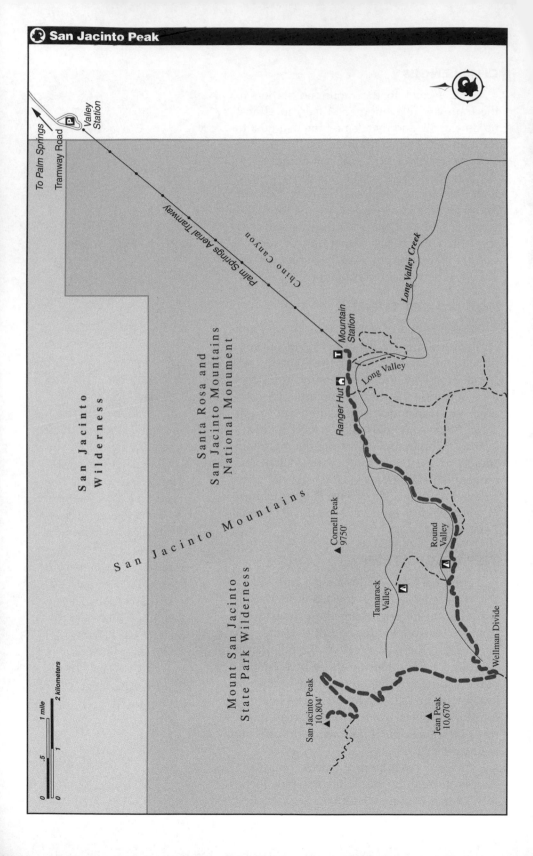

impressive view—south over tree-covered summits, foothills, and distant desert and coastal valleys. From Wellman Divide, continue a more leisurely uphill grind toward San Jacinto Peak. You traverse north for more than a mile across a boulder-strewn slope dotted with lodgepole pines and a carpet of low-growing alpine shrubs. Abruptly, you change direction at a switchback corner, climb southwest, and arrive (2 miles from Wellman Divide) in a saddle just south of the peak itself. Veer right and follow the summit path over stony ground, pass a stone hut, and then scramble from boulder to boulder for about 100 yards to reach the top.

If the weather cooperates, you can rest a spell in the warm sun, cupped amid the jumbo-sized rocks, and savor the lightheaded sensation of being on top of the world. The bald, gray (or white if covered by snow) ridge to the north is 11,499-foot San Gorgonio Mountain in the San Bernardino Mountains. The Pacific Ocean can sometimes be seen over many miles of coastal haze to the west. Eastward, where the air is usually most transparent, the tan and brown landscape of the desert rolls interminably toward a horizon near Arizona.

BUILD-UP AND WIND-DOWN TIPS ·

Perhaps this "easy opener" to the Southern California high country will whet your appetite for more lengthy routes in the San Jacinto Mountains. Other, more challenging routes to San Jacinto Peak originate near **Idyllwild**, a piney resort community at an elevation of about 5000 feet, south of the peak.

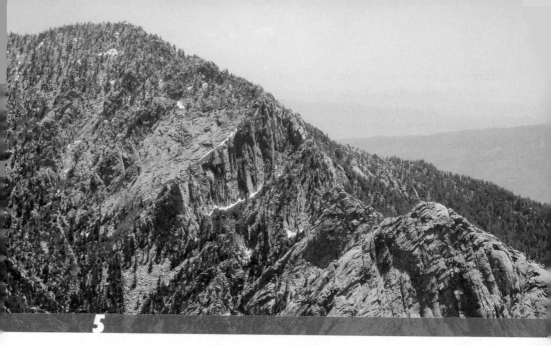

5

SAN JACINTO LOOP

David Money Harris

MILES: 17.6
RECOMMENDED DAYS: 2–3
ELEVATION GAIN/LOSS: 4500´/4500´
TYPE OF TRIP: Point-to-point or Loop
DIFFICULTY: Moderate
SOLITUDE: Crowded
LOCATION: Santa Rosa and San Jacinto Mountains National
          Monument, Mount San Jacinto State Park
MAPS: USGS 7.5-min. *San Jacinto Peak* or
          Tom Harrison's *San Jacinto Wilderness Trail Map*
BEST SEASON: Summer through fall

PERMITS ·

Permits are required for both dayhiking and backpacking. For more information, contact the Idyllwild Ranger Station, 54270 Pinecrest or P.O. Box 518, Idyllwild, CA, 909-382-2921 or Mt. San Jacinto State Park, P.O. Box 308 or 25905 Highway 243, Idyllwild, CA 92549, 951-659-2607. You can download the permit application at www.fs.fed.us/r5/sanbernardino/documents/san_jacinto_wilderness_permit_application.pdf.

Photo: Tahquitz Peak

CHALLENGES

Permits are free but quotas fill during summer weekends, so reserve your spot early. Campfires are not permitted. Dogs are permitted in the national forest but are prohibited in the state park section of the wilderness.

HOW TO GET THERE

From Highway 243 just below the Idyllwild Ranger Station, turn northeast on North Circle Dr. Continue 0.7 mile to a four-way intersection, and then turn right on South Circle Dr. Proceed 0.1 mile, and then turn left on Fern Valley Rd. After 1.8 miles, reach the large Humber Park Trailhead at the top of the road.

If you will be exiting on the Deer Springs Trail, arrange for a second vehicle at the trailhead 1 mile west of the ranger station on the north side of the road just above the County Park Nature Center.

TRIP DESCRIPTION

This trip follows the first recorded route on San Jacinto, pioneered by the mysterious Mr. F of Riverside in 1874. From 6420 feet in elevation in Humber Park, the Devil's Slide Trail climbs 1600 feet over 2.5 miles to Saddle Junction. The first cattle ranchers used to drive their herds up through the loose and dangerous slopes to summer pastures in Tahquitz Valley. The trail is now so well-graded that some hikers have rechristened it "Angel's Walk," but it nevertheless is a strenuous start with a heavy pack.

The five-way Saddle Junction delimits the west end of the spectacular Tahquitz Valley. Creeks flow through the meadows and open forest, and there is good camping at Tahquitz Valley and Skunk Cabbage Meadow. If you have an extra day, consider spending the night here and exploring the trails to Tahquitz Peak or the Caramba Overlook.

Otherwise, turn left at Saddle Junction and follow the Pacific Crest Trail (PCT) up the

TAKE THIS TRIP

At 10,804 feet, San Jacinto Peak is one of the three tallest major summits ringing the Los Angeles Basin. This loop from Humber Park in Idyllwild offers a grand tour of the mountain, taking you past sheer granite cliffs, shady forests of pine and fir, and cool alpine creeks to the stacked summit boulders. If a second vehicle is available, the easiest option is to emerge at the Deer Springs Trailhead and make a 4-mile shuttle. Otherwise, you have the option of dropping down a steep climber's trail next to Suicide Rock to return to Humber Park.

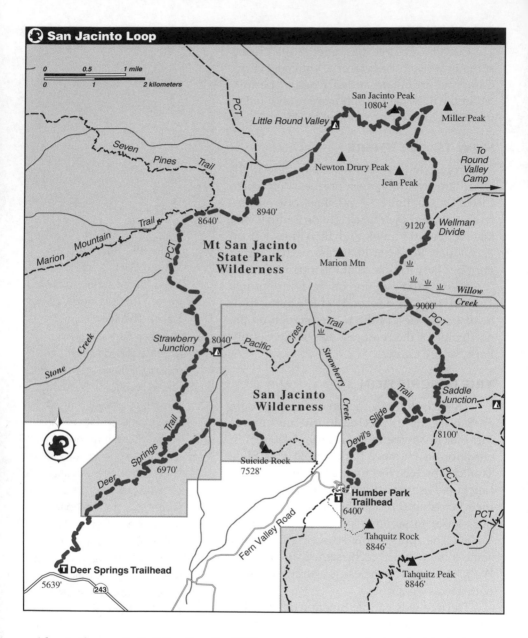

San Jacinto Loop

ridge to the north. In 1.9 miles, the PCT turns west across the head of Strawberry Valley but your route continues north. It passes the swampy Wellman Cienega and threads its way up past chaparral and boulders, reaching the Wellman Divide in another mile. Here, another trail branches off to the east, leading a mile to the fine but busy campsites of Round and Tamarack Valleys and out to the Palm Springs Aerial Tramway.

Your trip again continues north across a long slope clad in chaparral beneath Jean Peak. Look for the rocky pyramid of Cornell Peak on the north skyline. The trail switches back and in 2.4 miles climbs to a saddle immediately south of San Jacinto Peak. Scramble 0.3 mile up to the granite summit boulders. Along the way, look out for the stone hut that offers emergency shelter from storms.

Peer over the north edge of the summit to admire the cliffs of Snow Creek, which drops more than 8000 feet to the desert over scarcely 3 miles. The precipice is especially impressive when it's covered with snow in the spring and early summer. Snow Creek is only suitable for advanced mountaineers with ice and rock gear; more than one casual hiker has gotten lost and perished here.

After returning to the saddle, descend west for 1.3 miles to excellent camping at Little Round Valley, your last dependable source of water. The trail continues southwest for another mile to rejoin the PCT, where you turn left (south). In 0.5 mile, it passes junctions with the Seven Pines and Marion Mountain trails

On the PCT north of Saddle Junction

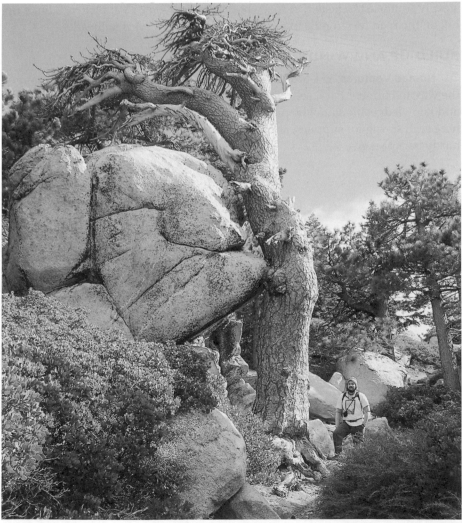

and then winds around the west flank of Marion Mountain for 2.3 miles to reach Strawberry Junction. The open forests of Jeffrey pine and white fir are some of the most beautiful in Southern California. Strawberry Junction Camp, situated immediately to the east, has good views but no running water.

Leave the PCT again and hike south down a ridge on the Deer Springs Trail. In 1.8 miles, reach the signed turnoff for Suicide Rock. If you left a vehicle at the Deer Springs Trailhead, you can continue down the ridge for 2.3 more easy miles past stands of enormous red manzanita to reach the road.

Otherwise, take the Suicide Rock Trail for a mile as it climbs up to the top of the granite outcrop. The way down is via a climber's trail on the northwest edge of the rock before you reach the true summit. Look for a path that skirts the edge of the rock. Do not be tempted to descend the cliffs directly; there is no safe route without a rope. Carefully follow the faint and confusing climber's trail, which is occasionally marked with cairns. After passing the base of the rock, it descends steeply southeast to meet dirt roads and eventually Fern Valley Road. Hike up-hill on the road for 0.4 mile to return to the Humber Park Trailhead.

BUILD-UP AND WIND-DOWN TIPS ·

Nomad Ventures, 951-659-4853, at 54415 North Circle Drive in Idyllwild on the way to Humber Park, sells almost any gear you might need and has friendly and knowledgeable staff who provide expert advice. Many PCT thru-hikers stop here each spring for supplies, and in the store you can admire snapshots of these hardy backpackers.

ART SMITH TRAIL

David Money Harris

MILES: 16.0
RECOMMENDED DAYS: 2
ELEVATION GAIN/LOSS: 3300´/3300´
TYPE OF TRIP: Out-and-back, with a point-to-point option
DIFFICULTY: Moderate
SOLITUDE: Moderate solitude
LOCATION: Santa Rosa and San Jacinto Mountains National Monument
MAP: USGS 7.5-min. *Rancho Mirage* (trail is not shown)
BEST SEASON: Fall through early winter

PERMITS

No permits are required, but the upper end of the trail is voluntarily closed from January 1 through September 30 to protect the endangered Peninsular bighorn sheep during lambing season.

CHALLENGES

Water is unavailable along this route, so carry all that you will need. The trail is not marked on the topo map, and there are several side trails to avoid. Respect the voluntary closure from January 1 to September 30. Dogs are never permitted

Photo: Oasis along the Art Smith Trail

TAKE THIS TRIP

The Santa Rosa Mountains are an undiscovered wonderland of cactus, yucca, palm oases, and outlandish rock formations located south of Palm Springs. The Art Smith Trail, named for the former trail boss of the Desert Riders equestrian group, invites you to lose yourself among varnished canyons, sandy washes, and boulder-studded slopes. If you are lucky, you might see one of the few remaining Peninsular bighorn sheep that roam the hills. This foray into the heart of the Santa Rosas explores one of the hidden gems of Southern California.
You can do this trip as an out-and-back with a camp at the Mike Dunn Desert Riders Oasis. Alternatively, with a shuttle, you can continue out any of numerous trails in the Palm Canyon area to reach Palm Springs.

in the Santa Rosa Wilderness. The temperature in the shade routinely exceeds 110°F during the summer.

HOW TO GET THERE

From Interstate 10, exit at Monterey and drive south for 6 miles to Highway 111 in Palm Desert. Monterey changes names to Highway 74. Continue south another 4 miles to the large paved Art Smith parking lot on the west side of Highway 74, directly across from the Santa Rosa Visitor Center.

TRIP DESCRIPTION

From the large signed Art Smith Trailhead at the bottom of the parking lot, the trail leads north along a levee and then gains the toe of a hill and turns west. In 0.3 mile, pass through a gate and hike west up the sandy wash in Dead Indian Canyon. The trail is indistinct at times but is marked with posts. In 0.4 mile, just before reaching a palm oasis at the head of the canyon, turn right (north) up a major side canyon. The train becomes well defined again and passes two more signs as it climbs out of the canyon through clumps of barrel and jumping teddybear cholla cactus.

Soon you arrive at a rocky saddle with views north into Palm Desert. Watch for a trail junction with the maze of trails overlooking the Bighorn development to the north, but keep left on the Art Smith Trail as it proceeds northwest. The trail climbs, then levels off in a maze of granite boulders glazed with brown desert varnish. For the next mile and a half, it passes a series of dry palm oases before staying left at a junction with the Schey Trail; at 3.2 miles from the start, this is the last of the confusing trail junctions.

Soon the trail traverses a plateau with views of the long flat-topped Haystack Mountain to the left. In 1.7 miles, it passes the top of another canyon dotted with palms. You are now in the heart of the Santa Rosa Mountains. Though endless subdivisions, golf courses,

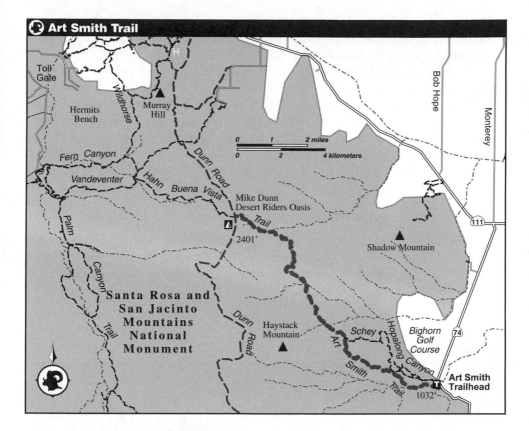

and swimming pools crowd the valley only a few miles away, you can enjoy the same sense of seclusion that a Cahuilla hunter must have known centuries ago.

In another 2.2 miles, the trail disappears into a sandy wash and passes through a narrow canyon. In 0.4 mile, it exits the wash on the left and climbs a ridge. From the crest of the ridge in a forest of agave, you can see the San Jacinto and San Gorgonio mountains towering to the west over the Santa Rosa Mountains, Palm Canyon, and the tan ribbon of Dunn Road. Descend 0.2 mile to reach the Mike Dunn Desert Riders Oasis marked by

MARATHON DAYHIKES

When you have a young family and tend to hike alone, long dayhikes can be a wonderful alternative to backpacking. Many of the trips in this book can be done in a day with a light pack and a bit of conditioning. Long dayhikes are a great physical and mental challenge and a way to see fabulous scenery. Hiking 30 miles is no more difficult for most people than running a marathon, and is easier on the joints. Besides, it's great to go enjoy the outdoors and still be home to help with the 2 AM feeding.

hitching posts, a lonely cluster of picnic tables, and a broken-down bulldozer. There is plenty of space for camping but no water. Dunn Road is closed to motorized vehicles and is popular among hardy mountain bikers.

When you're ready to return to the trailhead, retrace your steps to your car. Alternatively, there are many ways to continue west or north. The aptly named Hahn Buena Vista Trail continues west from Dunn Road down toward Palm Canyon and the southern limits of Palm Springs. Even if you are not going this way, consider hiking 0.5 mile west on the trail to a hilltop vista. Dunn Road leads north to Cathedral City. Bighorn Taxi, at 760-321-4599, can take you back to the trailhead (for a hefty fee) if you have not positioned a second vehicle in advance.

BUILD-UP AND WIND-DOWN TIPS· ·

Palm Springs offers countless dining opportunities for hungry hikers fresh off the trail. One of my personal favorites is **Thai Smile** at 651 N. Palm Canyon Dr., 760-320-5503, which serves outstanding yellow curry and doesn't object to grubby hikers.

California barrel cactus

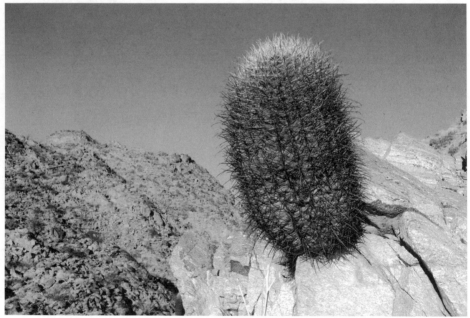

THE TRANSVERSE RANGES

The "transverse" in Transverse Ranges refers to the fact that this mountain province stretches west to east, athwart the general northwest-southeast structural grain of California. Movements along the San Andreas Fault are recognized as the cause of this anomaly. A bend in this fault has caused compression that has uplifted an entire zone consisting of (among some other lesser ranges) the coastal Santa Monica Mountains, the San Gabriel Mountains north of Los Angeles, and the San Bernardino Mountains north and east of San Bernardino.

Each range has its own character. The comparatively low Santa Monicas are dominated by chaparral and oak savannah. The sometimes-sheer slopes of the San Gabriel Mountains are clothed in dense chaparral, but higher up (up to 10,000 feet) coniferous forest thrives. The San Bernardinos botanically resemble the San Gabriels, but they are higher, culminating in 11,499-foot San Gorgonio Mountain, the highest summit in California south of the Sierra Nevada.

The San Bernardino Mountains are largely within San Bernardino National Forest territory, while the San Gabriels lie almost completely within Angeles National Forest. Several wilderness areas have been designated in the highest and most remote sections of both mountain ranges—the same areas that are most attractive to backpackers. The Santa Monica Mountains, on the other hand, are blanketed by an intricate patchwork of private and public lands (which collectively comprise the Santa Monica Mountains National Recreation Area) stretching from the western edge of the City of Los Angeles to Ventura County. Though dayhiking is the norm here, creative travelers can fashion overnight trips on the nearly completed Backbone Trail, which traverses the length of the range.

THE SAN BERNARDINO MOUNTAINS

From Cajon Pass and the slanted troughs of the great San Andreas Fault, the San Bernardinos rise, rather steeply at first, in chaparral-coated slopes, to the 5000-foot-high summits of Cleghorn and Cajon mountains. Eastward from here, for 30 miles, the crest of the San Bernardinos is remarkably uniform. Undulating ridges and tapered hillocks conceal within their folds forested glens and sparkling blue lakes. This is the Crestline-Lake Arrowhead-Running Springs-Big Bear country, the part of the mountains best known to thousands of Southern Californians. Near Big Bear Lake, the San Bernardinos veer southward, toward the majestic heights of the San Gorgonio Wilderness. Here, under granite spines hammered up against the sky, lodgepole and limber pines grow sturdy and weather-resistant, tumbling streams flow icy cold, and the thin air is crisp with the chill of elevation. Reigning over all is 11,499-foot San Gorgonio Mountain, the rooftop of Southern California.

The San Gorgonio Wilderness, which more or less centers on San Gorgonio Mountain, is by far the most popular destination for backpacking trips of two or three days. Due to the popularity of hiking and backpacking there, and possible trailhead quotas, it's wise to plan your trip well in advance. Depending on the amount of precipitation in any given year (which varies widely in Southern California), snow can remain on the north slopes for more than half the year—something to think about when planning a trip.

THE SAN GABRIEL MOUNTAINS

The San Gabriel Mountains cover an area stretching north from the edge of the Los Angeles metropolis to the western extremity of the Mojave Desert. This is fault-torn country: The San Gabriels are a conglomeration of rock units of various ages and origins, separated from the surrounding landscape by the San Andreas Fault zone on the north, the San Gabriel and Sierra Madre faults on the south, and the Soledad Fault on the west.

Throughout most of their length, the San Gabriels are made up of two, roughly parallel ranges. The southern, lower range, at about 5000 feet high, rises abruptly from the city of Pasadena and adjoining communities in the San Gabriel Valley. The northern range—farther inland, longer, and loftier—climaxes near its eastern end at 10,064-foot-high Mt. San Antonio (Old Baldy). Both ranges are incised with deep canyons whose slopes are notoriously steep and easily eroded. Inside many of these canyons, crystalline streams hasten through shady riparian woods, and backpackers find complete escape from sight and sound of the great suburban metropolis not far away.

The proximity of the San Gabriel Mountains to millions of city residents makes them particularly vulnerable to overuse. Most of this use, though, centers on picnic areas and the trails most easily accessible from Angeles Crest Highway—the main route through the mountain range. Any hiker or backpacker willing to hoof it far enough, however, is practically guaranteed a measure of solitude.

THE SANTA MONICA MOUNTAINS

The backdrop for countless movies and TV shows and home of the famous Hollywood sign and Griffith Park, the Santa Monica Mountains may seem like the least likely place in California for backpacking. Yet, particularly at its western end, the range offers solitude and pockets of wilderness that rival the more often-hiked San Gabriel Mountains to the north. The hills and mountains here tend to be rounded, the grades gentle, and the scenery more pastoral than spectacular. When the High Sierra and even the ranges ringing the Los Angeles basin are still covered with winter's white mantle, the Santa Monicas beckon with wildflower-dotted hillsides, cool green canyon bottoms, and mild temperatures.

At more than 150,000 acres, Santa Monica Mountains National Recreation Area, a unit of the National Park system, is the world's largest urban national park. From chaparral-drenched hillsides to cool, forested streams, to some of the last remaining native grasslands in Southern California, more than 500 miles of trails lace the region. The 70-mile Backbone Trail, comprising segments of many different trails, roughly follows the crest of the range from east to west, and completing it is a worthy goal for the serious hiker.

Most of the trail camps in the Santa Monicas are located in the western half of the range; as a consequence backpacking opportunities are limited primarily to this area. Point Mugu State Park offers the possibility of two- and three-day backpacking trips beyond the one described in this book. Additional sections of the Backbone Trail can be included in overnight trips, and it is possible to construct trips that include 3111-foot Sandstone Peak, the high point of the range.

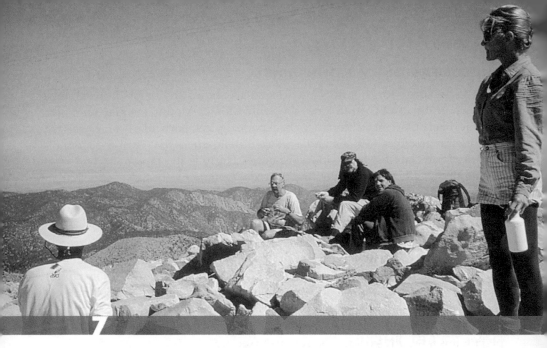

SAN GORGONIO MOUNTAIN

Jerry Schad

MILES: 9.6 round-trip to High Creek trail camp,
15.6 round-trip to summit of San Gorgonio Mountain
RECOMMENDED DAYS: 2
ELEVATION GAIN/LOSS: 3400´/3400´ to High Creek trail camp,
5700´/5700´ to summit of San Gorgonio
Mountain
TYPE OF TRIP: Out-and-back
DIFFICULTY: Moderately strenuous
SOLITUDE: Moderately populated
LOCATION: San Bernardino National Forest
MAPS: USGS 7.5-min. *Forest Falls* and *San Gorgonio Mountain* or
U.S. Forest Service *Guide to the San Gorgonio Wilderness*
BEST SEASONS: Late spring, summer, and fall

PERMIT ·
A wilderness permit is required for all entry into the San Gorgonio Wilderness. Get one at the San Gorgonio Ranger Station, or better yet, obtain one in advance. Call 909-382-2881 or visit www.fs.fed.us/r5/sanbernardino for information. Cars parked at the trailhead must display a National Forest Adventure Pass.

Photo: San Gorgonio Mountain summit, the highest in Southern California

CHALLENGES

Backpacking Gorgonio and bagging the peak squeezes a lot into a two-day weekend. In November, when the daylight period shortens to less than 11 hours and sunset occurs near 5 PM, be sure to get an early start to ensure that you will have enough light during the afternoon. Various three-day itineraries are possible on the route, too. There are three trail camps on the way up, and a fourth camp lies just below the summit. The season for the south-facing Vivian Creek route featured here begins in April or May with the melting of the snow, and ends sometime in November or December with the first heavy snowfall.

HOW TO GET THERE

From Interstate 10 just east of the city of San Bernardino, exit at Highway 38 (Orange Street) in Redlands. Turn left (north), proceed 0.5 mile north to Lugonia Avenue, and turn right (east), remaining on Highway 38. Continue 8 miles to an intersection with Bryant Street. (The San Gorgonio Ranger Station, where you can secure a wilderness permit, is located at this intersection.) Continue driving east on Highway 38, now signed Mill Creek Road, for 6.2 miles. Turn right at Valley of the Falls Boulevard, and proceed the remaining 4.3 miles to the road's end, where the Vivian Creek Trailhead is located.

TRIP DESCRIPTION

The Vivian Creek Trail is the original path to the top of San Gorgonio, built around the turn of the 20th century. Today, at least seven other routes (or variations on routes) culminate at the summit, but none is shorter and faster.

From the paved parking lot at the trailhead, walk east (uphill) past a vehicle gate and follow a dirt road for 0.6 mile to its end. Go left across the wide, boulder wash of Mill Creek and find the Vivian Creek Trail going

TAKE THIS TRIP

The rounded, talus-strewn summit of San Gorgonio Mountain (or "Greyback," as it was called long ago) crowns the San Bernardino Mountains and regally presides over thousands of square miles of varied Southern California terrain. The mountain's 11,499-foot elevation qualifies it as the highest peak in California south of the Sierra Nevada. No California peakbagger's long-term itinerary is complete without a visit to the top.

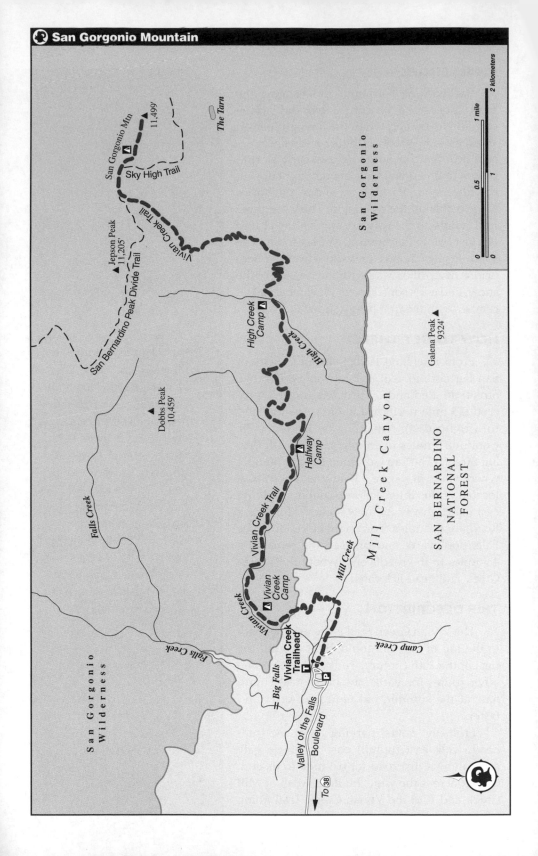

sharply up the oak-clothed canyon wall on the far side. The next half mile is excruciatingly steep, but not typical of the route as a whole.

After leveling momentarily, the trail assumes a moderate grade as it sidles alongside Vivian Creek. A sylvan Shangri-La unfolds ahead. Pines, firs, and cedars reach for the sky. Bracken fern smothers the banks of the melodious creek, which dances over boulders and fallen trees. After the first October frost, the bracken turns a flaming yellow, made all the more vivid by warm sunlight pouring out of a fierce blue sky.

Near Halfway Camp (2.5 miles) the trail begins climbing timber-dotted slopes covered intermittently by thickets of manzanita. After several zigs and zags on north-facing slopes, you swing onto a brightly illuminated south-facing slope. Serrated Yucaipa Ridge looms in the south, rising sheer from the depths of Mill Creek Canyon. Soon thereafter, the sound of bubbling water heralds your arrival at High Creek, 4.8 miles, and the trail camp of the same name. If you stay here overnight (your best choice on a one-night trip), be prepared for a chilly night. Cold, nocturnal air flows down along the bottom of this canyon from the 10,000-foot-plus peaks above.

When you're ready to dayhike to the summit, you plod upward on long switchback segments with a light load on your back through lodgepole pines, and attain a saddle on a rocky ridge. The pines thin out and appear more decrepit as you climb crookedly up along this ridge toward timberline. At 7.2 miles (from the trailhead), the San Bernardino Peak Divide Trail intersects from the left. Stay right and keep climbing on a moderate grade across stony slopes dotted with cowering krummholz pines. Soon, nearly all vegetation disappears.

On the right you pass Sky High Trail. Keep straight and chug upward into the thinning air. A final burst of effort puts you on the summit boulder pile, 7.8 miles from your starting point. From this airy vantage, even the soaring north face of San Jacinto Peak to the south appears diminished in stature. With the midmorning sunlight knifing downward from the southeast, your best views are likely to be of the vast Mojave Desert spreading north and east. Under ideal atmospheric conditions, you may be able to spot certain high peaks in the southern Sierra Nevada, plus Telescope Peak—the high point of Death Valley National Monument.

BUILD-UP AND WIND-DOWN TIPS ·

Just west of the trailhead for Vivian Creek is a short path leading across Mill Creek Canyon wash and up near the base of **Big Falls**, one of the highest cascades in Southern California. This is a worthwhile spot to visit in the spring, when there's enough runoff from melting snow.

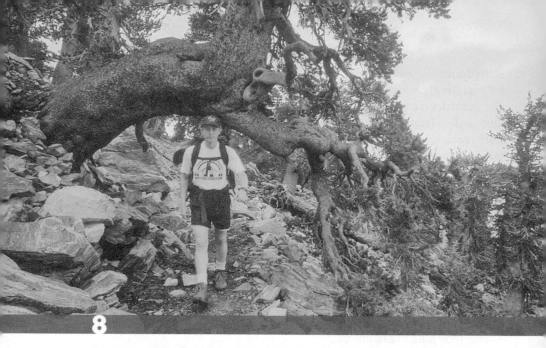

8

SAN BERNARDINO MOUNTAIN TRAVERSE

Jerry Schad

MILES: 21.6, add several more for side trips to various trail camps atop the San Bernardino Peak Divide

RECOMMENDED DAYS: 2–3

ELEVATION GAIN/LOSS: 5500´/4500´

TYPE OF TRIP: Point-to-point

DIFFICULTY: Moderately strenuous

SOLITUDE: Moderately populated

LOCATION: San Gorgonio Wilderness, San Bernardino National Forest

MAPS: USGS 7.5-min. *Moonridge, San Gorgonio Mountain, Forest Falls*, and *Big Bear Lake* or U.S. Forest Service *Guide to the San Gorgonio Wilderness*

BEST SEASONS: Late spring, summer, and fall

PERMITS

A wilderness permit is required for all entry into the San Gorgonio Wilderness. Get one at the San Gorgonio Ranger Station, or better yet, obtain one in advance. Call 909-382-2881 or visit www.fs.fed.us/r5/sanbernardino for information. Cars parked at any trailhead must display a National Forest Adventure Pass.

Photo: On the trail below San Bernardino Peak

CHALLENGES

This traverse is challenging and exhausting to anyone without recent altitude experience or training. The north-facing aspect of the ascent and descent combined with the 10,000-foot-plus elevation of the route's midsection shorten the season for backpacking to as little as six months. Lightning-struck pines atop of the divide speak of the violence of thunderstorms, which visit the area regularly and somewhat unpredictably in the summer. Alternately, intense July and August sunlight and heat can easily sap your energy. Pre-Memorial Day and post–Labor Day trips usually take advantage of the best weather.

HOW TO GET THERE

From Interstate 10 just east of the city of San Bernardino, exit at Highway 38 (Orange Street) in Redlands. Turn left (north), proceed 0.5 mile north to Lugonia Avenue, and turn right (east), remaining on Highway 38. Continue 8 miles to an intersection with Bryant Street. (The San Gorgonio Ranger Station, where you can secure a wilderness permit, is located at this intersection.) Continue driving another 11 miles east (up into the mountains) on Highway 38 to the small community of Angelus Oaks, where a large sign on the right directs you toward the San Bernardino Peak Trailhead, a short distance away via dirt road. Since this is a car-shuttle trip, drive your other car 5 miles farther east on Highway 38 to Jenks Lake Road on the right. Go 2.5 miles east on Jenks Lake Road to the spacious South Fork Trailhead on the left.

TRIP DESCRIPTION

From the San Bernardino Peak Trailhead, commence a relentless, switchbacking ascent south and east, up a timbered slope graced with fine, aromatic specimens of Jeffrey pine and sugar pine, plus large and small varieties of oak trees. A sign at 2 miles announces the

TAKE THIS TRIP

The peaked roofline of Southern California's highest watershed divide–San Bernardino Peak to San Gorgonio Mountain–features eight named summits–all over 10,000 feet in elevation. Four of the eight peaks lie no more than a few minutes scramble from the two-day backpack route described here. If you wish, schedule in an extra day for dayhiking to and from the other four peaks. Either way, you'll experience a good piece of the largest subalpine wilderness area south of the Sierra Nevada.

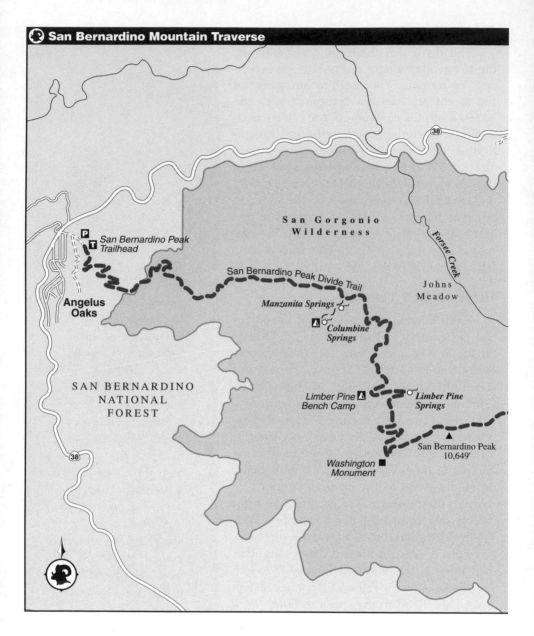

San Bernardino Mountain Traverse

San Gorgonio
Wilderness

San Bernardino Peak
Trailhead

San Bernardino Peak Divide Trail

Angelus
Oaks

Manzanita Springs

Columbine
Springs

Johns
Meadow

Forsee Creek

SAN BERNARDINO
NATIONAL
FOREST

Limber Pine
Bench Camp

Limber Pine
Springs

San Bernardino Peak
10,649'

Washington
Monument

boundary of San Gorgonio Wilderness. As you continue upward, the oaks rather suddenly disappear, and the trail climbs more moderately atop a rounded, linear ridge about 8000 feet in elevation. On that ridge you eventually emerge from parklike stands of Jeffrey pines into a sunny landscape of low-growing chaparral—mostly manzanita. Blocky San Bernardino Peak looms ahead on this plateau phase of the hike, and you clearly realize the magnitude of the remaining ascent ahead.

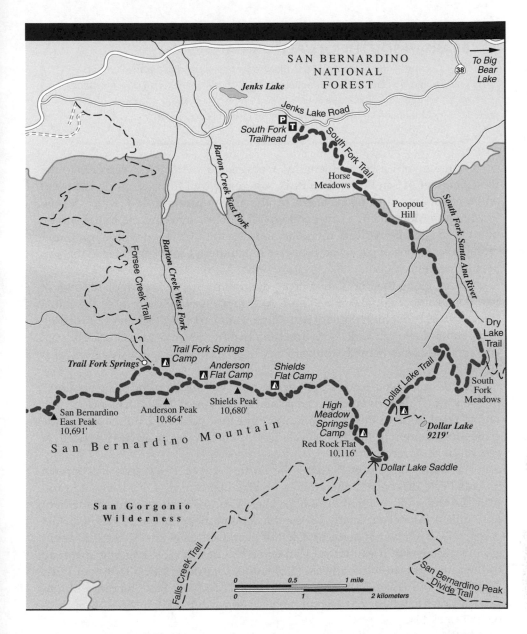

Amid the manzanita you come to a trail junction at 4.3 miles. Seasonal Manzanita Springs and Columbine Springs trail camp lie to the west, and an obscure, unmaintained trail meanders east toward Johns Meadow. Ahead at 5.7 miles and about 1000 feet higher on a spacious and viewful bench dotted with lodgepole pines is Limber Pine Bench trail camp—too short a destination for a first night's camp but fine if you intend to spend three days on the traverse. Cool water fairly dependably issues from a ravine (Limber Pine Springs) alongside the trail about 0.3 mile east.

BEARS IN SOUTHERN CALIFORNIA?

Yes, the range of the American black bear has expanded south into the San Gabriel and San Bernardino mountains, where these animals can be a nuisance in camping areas. Black bears have also been sighted as far south as the San Jacinto Mountains, and some remote parts of San Diego County.

Continue your ascent on lengthy, well-graded switchback segments to the west shoulder of San Bernardino Peak, where the trail turns abruptly left (east) and a panoramic view opens to the south. As you continue east, watch for the Washington Monument, a cairn and wooden debris marking the initial survey point of the San Bernardino meridian and baseline. To this day, township and range descriptions of surveyed property in Southern California refer to this important reference point.

Ahead, along the undulating crest, the trail passes just north of 10,649-foot San Bernardino Peak (8.0 miles) and even more narrowly north of the talus-strewn, 10,691-foot high point of San Bernardino East Peak (9.4 miles). From the latter summit you can look south into the yawning chasm of Mill Creek Canyon, and spot the unmaintained Momyer Peak Trail cutting precipitously across talus slopes below.

At 10.2 miles you reach a split in the trail. Both trails reconverge about 0.8 mile ahead. Trail Fork Springs camp (and the seasonal Trail Fork Springs in a ravine nearby) lie to the left, while the right fork passes 0.2 mile north of the 10,864-foot summit of Anderson Peak. Dry Anderson Flat camp lies just north of where the trails reconverge.

The trail continues east across the north slope of 10,680-foot rock-strewn Shields Peak, descends moderately to Shields Flat camp (12.0 miles), and rambles east and south to a trail turnoff for High Meadow Springs camp on the right (13.7 miles). Water can usually be found in a ravine near the camp. Red Rock Flat camp, with a number of perfectly flat if dry campsites, lies next to the trail about a half mile beyond. If you intend to spend a half day or more bagging any or all of the four peaks to the southeast (10,806-foot Charlton Peak, 10,696-foot Little Charlton Peak, 11,205-foot Jepson Peak, and 11,502-foot San Gorgonio Mountain), it's nice to set up your second night's camp at either High Meadow Springs or Red Rock Flat.

At the four-way trail junction atop Dollar Lake Saddle (14.5 miles), turn left and descend north past the trail turnoff for Dollar Lake and farther down to South Fork Meadows (17.0 miles). Even during the driest months of the driest years, the clear waters of the South Fork Santa Ana River tumble through this sylvan spot. Stay left at the trail intersection here and at every other trail junction ahead to remain on the descending course that takes you almost straightway to the South Fork Trailhead and your parked car.

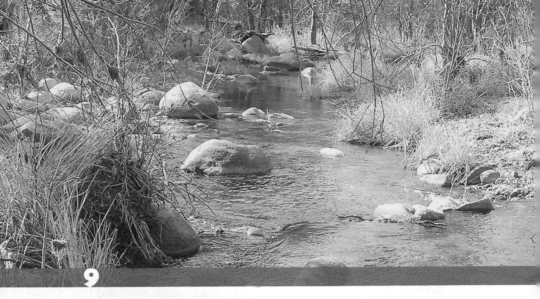

9

HOLCOMB CROSSING TRAIL CAMP LOOP

David Money Harris

MILES: 5.6
RECOMMENDED DAYS: 2
ELEVATION GAIN/LOSS: 900´/900´
TYPE OF TRIP: Loop
DIFFICULTY: Easy
SOLITUDE: Crowded
LOCATION: San Bernardino National Forest
MAP: USGS 7.5-min. *Butler Peak*
BEST SEASONS: Spring and fall

PERMITS

No permits are required for this trip.

CHALLENGES

Beware of the hunters and all-terrain vehicle riders who frequent the Crab Flats area and who may not be watching for backpackers. While deer hunting season lasts from October to November, most hunting in this area is done in autumn.

Photo: Holcomb Creek

TAKE THIS TRIP

The green forest meets the tawny desert on the north slopes of the San Bernardino Mountains. Holcomb Creek cuts a deep canyon through these slopes. Two trail camps are situated beneath shady pines on the banks of the creek. When the desert is sizzling and the high peaks are blanketed in snow, Holcomb Creek is an ideal destination for a short backpacking trip.

HOW TO GET THERE

From the Rim of the World Highway (State Highway 18), 2.9 miles northeast of the intersection with Highway 330 at Running Springs and just past mile marker 018 SBD 34.50, turn left (north) onto Green Valley Road. After 2.6 miles—shortly before you reach Green Valley Lake—turn left again onto Crabs Flat Road (3N16). This dirt road is usually in good condition, but may be impassible after winter snows and during high water. Descend toward Crab Flats Campground, passing several side roads and crossing Crab Creek. In 3.8 miles, reach a signed junction. The right fork leads to Big Pine Flat, but you veer left on 3N34, passing Crab Flats Campground after 0.2 mile. The road deteriorates and low-clearance vehicles may prefer to park outside the campground. In 1.1 miles, park at a clearing and large VISITORS TO DEEP CREEK sign near Tent Peg group camp.

TRIP DESCRIPTION

Look for the signed 2W08 trail leading north from the parking area. It begins as an all-terrain vehicle (ATV) track but soon narrows to a hiking trail, climbs over the forested ridge, and drops down to Holcomb Creek. Portions of the area were ravaged in the 2003 Old Fire, while others were left untouched. The trail offers fascinating insight into the process of regrowth. Oaks and Jeffrey pines are common in the unburned patches. The north slope across the creek offers a dramatic contrast, dotted with pinion pines, yucca, and other Upper Sonoran desert shrubs.

In 1.7 miles, 2W08 terminates at the Pacific Crest Trail (PCT) on the canyon bottom. Turn right (east) on the PCT and hike 0.6 mile to Bench Camp, where you can enjoy the shady flat above the creek. Or better yet, continue 0.8 mile, passing the ATV track 1W17, to Holcomb Crossing Trail Camp beneath magnificent Jeffrey pines beside the creek. From Holcomb

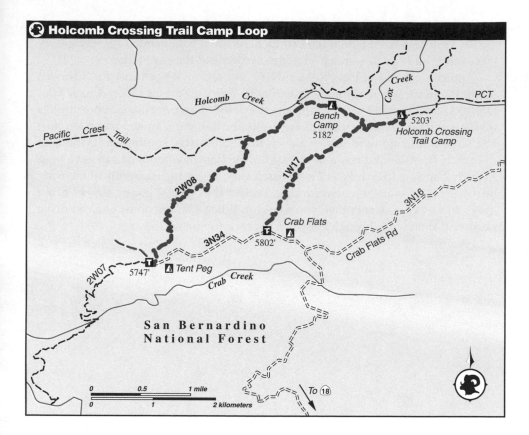

Holcomb Crossing Trail Camp Loop

Crossing Trail Camp, a pleasant side trip follows the PCT east to explore the upper reaches of the watershed.

To complete the loop trip, hike steeply up 1W17 for 1.3 miles to Crab Flat. Turn right (west) and follow the dirt road 3N34 0.8 mile back to your vehicle.

BUILD-UP AND WIND-DOWN TIPS •

After your trip, consider taking an excursion to **Deep Creek Hot Springs** and exploring the maze of dirt roads on the north slopes of the San Bernardino Mountains en route. The roads are usually in good condition and passable with a two-wheel-drive vehicle but can wash out in a wet winter. The U.S. Forest

THE SUN ALSO RISES

I love early starts on extended backpacking trips. I can only lay in a tent for a limited number of hours. At dawn, it is too chilly to goof around camp, but the temperature is ideal for walking and the light is gorgeous. I eat a cold breakfast, repack my gear, and *vamanos!* Best of all, miles beneath the boots before lunch are always easier than those in the heat of the day.

Service *San Bernardino National Forest* map or the *San Bernardino Mountains Recreation Topo Map* from Fine Edge Productions are recommended for navigating these roads and can be purchased at the Arrowhead Ranger Station.

Return to the Crab Flats Road (3N16) and follow it northeast for 8.3 miles to Big Pine Flat, where camping is available. Turn left on the Coxey Truck Trail (3N14) and follow it 12 miles down into the desert. There are more opportunities for car camping along the way among the jumbo boulders. Make a sharp left turn at a large BLM sign onto Bowen Ranch Road and drive southwest 3.3 miles to the ranch. Register and pay a use fee at Bowen Ranch, where you can get a map to the hot springs. The hike is 2 miles each way. The return is uphill all the way; bring plenty of water on a warm day. Protect this special place—do *not* bring glass, and leave it cleaner than you found it. When you are done, you can drive north and then west through Hesperia to reach Interstate 15.

10

BIG SANTA ANITA LOOP

Jerry Schad

MILES: 9.4 round-trip, 3.5 to Spruce Grove Trail Camp
RECOMMENDED DAYS: 2
ELEVATION GAIN/LOSS: 2100´/2100´
TYPE OF TRIP: Loop
DIFFICULTY: Moderately strenuous
SOLITUDE: Moderately populated
LOCATION: Angeles National Forest
MAP: USGS 7.5-min. *Mount Wilson*
BEST SEASONS: Fall, winter, and spring

PERMITS

A wilderness permit is not required. Campfires are prohibited outside of designated campgrounds in the Angeles National Forest. A fire permit is required for the use of self-contained camp stoves, which may be used at remote sites whenever the wildfire potential is not deemed too great. Cars parked at the trailhead must display a National Forest Adventure Pass. Contact San Gabriel River Ranger District, Angeles National Forest at 626-335-1251 or visit www. fs.fed.us/r5/angeles.

Photo: Bigleaf maples showing autumn color, Big Santa Anita Canyon

53

TAKE THIS TRIP

In the lush and shady re-
cesses of the "front range"
of the San Gabriel Moun-
tains you can easily lose
all sight and sense of the
hundreds of square miles
of dense metropolis, and
the millions of Angelenos,
that lie just over the ridge
to the south. With easy access from the San Gabriel
Valley by city street and
mountain road, you can be
laying bootprints down a
fern-lined path less than a
half hour from the freeway.

CHALLENGES

Avoid days when a strong temperature
inversion exists and stagnant, smoggy air
drifts into the lower canyons of the San Gabriel Mountains. On weekends, parking at the
trailhead is scarce, and the remote camping
spots are often filled. Consider making this
trip on weekdays.

The curvy mountain road that services
the trailhead is notoriously susceptible to
washouts in wet weather, and repairs can take
weeks or months. The road can also close on
short notice due to fire danger in very dry
summer or fall seasons.

HOW TO GET THERE

Exit Interstate 210 at Santa Anita Avenue in Arcadia and drive 6 miles north (first
through the suburbs and then up the curvy
road) to the large trailhead parking area at
Chantry Flat.

TRIP DESCRIPTION

In this scenic and varied loop trip from
Chantry Flat, you climb by way of the Gabrielino National Recreation Trail to historic Sturtevant Camp, and return by way of the Mt.
Zion and Upper Winter Creek trails. You can
stay overnight at Spruce Grove Camp, about
one-third of the way around the loop; or opt
for a very leisurely three-day trip by staying
a second night at Hoegees Camp, about two-
thirds of the way around the loop.

From the lower parking lot at Chantry
Flat, hike the first, paved segment of the Gabrielino Trail down to the confluence of Winter
Creek and Big Santa Anita Canyon at 0.6 mile.
The pavement ends at a metal bridge spanning Winter Creek. Pass the restrooms and
continue up alder-lined Big Santa Anita Canyon on a wide path following the left bank.
The trail edges alongside a number of small
cabins and various flood-control check dams
built with concrete "logs" and soon assumes
the proportions of a foot trail.

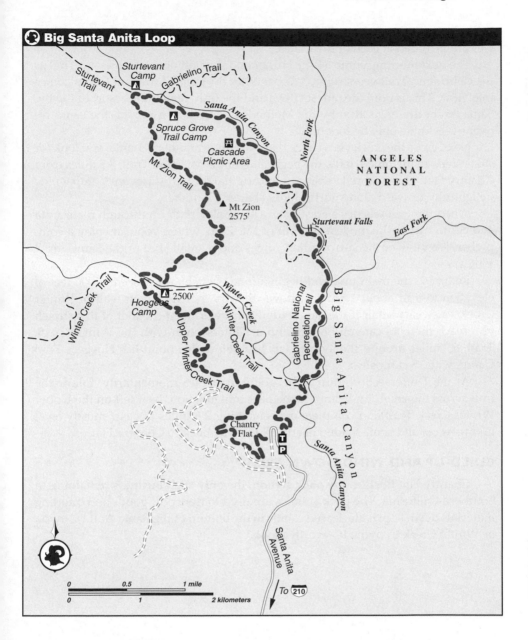

Big Santa Anita Loop

Sturtevant Camp

Gabrielino Trail

Sturtevant Trail

Santa Anita Canyon

North Fork

ANGELES NATIONAL FOREST

Spruce Grove Trail Camp

Cascade Picnic Area

Mt Zion Trail

Mt Zion 2575'

Sturtevant Falls

East Fork

Winter Creek Trail

Winter Creek

2500'

Hoegees Camp

Winter Creek

Winter Creek Trail

Upper Winter Creek Trail

Gabrielino National Recreation Trail

Big Santa Anita Canyon

Chantry Flat

Santa Anita Canyon

Santa Anita Avenue

To 210

0   0.5   1 mile

0   1   2 kilometers

At 1.4 miles, amidst a beautiful oak woodland, you come to a three-way split. The right branch goes up-canyon to the base of 50-foot-high Sturtevant Falls, a worthy side trip during the wet season. The middle and left branches join again about a mile upstream. The middle, more scenic trail slices across a sheer wall above the falls and continues through a veritable fairyland of miniature cascades and crystalline pools bedecked with giant chain ferns.

You pass Cascade Picnic Area (2.8 miles), and arrive at Spruce Grove Trail Camp, 3.5 miles from the start, named for the bigcone Douglas fir (bigcone spruce) trees that attain truly inspiring proportions hereabouts. Stoves and tables are included at each of the 7 sites.

The next morning climb a little farther and stay left on the Sturtevant Trail as the Gabrielino Trail veers right. After another 0.1 mile, Sturtevant Camp comes into view. This is both the oldest (1893) and the only remaining resort in the Big Santa Anita drainage. Run by the Methodist Church as a retreat, the camp remains accessible only by foot trail.

Next, cross the creek via a check dam, continue another 0.1 mile, and look for stone steps rising on the left—the beginning of the Mt. Zion Trail, 3.9 miles from Chantry Flat. This restored version of the original trail to Sturtevant Camp winds delightfully upward along north slopes shaded by timber.

When the trail reaches a crest, take a short side path up through manzanita and ceanothus to the modest summit of Mt. Zion, where you can enjoy a comprehensive view of the surrounding ridges and a small slice of the San Gabriel Valley.

Return to the main trail and begin a long, switchback descent (1000 feet of elevation loss in about 1.5 miles) down the dry, north canyon wall of Winter Creek—a sweaty affair if the day is sunny and warm. At the foot of this stretch you reach the cool canyon bottom and a T-intersection with the Winter Creek Trail, 6.7 miles around the loop so far. Just below this point lies Hoegees Trail Camp, with 15 campsites.

At the T-intersection, turn right, going upstream momentarily, follow the trail across the creek, and climb to the next trail junction. Bear left on the Upper Winter Creek Trail and complete the remaining 2.6 miles of easy, mostly level hiking—cool and semi-shaded nearly all the way back to Chantry Flat.

BUILD-UP AND WIND-DOWN TIPS ·

Chantry Flat hosts a tiny **pack station**, the only such business remaining in Southern California. The pack animals are used to transport goods and building materials down to private, leased cabins in the bottom of Big Santa Anita Canyon or Winter Creek Canyon. It's worth a look.

11

DEVILS CANYON

Jerry Schad

MILES: 5.4 round-trip to canyon-bottom campsite
(options for dayhiking farther)
RECOMMENDED DAYS: 2
ELEVATION GAIN/LOSS: 2100´/2100´ to top of falls
TYPE OF TRIP: Out-and-back
DIFFICULTY: Moderately strenuous
SOLITUDE: Moderate solitude
LOCATION: San Gabriel Wilderness
MAPS: USGS 7.5-min. *Chilao Flat* and *Waterman Mtn.*
BEST SEASONS: Fall, winter, and spring

PERMITS

A wilderness permit is not required. Campfires are prohibited outside of designated campgrounds in the Angeles National Forest. A fire permit is required for the use of self-contained camp stoves, which may be used at remote sites whenever the wildfire potential is not deemed too great. Cars parked at the trailhead must display a National Forest Adventure Pass. Contact San Gabriel River Ranger District, Angeles National Forest at 626-335-1251 or visit www. fs.fed.us/r5/angeles.

Photo: *Looking down into the wilds of the San Gabriel Wilderness*

TAKE THIS TRIP

The varied, rough, and remote habitat of the San Gabriel Wilderness harbors mule deer, Nelson bighorn sheep, black bears, and mountain lions—facts that hint at the quality of the wilderness experience you can get here. Only one trail stabs deeply into the corrugated heart of this wilderness: the Devils Canyon Trail. It leads you to a clear, cascading stream fringed by a green ribbon of vegetation hidden in the crease of a 2000-foot-deep canyon. Splash around in shallow pools, watch ducks and water ouzels at work or play, fish for trout, or trek down-canyon to visit the upper lip of a waterfall.

CHALLENGES

Rare, torrential floods may visit Devils Canyon after heavy winter rains, rendering the canyon stream impossible to ford. The hike into and along the canyon is entirely downhill on the way in and uphill on the way out. If the weather is warm and sunny, you may want to wait until afternoon before you start the steep climb out to ensure that you get plenty of shade.

HOW TO GET THERE

From Interstate 210 in La Canada-Flintridge, drive up Angeles Crest Highway (State Highway 2) for 27 miles to the Devils Canyon Trailhead. The well-marked trailhead is 3 miles past the Charlton Flats Picnic Area. If you reach the turnoff for the Chilao Visitor Center, you have gone about 200 yards too far.

TRIP DESCRIPTION

The zigzagging descent on the trail takes you across slopes clothed alternately in chaparral and mixed conifer forest. By 1.5 miles you reach a branch of what will soon become a trickling stream—one of the several tributaries that contribute to Devils Canyon's ample springtime flow. The deeply shaded trail leads to the main canyon at 2.6 miles. (Be sure to mark this spot or take note of surrounding landmarks so you can recognize this place when it's time to head back up the trail.) The trail continues a bit farther downstream to reach the site of a former trail camp on a flat bench west of the Devils Canyon stream. In accordance with the philosophy of returning wilderness areas to as natural a condition as possible, this former trail camp has had its stoves and tables removed.

Downstream, some real fun ensues if you're sure-footed and adventurous. Here and there, you follow a pathway alongside the stream; otherwise you boulder-hop and wade. Mini-cascades feed pools 3–4 feet deep

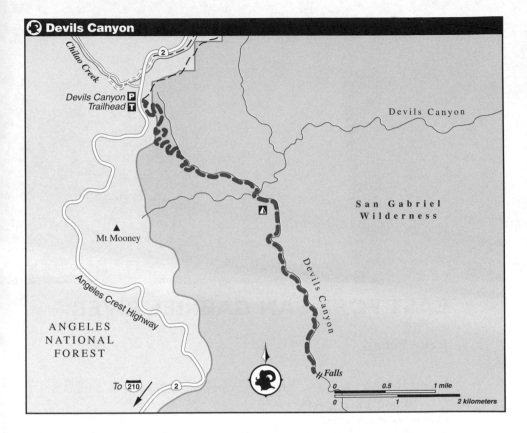

harboring elusive brook trout. Water-loving alders and sycamores cluster along the stream, while patriarchal live oaks and bigcone Douglas firs stand on higher and dryer benches and slopes, waiting in the wings, as it were, for the next big flood to sweep the upstarts away. Watch for poison oak as the canyon walls narrow; and keep an eye out for a silvery, two-tier waterfall at the mouth of a side canyon coming in from the east, nearly 2 miles down from the campsite.

Beyond the two-tier fall, 0.4 mile of rock scrambling and wading takes you to a constriction in the canyon where water slides down a sheer incline some 20 vertical feet. Avoiding the slippery lip of these falls, you might try scrambling up the rock wall to the right for an airy view of the cascade and shallow pool below. Without rappelling gear, this is basically the end of the line for downstream travel through the canyon. At this point you've come 4.9 miles from the Devils Canyon Trailhead and descended some 2100 feet. Your return trip will be entirely uphill.

BUILD-UP AND WIND-DOWN TIPS ·

Either before or after your journey, visit the **Chilao Visitor Center**, open daily and just north of the Devils Canyon Trailhead. This is the major interpretive facility for Angeles National Forest, which has exhibits, free printed information, books for sale, and rangers on duty.

12

EAST FORK SAN GABRIEL RIVER

Jerry Schad

> **MILES:** 14.5; 7.3 and 8.4 to wilderness campsites at Fish Fork and
>   Iron Fork, respectively
> **RECOMMENDED DAYS:** 2
> **ELEVATION GAIN/LOSS:** 200´/4800´
> **TYPE OF TRIP:** Point-to-point
> **DIFFICULTY:** Moderately strenuous
> **SOLITUDE:** Moderate solitude
> **LOCATION:** Sheep Mountain Wilderness, Angeles National Forest
> **MAPS:** USGS 7.5-min. *Crystal Lake, Mount San Antonio,* and *Glendora*
> **BEST SEASONS:** Late spring, summer, and fall

PERMITS

A wilderness permit is not required, although there is a self-registering wilderness permit kiosk at the East Fork Trailhead at the finish point (East Fork Ranger Station). Campfires are prohibited outside of designated campgrounds in the Angeles National Forest. A fire permit is required for the use of self-contained camp stoves, which may be used at remote sites whenever the wildfire potential is not deemed too great. Cars parked at both trailheads must display a National Forest Adventure Pass. Contact San Gabriel River Ranger District, Angeles National Forest, 626-335-1251, www.fs.fed.us/r5/angeles.

Photo: Fish Fork, a tributary of the East Fork San Gabriel River

CHALLENGES

The upper trailhead at Vincent Gap may not be accessible through early spring due to snow. High water levels in the East Fork after a rainy winter or spring may make this route impassable or dangerous. Contact the U.S. Forest Service (or check out water levels in the lower canyon for yourself) before attempting this one-way, downhill trip. Long and hot June and July days are fine as long as you keep cool by getting wet at frequent intervals.

HOW TO GET THERE

It's best to have someone drop you off at the start (Vincent Gap) and later pick you up at the end (East Fork Station), an 85-mile drive around by way of Interstate 15 to the east. The Vincent Gap Trailhead is on Angeles Crest Highway, 9 miles west of Wrightwood. To reach East Fork Station, drive north from Azusa on Highway 39 for 10 miles to East Fork Road, and then go east 6 miles to the end of the road.

TRIP DESCRIPTION

From the parking area on the south side of Vincent Gap, walk down the gated road to the southeast. After only about 200 yards, a footpath veers left, into Sheep Mountain Wilderness. Take it; the road itself continues toward the posted, privately owned Big Horn Mine, an inholding in the national forest.

You're intermittently shaded by bigcone Douglas firs, white firs, Jeffrey pines, and live oaks as you follow the descending path along the south slope of Vincent Gulch. The gulch itself follows the Punchbowl Fault, a splinter of the San Andreas Fault. After a few switchbacks, the trail crosses Vincent Gulch (usually dry at this point, wet a short distance below) at 1.6 miles. Thereafter it stays on or above the east bank as far as the confluence of Prairie Fork, 3.8 miles. At Prairie Fork a trail heads east to Cabin Flat. You veer right (west) down

TAKE THIS TRIP

On this epic journey along the banks of the East Fork San Gabriel River, you'll descend nearly a mile in elevation, traveling from high-country pines and firs to sun-scorched chaparral. On the first day of hiking, you could experience a temperature fluctuation of as much as 50°F. At one spot called the Narrows in the East Fork canyon, the stream lies 5200 feet below Iron Mountain to the east and 4000 feet below the ridge to the west—making this the deepest gorge in Southern California.

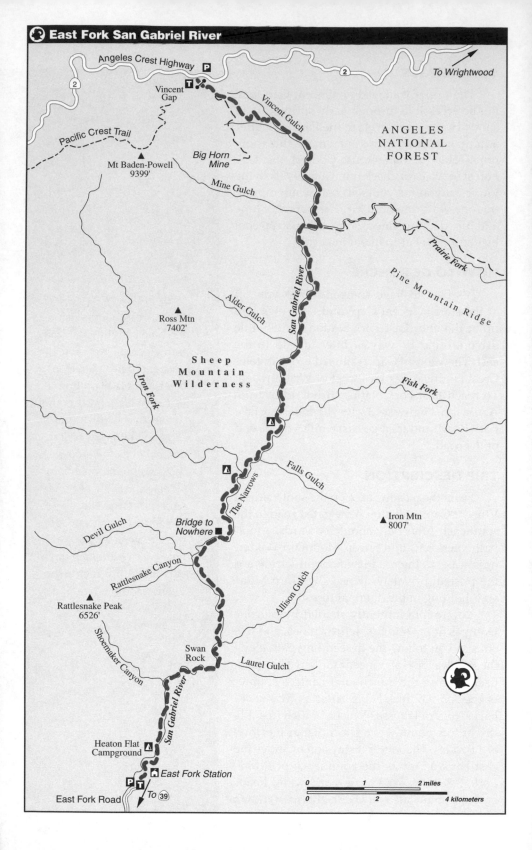

Angeles Crest Highway

P

2

To Wrightwood

2

Vincent
Gap

T

Vincent Gulch

ANGELES
NATIONAL
FOREST

Pacific Crest Trail

Big Horn
Mine

Mt Baden-Powell
9399'

Mine Gulch

Prairie Fork

San Gabriel River

Pine Mountain Ridge

Alder Gulch

Ross Mtn
7402'

Sheep
Mountain
Wilderness

Fish Fork

Iron Fork

Falls Gulch

The Narrows

Iron Mtn
8007'

Devil Gulch

Bridge to
Nowhere

Rattlesnake Canyon

Allison Gulch

Rattlesnake Peak
6526'

Shoemaker Canyon

Swan
Rock

Laurel Gulch

San Gabriel River

Heaton Flat
Campground

East Fork Station

P

T

To 39

East Fork Road

0		1		2 miles
0		2		4 kilometers

a gravelly wash, good for setting up a camp. Shortly after, at the Mine Gulch confluence, you bend left (south) into the wide bed of the upper East Fork. For several miles to come, there's no well-defined trail and it is here that any swiftly flowing water would present possible insurmountable challenges.

Proceed down the rock-strewn flood plain, crossing the creek (and battling alder thickets) several times over the next mile. The canyon becomes narrow for a while starting at about 5.0 miles, and you must wade or hop from one slippery rock to another. Fish Fork, on the left (east) at 7.3 miles, is the first large stream below Prairie Fork. Flat sites suitable for camping are nearby. The mouth of Iron Fork, on the right (west) at 8.4 miles, has more possible campsites.

If you have the time for an intriguing side trip, Fish Fork Canyon is well worth exploring. Chock full of alder and bay, narrow with soaring walls, its clear stream tumbling over boulders, the canyon boasts one of the wildest and most beautiful settings in the San Gabriel Mountains. About 1.6 miles upstream lies a formidable impasse: There, the waters of Fish Fork drop 12 feet into an emerald-green pool set amid sheer rock walls.

Below Iron Fork you enter the Narrows. A rough trail, worn in by hikers, traverses this one-mile-plus section of fast-moving water. You'll pass swimmable pools cupped in the granite and schist bedrock, and cross the stream when necessary. Listen and watch for water ouzels by the edges of the pools.

At the lower portals of the Narrows (9.7 miles), you come upon the enigmatically named Bridge to Nowhere. During the 1930s, road builders managed to push a highway up along the East Fork stream to just this far. The arched, concrete bridge, similar in style to those built along Angeles Crest Highway, was to be a key link in a route that would carry traffic between the San Gabriel Valley and the desert near Wrightwood. Fate intervened. A great flood in 1938 thoroughly demolished most of the road, leaving the bridge stranded.

Below the bridge, on remnants of the washed-out road, you'll run into more and more hikers, people fishing, and other travelers out for the day. At 12.0 miles, Swan Rock—an outcrop of metamorphic rock branded with the light-colored imprint of a swan—comes into view on the right. At 14.0 miles you come upon Heaton Flat Campground. From there a final, easy 0.5-mile stroll takes you to the East Fork Trailhead at the end of East Fork Road.

BUILD-UP AND WIND-DOWN TIPS

The West Fork San Gabriel River, considerably tamer in topography than the East Fork, contains the popular **West Fork National Recreation Trail**. The trail is a paved path (closed to motor vehicles) that runs for 7.5 miles from Highway 39 to the dam of Cogswell Reservoir. Fishing, bicycling, and picnicking are popular activities along this trail—something to consider for the person or persons who may be assisting you with transportation.

13

POINT MUGU STATE PARK LOOP

Doug Christiansen

MILES: 23.2
RECOMMENDED DAYS: 2–3
ELEVATION GAIN/LOSS: 5050´/5050´
TYPE OF TRIP: Loop
DIFFICULTY: Moderate
SOLITUDE: Crowded
LOCATION: Point Mugu State Park
MAPS: USGS 7.5 min. *Pt. Mugu* and *Triunfo Pass*
BEST SEASON: Winter through spring

PERMITS

A permit is not required for a backcountry trip, but first-come, first-served La Jolla Valley Walk-In Camp charges a $3 fee per person per night, which you'll need to deposit in the "iron ranger" fee collection box at the campground itself. A host of agencies at the city, county, state, and national level are charged with oversight of the area; an excellent visitor center (805-370-2301) at 401 West Hillcrest Drive in Thousand Oaks offers maps, books, pamphlets, and advice.

Photo: *La Jolla Valley in summer, Santa Monica Mountains*

CHALLENGES

This is not summer hiking country! Although it's near the coast, temperatures skyrocket a ridge or two inland. Water is scant or nonexistent, and there's little shade on most sections of the hike.

HOW TO GET THERE

From Santa Monica, drive west on Pacific Coast Highway (Highway 1), past the Ventura County Line, to the Ray Miller Trailhead at the mouth of La Jolla Canyon, some 32 miles from Santa Monica. You'll see the Thornhill Broome Beach campground on your left along the immediate shore. Take the narrow road a few hundred yards inland to a small parking area adjacent to the trailhead.

TRIP DESCRIPTION

As you travel west on the Pacific Coast Highway, past the condos and the markets and beachfront palaces, you cross into Ventura County and finally reach the point where you feel you've left L.A. behind you—welcome to Pt. Mugu State Park. While most of the rest of the Santa Monica Mountains give the appearance of being little more than a large city park, the Pt. Mugu area provides a touch of wilderness at the extreme western end of the range. This is ideal winter and early-spring hiking country, when water is still running in the canyon-bottoms, the grass is green, and wildflowers dot the landscape. This three-day trip uses La Jolla Valley as a base camp. Although there are water faucets at various points near the campground, they're not dependable. Plan to carry all the water you'll need, at least 3 quarts per day per person.

From the Ray Miller Trailhead, walk past the sign for the Backbone Trail, which will be your return route, and take the wide trail that heads up La Jolla Canyon. After a short distance the trail climbs up and around a small waterfall, impressive in season, and soon (1.2

TAKE THIS TRIP

Simply put, this trip gives you the best bang for your buck in the Santa Monica Mountains. The Pt. Mugu area is the most remote, least traveled, and closest thing to wilderness in the range. With so many trails in the area, this loop hike is only one of several options. In spring after a wet winter, this is one of the most beautiful areas in Southern California. And it's all within an hour's drive of Los Angeles!

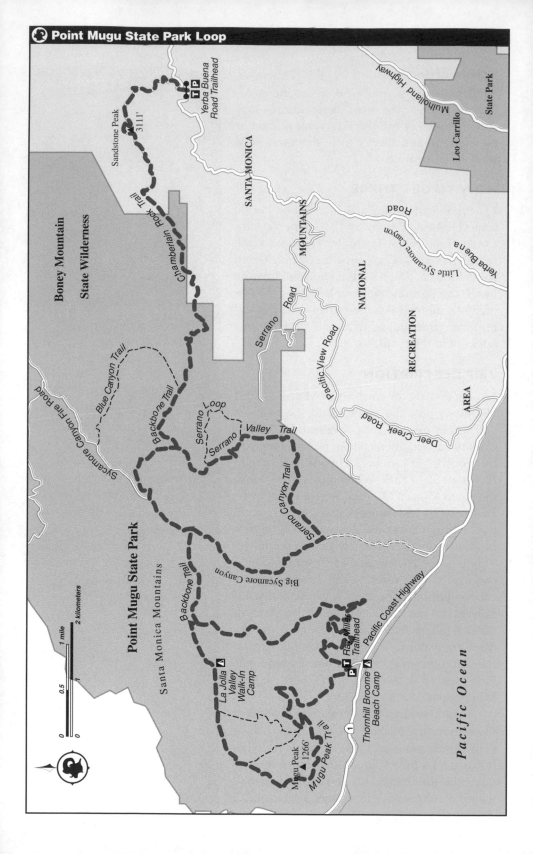

miles from the trailhead) you meet the narrow La Jolla Valley Loop Trail on your left; take this as it begins climbing up the west side of the canyon 0.4 mile to a junction with the Mugu Peak Trail where you bear left. You contour around the east and south flank of 1266-foot Mugu Peak until in just under a mile you reach a saddle; the steep five-minute scramble to the summit is well worth the effort. Below, to the south, stretches the vast Pacific. To the north is La Jolla Valley where you'll be camping later in the day.

Retrace your steps down the trail back to the saddle and continue west along the south face of Mugu Peak to an intersection with the Chumash Trail and more great views of the Pacific, 1.8 miles from where you joined the Mugu Peak Trail. Turn right here and head north along the trail as it descends into lovely La Jolla Valley, turns to the northeast, and finally deposits you at La Jolla Valley Walk-In Camp, 5.8 miles from the trailhead. Here among the spreading branches of oaks and some of the last remaining native grassland in Southern California, you make your base camp. If it's winter or spring in a season of normal-or-greater rainfall, you'll find a small, delightful pond at the southern end of the campground. Be sure to camp in the walk-in/hike-in campground and not the slightly more northern group campground intended for parties of 10 or more. Use the "iron ranger" to pay your fee. There's piped water at the campground, but, depending on conditions, the faucets may or may not deliver any water.

To begin the most strenuous day of the trip, 11.9 miles, walk northeast past the La Jolla Group Campground about 0.6 mile to a junction with the Overlook Fire Road, where you turn right; after a very short distance you turn left onto the Backbone Trail. The Backbone Trail loosely follows the crest of the range from east to west for nearly 70 miles from its beginning at the Ray Miller Trailhead to its end at Will Rogers State Historic Park. For this segment you follow the trail east 1.8 miles to a junction with Sycamore Canyon Fire Road. Later you'll explore the more southern portion of this beautiful valley; for now turn left and hike up-canyon 0.6 mile to a junction with the Old Boney Trail where you may want to pause and take a drink and catch your breath; you're about to climb 1000 feet in a little over a mile! The Boney Mountain State Wilderness comprises 6000 wild and lonely acres in the eastern portion of Pt. Mugu State Park. Here you're on the western flank of the main ridge as it undulates eastward to 3111-foot Sandstone Peak, the highest point in the Santa Monicas.

TEST YOUR EQUIPMENT

Test all your vital equipment at home before your trip. Check your flashlight or headlamp batteries. Test your lighter. Fire up your stove someplace outdoors. If your tent is new or it's been a while since you've used it, practice setting it up and taking it down. It never hurts to check it to make sure all the parts are included and in working order. Be prepared!

MAKING SURE YOU CAN SEE

If you wear eyeglasses or contacts, consider bringing a backup pair. Of course, it never hurts to bring a pair of glasses if you wear contacts or vice versa. You certainly don't want to find yourself unable to see in the middle of a backpacking trip. And don't forget to bring the requisite lens fluids and a mirror if you need one.

Back to the trail; 1.2 miles from Sycamore Canyon Road you reach a junction; the Boney Trail bears left where it soon meets up with the Backbone Trail. A worthwhile option here would be to take this trail for 6.5 miles, all the way east to Sandstone Peak and then down to the Yerba Buena Road, which would involve a 10-mile car shuttle from the Ray Miller Trailhead and would reduce the trip to two days. The three-day hike continues straight ahead on the Serrano Valley Trail. Serrano Valley is a quiet, sylvan glen with groves of oak, bay, and sycamore. You'll be tempted to stop by one of the many pools along the stream and cool your feet under the shady green canopy above. This is one of the hidden treasures of the Santa Monicas and well worth the effort you've already expended to get here.

Continue on the Serrano Valley Trail and bear right at three trail junctions in quick succession; they're part of the Serrano Loop Trail. At 3.5 miles from where you left the Old Boney Trail, 7.7 miles from the start, you rejoin Sycamore

Ray Miller Trailhead, Pt. Mugu State Park

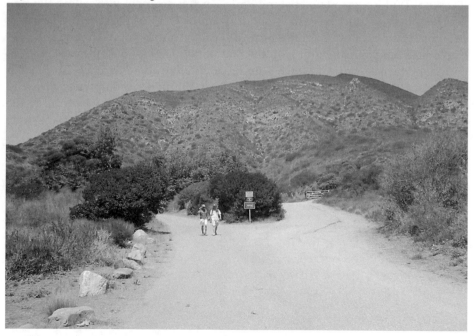

Canyon Road. Sycamore Canyon is another gem of the Santa Monicas. An easily-graded road passes through native grasses and stately sycamore trees as it meanders from Pacific Coast Highway through the heart of the range to near Highway 101 in the San Fernando Valley. From mid-October through February the canyon is home to large numbers of migrating monarch butterflies, and in any season it's prime birdwatching habitat. This very pleasant portion of the hike travels 1.8 miles north to the intersection of the Backbone Trail that you hiked earlier in the day. Turn left here and retrace your steps 2.4 miles back to La Jolla Valley Campground for a much needed rest!

It's 5.5 miles back to the Ray Miller Trailhead; start by once again walking northeast through the campground to the Overlook Fire Road. Turn right and follow the wide dirt road south; it follows the ridge and affords fine views of the country you've been hiking, Sycamore Canyon on your left and La Jolla Valley on your right. In 2 miles you meet the Backbone Trail as it climbs steeply up from the trailhead. From here it's a 2.7-mile, 950-foot descent back to the parking lot and your car.

BUILD-UP AND WIND-DOWN TIPS ·

After three days on the trail you're bound to be famished; on your way back to civilization stop in at **Malibu Seafood**, at 25653 Pacific Coast Highway, about 1.5 miles west of Pepperdine University. It's an unpretentious, funky little eatery with patio seating and a wide variety of fresh fish that won't leave your wallet too much lighter.

THE COAST RANGES

C alifornia's Coast Ranges stretch from San Diego to the Oregon border, a near-continuous line of rugged subranges that runs parallel to the coastline and extends inland for roughly 100 miles. The overall topography consists of closely packed ridgelines and peaks separated by narrow, often deep valleys. Unlike the hard granite bedrock of the Sierra Nevada, the underlying geology consists primarily of the Franciscan Formation, a collection of mudstones, sandstones, and other loosely consolidated sedimentary rock. Annual precipitation increases as you travel from the chaparral slopes of southern California to the redwood forest of the central and northern coastlines. Rainfall is highest along the coastline, but diminishes rapidly as you move inland.

In southern California, the San Bernardino and San Gabriel mountains arc east-west around the Los Angeles metropolitan area, transitioning into the San Rafael and Sierra Madre Mountains to the north. These mountains then merge into the Santa Lucia Range, which rises abruptly from the ocean to form the precipitous interior terrain of the Big Sur region. A break in the Coast Ranges occurs inland from Monterey Bay before the land rises upward again to form the many subranges of the San Francisco Bay Area, including the redwood-cloaked Santa Cruz Mountains, oak-studded Diablo Range of the East Bay, and peaks of Marin County and Point Reyes National Seashore. From here north, the mountains widen into the broad expanse of Mendocino National Forest and eventually transition into the peaks of northwest California's Klamath Mountains. The topography remains sheer and severe along the coastline, however, reaching a rugged crescendo along the Lost Coast—the wildest stretch of coastline in the Lower 48 states.

BIG SUR

The name Big Sur evokes images of a wild coast nestled along the base of the rugged Santa Lucia Range. California's Big Sur country stretches from Carmel south to San Simeon, and from the Pacific Ocean east into the Santa Lucias. This dramatic landscape was home to the Native American Esselen, Ohlone, and Salinian tribes until the mid-1800s, when a handful of homesteaders, fur traders, ranchers, and entrepreneurs settled the area, building steep, narrow wagon roads.

Today, Big Sur shelters a wealth of natural treasures, from steep, redwood-lined canyons to headlands that tumble precipitously into the sea. It is still incredibly remote, with few roads crossing the Santa Lucia Range, and remains one of the largest roadless areas along the continental U.S. coastline. Though its attributes are many, Big Sur's inner beauty eludes most travelers who never venture far from Highway 1. The result is a vast, remote wilderness for backpackers to explore.

The trips into the Ventana Wilderness included in this book visit wildflower-strewn hillsides, oak woodlands, towering redwoods, fragrant coastal scrub, and pine-studded ridges. The higher you climb, the more rewarding the views become, with glimpses east into the sheer Santa Lucias and west to the rugged coast. Whatever you choose you're bound to return.

DIABLO RANGE

On the southeast edge of the Bay Area, a broad swath of landscape has been wrinkled upward to form the Diablo Range. A multitude of north-south ridges pack closely together to compose this wild and seldom-trod landscape, cloaked by rolling oak woodlands, sun-baked chaparral, and a riot of spring wildflowers. It is the Bay Area's most remote, challenging, and enticing backcountry destination.

Near the northern end of the range, the long-distance Ohlone Trail crosses the breadth of the mountains, traveling from Sunol Regional Wilderness to Del Valle Regional Park. A series of designated backcountry camping areas nestle beneath rustling oaks along the way, and the route winds past myriad viewpoints that encompass nearly the entire Diablo Range. Rose Peak looms near the middle of the hike, only 32 feet lower than Mount Diablo, offering views that span from San Francisco to the Sierra Nevada.

Farther south is Henry Coe State Park, the state's second largest state park and the largest parcel of protected land in the Bay Area. Its 85,000 acres include some of the most remote backcountry in the Bay Area, including the 23,300-acre Orestimba Wilderness in the park's northeast corner. This idyllic wilderness is truly out there; just to reach it requires a 15-mile hike. In September 2007, a large wildfire scorched 47,760 acres of the Diablo Range. Known as the Lick Fire, the conflagration burned 40,000 acres within Henry Coe State Park, including most of the park's eastern half and the entire Orestimba Wilderness. While the damage was not cataclysmic—most of the park's oak trees survived the blaze—trails and large swaths of the landscape were significantly affected. Wildfires are a natural part of the park's ecosystem, and the backcountry is expected to fully recover over the next few years.

The Diablo Range is primarily a spring destination, though fall trips are also a possibility along the Ohlone Trail and in some portions of Henry Coe. The heat of the summer sun on miles of unshaded trail can be oppressive, while the cold heights—and possibility of snow—make winter less appealing. Spring is prime time for this hike as wildflowers explode in one of the Bay Area's most dazzling and diverse displays. Wildflowers are extraordinary from March through May, and dozens of different species can be seen along the trail. Water becomes scarce to nonexistent throughout much of Henry Coe from late May until the winter rains have replenished the area.

SANTA CRUZ MOUNTAINS

The Santa Cruz Mountains are located between San Francisco and the Monterey Bay, extending south from Half Moon Bay to Santa Cruz and then west to the Santa Clara Valley south of San Jose. A multitude of creeks incise the rugged, ridge-lined landscape; stately redwood forests cloak the moist stream and river valleys. The geography is largely defined by the axis of long, northwest-trending Skyline Ridge. Stretching more than 50 miles from near Gilroy to Highway 92 above Half Moon Bay, it rises some 3000 feet and separates the developed Bay Area from the wild heart of these mountains. A multitude of creeks and rivers tumble west from Skyline Ridge toward the ocean, the largest of which are (from north to south) Pescadero Creek, Waddell Creek, and the San Lorenzo River.

In the heart of the Santa Cruz Mountains lies a large complex of contiguous and interconnected parks, centered around the Pescadero and Waddell creek drainages. The centerpiece is Big Basin Redwoods State Park, which protects the largest stand of old-growth redwood forest south of Humboldt County. Miles and miles of trail explore the park's primeval majesty, but perhaps none are as varied or compelling as the Skyline-to-the-Sea Trail.

This long-distance route begins atop Skyline Ridge in Castle Rock State Park and then travels west to reach the Pacific Ocean at Waddell Beach. En route it winds through Big Basin Redwoods State Park, including a 10-mile section of continuous old-growth redwood forest. A series of backcountry camping areas make this an ideal two- to three-day backpacking journey through the best of the Santa Cruz Mountains.

POINT REYES NATIONAL SEASHORE

An isolated world of forest and sea, Point Reyes National Seashore protects 30,000 acres of wild California within the boundaries of Philip Burton Wilderness. More than 100 miles of trail interlace through this protected landscape, a web of adventure spread among four distinct backcountry campgrounds. Come here to camp on a wild shoreline, commune with haunting old-growth forest, and experience a vast tract of coastal wilderness unlike any other in California. Along the coast, sandy beaches intersperse inaccessible cliffs. Salty spray and ocean winds combine to create low-lying coastal scrub along the immediate shoreline, providing far-reaching views of the Pacific Ocean. Inland, a moist and ferny forest of Douglas fir blankets the slopes and crest of Inverness Ridge. Point Reyes is a year-round destination, though summer is perhaps the least desirable season due to the thick fog that regularly smothers the landscape.

Philip Burton Wilderness lies in the rugged southern half of the Point Reyes Peninsula and encompasses a rectangular swath of land that stretches from the Pacific Ocean east over 1,200-foot Inverness Ridge to the Olema Valley, and is bordered to the north and south by Limantour Road and the town of Bolinas, respectively. Backcountry camping is confined to four designated hike-in camp-grounds—Coast, Sky, Glen, and Wildcat camps—each of which has its unique appeal.

LOST COAST

The Lost Coast can hardly be considered undiscovered. Ranchers, loggers, railroads, mills, and sea ports have all left their mark on the land. But it is remote, too rugged for Highway 1, keeping all but the adventurous away. The Lost Coast stretches from the Eel River Delta near Ferndale south to Highway 1, a distance of more than 70 miles. It is the most seismically active region in the state. Off-shore lies the Mendocino Triple Junction, the point where three tectonic plates meet. The San Andreas Fault reaches its terminus here, shearing the landscape with a multitude of faults. All this geologic activity causes dramatic uplift of the land, forming towering cliffs and summits that rise abruptly from the crashing sea. The dark cliffs weather to form unusual black sand beaches. Small creeks carve deep gullies on the mountainsides and provide entry points into the otherwise inaccessible interior.

The town of Shelter Cove—and the paved road that reaches it—neatly divides the Lost Coast. Sinkyone Wilderness State Park encompasses most of the southern section, including more than 22 miles of shoreline. To the north, the King Range Conservation and Wilderness areas protect the lofty King Range and a 23-mile stretch of continuous beach. Hiking in the two areas is markedly different. In Sinkyone, a point-to-point journey on the Lost Coast Trail involves nearly 4000 feet of elevation gain and loss as the route scrambles in and out of severe coastal drainages. In the King Range, you can walk for miles directly along the beach and then turn inland to tour the mountains and ridges surrounding King Peak, which rises to 4088 feet less than 3 miles from the ocean.

14

SYKES HOT SPRINGS

Analise Elliot Heid

MILES: 23.8
RECOMMENDED DAYS: 2–3
ELEVATION GAIN/LOSS: 2380´/1490´
TYPE OF TRIP: Out-and-back
DIFFICULTY: Moderately strenuous
SOLITUDE: Crowded
LOCATION: Pfeiffer Big Sur State Park, Ventana Wilderness
MAPS: USGS 7.5-min. *Big Sur* and *Ventana Cones*;
        Big Sur and Ventana Wilderness by Wilderness Press
BEST SEASON: Late spring through early fall

PERMITS

No wilderness permits are required in Ventana Wilderness. However, if you plan to use an open flame (campfire or cooking stove), you need a free fire permit from Big Sur Station. Campfires are permitted from late November through April (fire season information is posted at the trailhead).

Big Sur Station (831-667-2315) is located a half mile south of the park entrance on Highway 1. From Memorial Day through Labor Day, it is open daily, 8 AM to 6 PM; the rest of the year, it is open daily from 8 AM to 4:30 PM.

Photo: *A tempting oasis along the Big Sur River*

Pfeiffer Big Sur State Park charges an overnight parking fee of $4 per day. No dogs are allowed on state park trails; however, dogs are allowed in Ventana Wilderness.

For more information, visit www.parks.ca.gov or www.fs.fed.us/r5/lospadres.

CHALLENGES

Expect plenty of foot traffic in summer and over spring break (usually the first two weeks in April). If you crave solitude, hike the trail in winter. Be aware, however, that the river can rise swiftly during winter storms, making crossings deep and treacherous. The only ford along this trail is at Sykes Camp, and you can avoid this crossing since the hot springs are all located on the same side of the river. Overall, the trail is well-maintained to clear, but beware of poison oak.

HOW TO GET THERE

Pfeiffer Big Sur State Park is on the east side of Highway 1, 26 miles south of the Carmel Valley Road (County Road G16) junction in Carmel, and 28 miles north of the Nacimiento-Fergusson Road junction near Kirk Creek Campground. Big Sur Station is also on the east side of Highway 1, a half mile south of the state park entrance. The complex serves the U.S. Forest Service, CalTrans, and California State Parks.

The Pine Ridge Trailhead is at Big Sur Station, at the end of the parking lot beyond the visitor center. Self-pay parking is $4 per night. Water, flush toilets, and maps are available at the visitor center.

TRIP DESCRIPTION

The well-marked and heavily used Pine Ridge Trail starts at the southeastern end of the parking lot and briefly skirts a fenced-in pasture, before heading east to enter the cool, damp redwood- and fern-lined gullies high above Pfeiffer Big Sur State Park Campground.

TAKE THIS TRIP

A trip to Sykes Hot Springs is unquestionably the most popular route into the Ventana Wilderness. The trek leads to three rock-lined 100°F hot springs along the crystalline waters of the Big Sur River. Just 4 miles into this trip, you can also take a side excursion to one of Ventana's finest swimming holes, at Ventana Camp. Beyond this junction, the trail leads you high above the Big Sur River and the canyon floor, linking spacious riverside camps, refreshing swimming holes, and sought-after thermal pools at Sykes Camp.

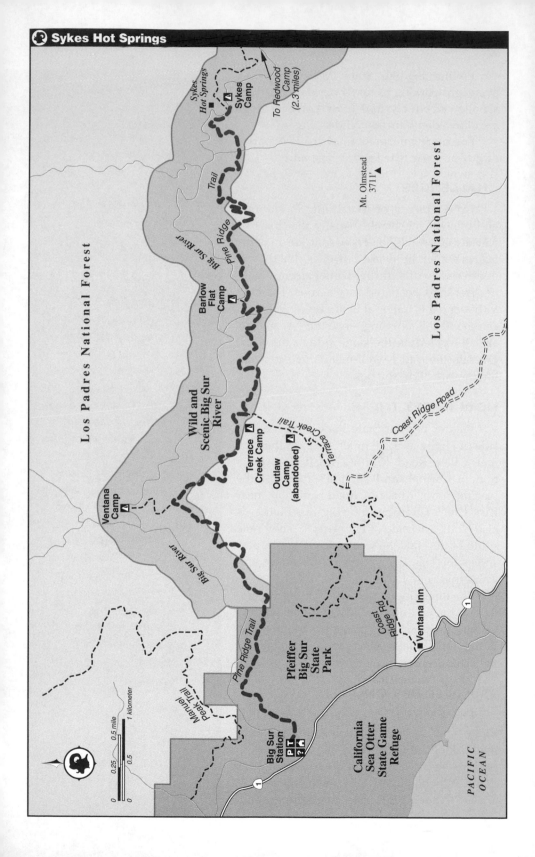

Sykes Hot Springs

Sykes Camp

To Redwood Camp (2.3 miles)

Mt. Olmstead 3711

Los Padres National Forest

Los Padres National Forest

Pine Ridge Trail

Big Sur River

Barlow Flat Camp

Wild and Scenic Big Sur River

Ventana Camp

Terrace Creek Camp

Outlaw Camp (abandoned)

Terrace Creek Trail

Coast Ridge Road

Big Sur River

Pine Ridge Trail

Manuel Peak Trail

Pfeiffer Big Sur State Park

Coast Ridge Rd.

Ventana Inn

Big Sur Station

California Sea Otter State Game Refuge

PACIFIC OCEAN

1

1

0.25   0.5 mile
0.5   1 kilometer
0
0

After a gradual descent and crossing of perennial Post Creek at 0.7 mile, the trail steadily switchbacks up a steep ridge to 850 feet in elevation. Pause to take in the view down-canyon, where the Big Sur River abruptly turns from southwest to northwest on its final stretch to Molera Beach. Also notice the flats where the river meets the major fault of the Big Sur drainage, the Sur Thrust Fault, which steadily slips, compresses, and erodes rocks in its path. The river closely follows this swath of destruction to the Pacific.

Onward, the tread turns to loose gravel along sunny slopes with scattered views into the steep-walled river gorge below. Across the canyon are the exposed south-facing slopes of Manuel Peak, clearly marked by the Manuel Peak Trail, which slices through dense chaparral thickets.

Continue through shady redwood gullies and tanoak groves devastated by sudden oak death, a funguslike pathogen responsible for killing California oaks in epidemic proportions. At 2.3 miles from the trailhead, reach a sign marking the state park boundary and your entry into the Ventana Wilderness.

From here, climb north nearly 300 feet in the next 0.3 mile to the trail's high point, and then turn east for a quick descent through two gullies. The second gully (at 3.3 miles and 1240 feet in elevation) boasts a seasonal, 40-foot waterfall that cascades from trailside cliffs in winter and spring, though by summer is barely a trickle. The trail climbs 0.5 mile past several overlooks and then descends to a nearby ridge and the Ventana Camp Trail junction, marked by a dilapidated sign, at 3.9 miles from the trailhead.

SIDE TRIP: VENTANA CAMP

Ventana Camp Trail is a strenuous 1.2-mile spur trail that drops 840 feet down a series of short switchbacks to a summertime swimming hole at the river. From the junction, turn left (north) down the trail and quickly reach an unofficial campsite. Though waterless and not as scenic as Ventana Camp, this is a good place to camp if you want to avoid hauling heavy gear down (and back up) the steep grade. It can hold up to two tents on sloping ground. After a series of 14 switchbacks, the trail emerges at Ventana Camp, perched atop a broad terrace on the upper Big Sur.

Shaded by oaks, madrones, and redwoods, the camp can accommodate large groups at 10 sites that flank the river. The large swimming hole in the river bend offers respite from the heat. Just past this bend, the river turns south-southwest through a steep-walled gorge, where the collective flow of the watershed's tributaries and runoff funnel through a notch less than 10 feet wide and plunge into one of Ventana's most alluring swimming holes. Depending on water levels, the swimming hole is accessible after a series of boulder hops to the base of the pool. Be aware of swift currents and slippery rocks.

Continue east past the Ventana Camp Trail junction for the remaining 5.7 miles to Sykes Camp. The trail winds deep into the heart of the Big Sur River drainage, ascending 70 feet and descending 260 feet over the next 1.4 miles to Terrace Creek Camp. Ventana (Spanish for "window") is an apt description for this section of trail, which offers framed glimpses down the Big Sur drainage to the sheer peaks and ridges of the Ventana Wilderness and distant Pacific. Look to the northeast for views of notched and barren Ventana Double Cone. According to local legend, a rock bridge once connected its twin peaks, forming a window-like frame of the ocean view nearly 5000 feet above the sea. Whether or not that's true, the double summit served as a prominent landmark for Spanish vessels in the 18th and 19th centuries.

Enjoy the vista, as the trail soon enters shady, viewless gullies laced with ferns and moss-covered boulders amid seasonal springs. After a brief climb to a nearby ridge, descend south into steep, redwood-lined Terrace Creek canyon to Terrace Creek Camp and the Terrace Creek Trail junction, at 5.3 miles from the trailhead.

Visible from the junction, the small camp, which can accommodate up to eight tents, flanks the creek just upstream from the junction. Don't expect solitude, as hikers stream past en route to Sykes Camp or Big Sur Station. You'll find one large main site for up to three tents along the east bank a few yards from the junction, just below a pit toilet. Three smaller sites lie upstream, two downstream. The steep canyon remains cool even in summer heat. In spring, carpets of redwood sorrel, mats of ferns and mosses, and delicate fairy bells line the babbling creek to its confluence with the Big Sur.

Beyond the junction, continue east on the Pine Ridge Trail to ascend 510 feet and descend 210 feet in the next 1.4 miles to Barlow Flat Camp. You'll skirt a ridge and head east along its marble slopes to two seasonal springs. Past the second spring, the trail enters a damp redwood glen. Microclimates vary dramati-

USE A WILDERNESS ETHIC

Part of backpacking is about preserving our land and its inhabitants for future generations, and that means adopting a healthy wilderness ethic:

- Leave no trace: Follow the principles of Leave No Trace—from planning ahead to minimizing your impact on the land. For details on how to do this, see www.lnt.org.
- Travel in small groups: The wilderness experience is about peace and quiet—two qualities that are easier to maintain with fewer people.
- Camp at an established site, or if one isn't available, camp away from the trail and at least 200 feet away from any water source.
- If campfires are allowed, use only established fire rings and keep your fire small, with dead and downed wood for fuel. Always make sure your fire is completely extinguished before you break camp.
- Don't infect the water: Pee, poop (in a toilet or in a hole at least 6 inches deep), and wash (biodegradable soap only) at least 200 feet from all natural water sources.
- Pack it out: As the saying goes, if you pack it in—including any toilet paper you use—pack it out.
- Respect wildlife: Do not feed wild animals or disrupt their habitat.

cally along the trail, which climbs to more arid slopes and sun-drenched ridges. Across the canyon, sheer granite walls reflect the sound of roaring rapids of the Big Sur River in the steep canyon far below.

Beyond a second ridge, the trail switchbacks north down to Logwood Creek canyon, 6.5 miles from the trailhead. The creek is an easy boulder hop in all but the wettest months. After the crossing, ascend 0.1 mile to a saddle, from which you can take a short, steep detour on a spur that climbs 200 feet south offering far-reaching views deep into Pfeiffer Big Sur State Park. Past the spur, the trail descends 0.1 mile to the signed Barlow Flat Camp Trail junction, 6.7 miles from the trailhead.

SIDE TRIP: BARLOW FLAT CAMP

From the junction, take the Barlow Flat Camp Trail north to descend steep switchbacks 150 feet in 0.2 mile to the outskirts of Barlow Flat Camp, the most spacious camp along the Pine Ridge Trail, often welcoming large groups in summer. The first three sites sit atop a flat, redwood-shaded bench above the south bank of the Big Sur River. Three more open sites are nestled amid fragrant bays, maples, alders, and sycamores closer to the water's edge. Five more sites lie beneath redwoods, tanoaks, and peeling madrones along the north bank. The crossing is often wet until summer and may be impassable during or after heavy winter rains. A narrow trail leads upstream, past the fifth site, to an 80-foot-long swimming hole and sandy beach.

The swimming opportunities at Barlow Flat are excellent. Its sun-drenched rocky outcrops are perfect for basking in the sun or diving into some of the deeper pools. Water temperatures are in the low 50s in spring and fall and the low 60s on warm summer days, though the temperatures may rise 10°F on a hot summer day.

A cross-country route northwest leads to more alluring swimming holes downstream (passage can be treacherous in the rainy season). The first pool is adjacent to the campsite farthest downstream along the south bank. Downstream another 150 yards, cascades plunge through the narrow gorge into deep, hidden pools. From late spring through fall, it's best to wade rather than scale the sheer canyon walls. Don't attempt passage in winter, as the frigid river can be swift and dangerous. Beyond an Olympic-sized pool, a gossamer 80-foot fall plunges from a small tributary into the Big Sur. If you're willing to swim and wade farther downstream, you'll reach another emerald pool.

Beyond the signed camp junction, the Pine Ridge Trail heads east toward Sykes Camp, 2.9 miles away. The trail starts out on a moderate, 500-foot climb past a wall of fragile ferns, fed in the wet season by a 40-foot waterfall above the trail. You may miss it entirely in summer. Climb through two increasingly large redwood gullies and emerge amid arid slopes cloaked with fragile wild irises beneath oaks, madrones, and a few pine saplings. As you crest a minor ridge (8.2 miles from the trailhead, at 1640 feet in elevation), the vegetation changes to a chaparral community of chamise, ceanothus, and poison oak.

POISON OAK

Common on stream banks, rocky canyons, mountain flanks, and coastal bluffs from sea level to about 5000 feet, this low-lying bush, shrub, or vine is identifiable by its cluster of three leaves that usually range from a half inch to 2 inches long. In fall, the leaves turn a brilliant red, while branches are bare in winter. Unfortunately, all parts of the plant are toxic year-round. Avoid the dreaded itchy rash by wearing long pants and long-sleeved shirts in poison oak areas. If you come into contact with it, wash your skin thoroughly with a product designed to remove the plant's toxic oil, such as Tecnu. If you get the rash and your symptoms are severe, see a physician.

Beyond this exposed ridge, descend 200 feet to a cool, damp redwood gully that provides habitat for six-fingered ferns, which bear delicate palmate fronds. Beyond the gully, the route contours 0.2 mile along Dolores Creek canyon to a small knoll and dips directly above hidden Sykes Hot Springs. Continue your descent southeast, switchback northwest, and then descend 150 feet to the Big Sur. The trail emerges at Sykes Camp and the Sykes Hot Springs Trail junction, at 9.6 miles from the trailhead. Sprawled along a 0.1-mile stretch of the Big Sur, Sykes Camp offers campers their choice of 10 sites. The best ones lie upstream from the Pine Ridge Trail.

Heading to camp from the trail junction, cross the river and head east upstream to a sandy beach and adjacent emerald pool. (This wet ford can be swift and treacherous as the river swells in the winter.) From here, you will soon reach the first of six sites, with room for up to two tents beneath live oaks and madrones. Fifty feet upstream is a pit toilet amid three large redwoods. The second and third sites lie nearby, along a narrow gravel bench. Each can accommodate up to three tents. A larger fourth site is perched above the rocky bank in the shade of fragrant bays, madrones, and live oaks, whose roots grasp riverside boulders. Secluded pools below this site are often less crowded than pools closer to the hot springs. Perch atop the sun-baked boulders and watch small trout dart between the whitewater cascades and calm pools.

Beyond the fourth site, the camp trail leads 60 feet upstream, crosses the river, and emerges on a sandy beach beside another attractive pool. Just above this pool is the fifth site, which can accommodate up to two tents. Eighty feet past a bend is the similarly small sixth site, atop a sandy flat bordered by a smooth rock face and alders.

Downstream from the junction with the Pine Ridge Trail, the unmarked 0.4-mile spur to Sykes Hot Springs heads west along the southern banks of the Big Sur. It is heavily used and easy to follow. Those who want to keep their feet dry will have to navigate sheer rock faces laced with poison oak. The preferred route requires a few boulder hops or a wade that may be difficult or impassable in the rainy season.

Assuming water levels are safe for the latter route, the spur trail from the Pine Ridge Trail junction heads downstream along the south bank 25 feet to the first crossing. After the crossing, pass a small, single-tent site along the northern bank, recross the river, and reach two more sites, equipped with a pit toilet. Beyond the third site, the trail crosses the river twice in 100 feet and arrives at a fourth site. About 0.3 mile downstream, you'll catch a whiff of sulfur from the first of several small hot seeps.

Along the southern banks of the Big Sur River, the trail ascends 60 feet from the water's edge to the first of three small pools (all located on the same side of the river), each large enough for up to four adults. Directly below the pool is a stone- and sandbag-lined hot tub, 6 feet across and 2 to 3 feet deep. Perched beside the clear, bracing waters of the Big Sur, these mineral-rich 100°F pools are among Ventana's most popular destinations. Don't expect a private soak in summer or on weekends and holidays in spring and fall.

Retrace your steps to return to the trailhead.

BUILD-UP AND WIND-DOWN TIPS ·

After more than 20 miles of hiking the Wild and Scenic Big Sur River canyon, renew your spirits and your feet at the **Big Sur River Inn** restaurant and bar (Big Sur River Inn, Highway 1 at Pheneger Creek, Big Sur, CA 93920, 831-667-2700, www.bigsurriverinn.com). You can enjoy a meal served along the banks of the Big Sur River as you dip your feet in the smooth, cool current under your willow chair. The place is steeped in local history, founded in 1934 by Ellen Brown, daughter of John Pfeiffer, and member of one of Big Sur's most prominent pioneering families. Relax, renew, and rejuvenate after a memorable trip!

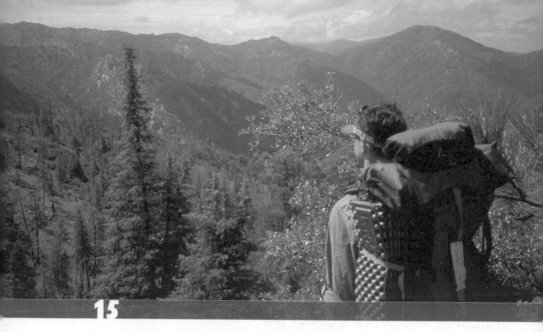

15

BLACK CONE TRAIL

Analise Elliot Heid

MILES: 30.2
RECOMMENDED DAYS: 3
ELEVATION GAIN/LOSS: 2900´/2900´
TYPE OF TRIP: Out-and-back
DIFFICULTY: Moderately strenuous
SOLITUDE: Solitude
LOCATION: Ventana Wilderness, Los Padres National Forest
MAPS: USGS 7.5-min. *Chews Ridge, Ventana Cones,* and *Tassajara Hot Springs; Big Sur and Ventana Wilderness* by Wilderness Press
BEST SEASON: Spring and fall

PERMITS

No wilderness permits are required. If you plan to use an open flame (campfire or cooking stove), you need a free fire permit from Big Sur Station. Campfires are permitted from late November through April (fire season is posted at trailhead). From the west side, obtain your permit at Big Sur Station (831-667-2315), a half mile south of the park entrance on Highway 1. From Memorial Day through Labor Day, it is open daily, 8 AM to 6 PM; the rest of the year, it is open daily, 8 AM to 4:30 PM. From the east side, obtain your fire permit at the U.S. Forest Service Monterey District Headquarters in King City (831-385-5434), open

Photo: The rare Santa Lucia fir grows on the Black Cone Trail's steep, rocky slopes.

Monday through Friday, 8 AM to 4:30 PM. For more information, visit www.parks.ca.gov or www.fs.fed.us/r5/lospadres.

CHALLENGES ·

As is the case with most wilderness trails in Ventana Wilderness, this trail suffers from overgrowth, washouts, and annoying ticks, flies, and mosquitoes. Fortunately, there's little poison oak above 3500 feet on the northern section of the trail, though it fills in again near Strawberry Camp. Bring a walking stick to help navigate the steep and slippery sections. Water can be scarce along much of the route. Fill up at Mosquito Springs, White Cone Springs (0.4 to 0.8 mile past Venturi Camp), the headwaters of the North Fork Big Sur (not reliable by late summer), Black Cone Camp, and Strawberry Creek.

HOW TO GET THERE · · · · · · · · · · · · · · ·

Heading south on Highway 1 from Monterey: Turn left on Carmel Valley Road (County Road G16) in Carmel and head east for 11.7 miles to Carmel Valley Village, your last opportunity for gas, food, and supplies. Drive through the village and continue another 11.3 miles to the Tassajara Road junction.

Heading north on Highway 101 from Southern California: Take Route 101 Business, Greenfield's southernmost exit. In a half mile, turn left on Elm Avenue (County Road G16) and head southwest for 5.8 miles to Arroyo Seco Road (County Road G17). The two roads merge for 6.5 miles and then fork. Take the right branch and continue 17 miles northwest on Carmel Valley Road to the Tassajara Road junction.

From the Tassajara Road junction: Turn southwest and drive 1.3 miles to a fork with Cachagua Road. Take the left branch to continue on Tassajara Road for 10.7 miles to the China Camp entrance. If you plan to camp here, make a sharp right turn into the campground entrance off Tassajara Road and drive

TAKE THIS TRIP

Following the 1977 Marble-Cone Fire, the Forest Service abandoned the Black Cone Trail, which was quickly reclaimed by dense thickets of chaparral. In 1999, Kirk Complex Fires raged along most of the trail, and like a phoenix rising from the ashes, the residual tread of the once lost Black Cone Trail was once again exposed. This now-restored 7.8 mile-route traverses some of Ventana's highest ridges and mountains, connecting the trails of the Arroyo Seco drainage with the trails of the Big Sur River and Carmel River drainages. Enjoy epic views of the Big Sur watershed and some of the best views of the Big Sur backcountry. Without the dedication of dozens of volunteers, it's feasible the trail could be reclaimed by encroaching brush in just a few years.

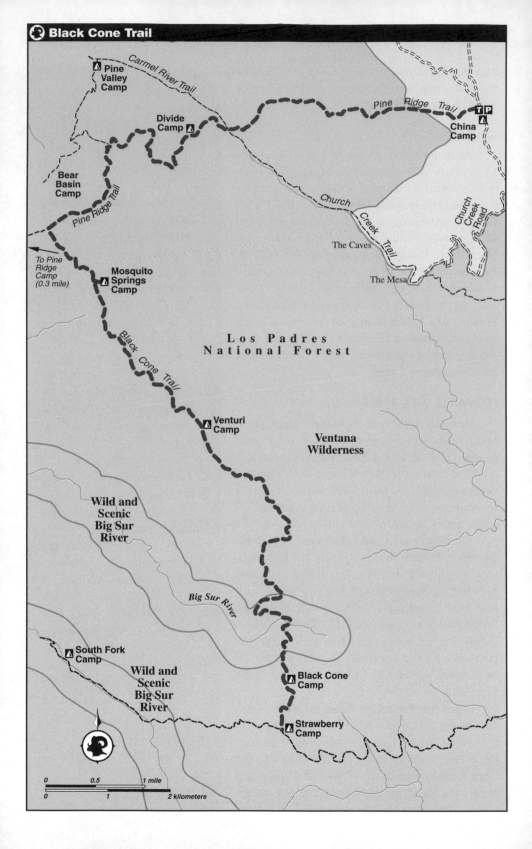

Black Cone Trail

Pine Valley Camp

Carmel River Trail

Divide Camp

Pine Ridge Trail

China Camp

Bear Basin Camp

Pine Ridge Trail

Church Creek Trail

Church Creek Road

The Caves

The Mesa

To Pine Ridge Camp (0.3 mile)

Mosquito Springs Camp

Black Cone Trail

Los Padres National Forest

Venturi Camp

Ventana Wilderness

Wild and Scenic Big Sur River

Big Sur River

Wild and Scenic Big Sur River

South Fork Camp

Black Cone Camp

Strawberry Camp

0   0.5   1 mile

0   1   2 kilometers

200 feet to the campground. If you're not camping, park in the small lot across Tassajara Road from the camp entrance. The trailhead is on the same side of the road as the campground, 100 feet south of the parking lot and 150 feet south of the campground entrance. There's no water at the trailhead. There's no fee if you park at the turnout on Tassajara Road directly across from the China Camp entrance; parking at the campground costs $5 per night.

TRIP DESCRIPTION··

The trail—which is marked, though encroaching brush often obscures the sign—begins on a saddle above China Camp. Like most trails in the Ventana Wilderness, this one is not regularly maintained. In 1999, fire scorched the area, allowing fire-adapted species to thrive. As a result, trail sections over the first 1.2 miles are heavily overgrown.

From the trailhead, head west to gradually climb 400 feet, and then descend the same elevation through shoulder-high brush dominated by ceanothus and tanoak. In 0.6 mile, you'll emerge from the worst of the overgrown sections at the route's high point (4750 feet). Views stretch south to the Black Cone Trail ridgelines and the Church Creek and Tassajara Creek drainages, west along the Coast Ridge, and southeast toward Cone and Junipero Serra peaks. Rising nearly a mile above the Pacific, Cone Peak rises above the farthest visible ridge, 17 miles south. Dominating the horizon to the southeast is 5862-foot Junipero Serra, above the unseen Salinas Valley.

The trail gradually descends a scenic ridge across golden grasslands and past thickets of new growth sprouting from the remains of the charred forest. The ridge separates the Miller Creek and Church Creek drainages. Continue through oak woodlands and grasslands speckled with stalks of Our Lord's candle, top a minor saddle, and climb the ridge to a prominent saddle. Views vanish briefly as the trail switchbacks southwest and then climbs north to the second-highest point (4740 feet) along the route, at 2.1 miles from the trailhead. From here the route is all downhill to Pine Valley.

Pause for glimpses through the bare branches of burned snags. Look west to spot the sandstone formation that parallels Church Creek Fault. The trail turns southwest on a steep grade, dropping 850 feet through open oak woodlands carpeted with vibrant spring wildflowers. After 1.5 miles, the trail switchbacks down to Church Creek Divide, which marks the four-way junction of the westbound Pine Ridge Trail, the southeast-bound Church Creek Trail, and the northwest-bound Carmel River Trail to Pine Valley.

Forming a deep saddle between two west-trending ridges, the divide sits atop the 29-mile east-west Church Creek Fault. For millions of years, the North American and Pacific plates have ground past one another, creating Church Creek canyon. From the divide, the fault continues northwest, following the Carmel River Trail to Hiding Canyon Camp, ascending the Puerto Suelo Trail to the prominent Puerto Suelo saddle, and emerging at the Pacific near Kaslar Point. To the northwest lie the headwaters of the Carmel River, while to the southeast are the headwaters of the Salinas River along Church Creek. Oddly enough, the latter winds some 80 miles north of the Carmel River before finding its way to the sea.

SIDE TRIP: PINE VALLEY

To reach the wildflower-strewn meadows and tall trees of Pine Valley, turn right and head northwest on the Carmel River Trail and walk 1.7 miles to this excellent camping destination with scenes reminiscent of the Sierra. Ponderosa pines rise from an open meadow beside steep, sandstone cliffs, and you can also take a refreshing dip in Pine Valley Falls at the headwaters of the Carmel River. Although the Bear Basin Trail leads back to the Pine Ridge Trail, it is in poor condition. You would be better off retracing your steps to the junction with the Pine Ridge Trail at Church Creek Divide.

If you're not bound for Pine Valley, continue straight (west) along the Pine Ridge Trail. Immediately past the saddle, the trail climbs past heavily overgrown madrones, manzanitas, and ceanothus—fire-adapted species that thrive on this scarred hillside. Cross two small gullies laden with blackberries, horsetails, and fragrant hedge nettles. These seasonal creeks run dry by summer.

Walk about 0.5 mile past head-high brush and scattered black oaks, madrones, and ponderosa pines, and round a minor ridge to reach the Divide Camp Trail junction, 4.1 miles from the trailhead. The spur leads 200 feet north to the first of two sites in the shade of large pines, oaks, and alders. Each can accommodate up to two tents. About 100 feet west of camp is a small spring that dwindles to a muddy seep by midsummer and early fall.

Past the spur junction, the Pine Ridge Trail climbs above camp, meanders southwest past two small seeps, and leads 100 feet farther to a spring-fed creeklet lined with enormous chain ferns. A large fallen oak blocks the trail, requiring careful footing, especially if you're carrying a heavy pack. Past the creeklet, trail conditions worsen, and you must forge through thickets of ceanothus. Fortunately, there's very little poison oak, and the trail is well graded. In spots, the brush clears, offering glimpses of Ventana's high peaks. Flat-topped Uncle Sam Mountain is 6 miles to the northwest, rising above the Puerto Suelo saddle. A long ridge leads left (south) from the saddle up to Ventana Double Cone.

Ascending toward Pine Ridge, cross a small, spring-fed creek, the most reliable water source in the 3.6 miles between Divide Camp and Pine Ridge Camp. The route contours past an unnamed 4751-foot peak to the south, then reaches the Pine Valley-Pine Ridge Trail junction, 5.8 miles from the trailhead. Westbound hikers who spend the night in Pine Valley can rejoin the Pine Ridge Trail here, but would have an easier time going out-and-back to Church Creek Divide (see side trip).

Past the junction, the trail becomes increasingly overgrown with bay laurel, ceanothus, manzanita, and scrub oak, more fire-adapted species. Press on through the encroaching brush to ascend a minor saddle offering good views southeast along Tassajara Creek canyon to the highest point in the Santa Lucia Range, 5862-foot Junipero Serra Peak.

FIRE AS A SHAPING FORCE

Over just two days in the fall of 1999, the Ventana Wilderness was hit by some 1200 lightning strikes, as a subtropical system from the Gulf of California unexpectedly formed a massive electrical storm over the Santa Lucia Range. This awe-inspiring display ignited the Kirk Complex Fires, a series of 47 wildfires that, over three months, swept across more than 90,000 acres of the wilderness, sparing only the most protected canyons and barren ridges.

The region is no stranger to fire. Every acre of the wilderness has been scorched at least twice in this century alone. As a result, many plants are well adapted to fire. Since the Kirk Complex Fires, aggressive brush has overrun the eastern section of the Pine Ridge Trail, rendering it impassable by many hikers' standards. Without maintenance, this section may be completely overgrown within the next couple of years.

From the saddle, the trail gently ascends 200 feet and then quickly descends to Pine Ridge, 7.3 miles from the trailhead. Listen for woodpeckers at work on the enormous charred pine snags atop the ridge. This ridge separates the three major drainages of the northern Santa Lucia Range: The Carmel River headwaters of Blue Creek lie just north of the ridge, the Big Sur River headwaters of Cienega Creek flow southwest, and Tassajara Creek runs southeast into the Arroyo Seco, then north to the Salinas River, and finally out to sea. From Pine Ridge, the major climbing is behind you. Unfortunately, the major bushwhacking is not.

After a few minutes along the ridge, reach the Black Cone Trail junction, where a metal plaque nailed to a charred snag points the way south along the western flanks of 4965-foot South Ventana Cone. Over 0.8 mile, the loose-packed trail passes low-lying thickets of manzanita, scrub oak, ceanothus, yerba santa, and a few yuccas. The first prominent saddle marks the Mosquito Springs Camp Trail junction, at 8.1 miles from the trailhead.

SIDE TRIP: MOSQUITO SPRINGS CAMP

The Mosquito Springs Camp Trail leads east, dropping 500 feet in a half mile to eventually reach Mosquito Camp. This can be a slippery half-mile descent over loose tread obscured by overgrowth. Fortunately, someone has placed yellow flagging at the major switchbacks. As the trail levels off, you reach the camp, which offers a few flat tent sites nestled between granite talus and aggressive brush growth stemming from the 1999 Kirk Complex Fires. Be aware that the one or two decent sites lie along the runoff path for winter storms. True to the camp name, mosquitoes thrive here in spring and early summer, diminishing again by fall. Water is reliable here in all but the driest years.

From the junction, the Black Cone Trail contours just west of the ridgelines that separate the Big Sur and Arroyo Seco drainages. You'll meander on and off the spine, eventually arriving at a saddle atop a steep, narrow canyon that holds the western headwaters of Tassajara Creek. The saddle hosts Venturi Camp (10.7 miles from the trailhead, at an elevation of 4100 feet), which has enough room for two tents. The nearest water is 0.4 mile west downslope along the trail at White Cone Springs. The sheer topography exposes the camp to strong, cold winds that funnel up from the canyon.

Beyond camp, the trail skirts the western flanks of an enormous white granite peak known locally as White Cone. Over the next 0.3 mile, you pass two impressive peaks—4721 feet and 4719 feet, respectively (the trail doesn't thread the peaks, but remains well below them on the contour). You'll soon reach the first of three reliable springs at 11.1 miles from the trailhead; however, this one may run dry in drought years. In just 0.1 mile, White Cone Springs gushes over moss-covered, white granite cliffs. Head east 0.4 mile toward a massive granite face to find the third spring.

Beyond the springs, the trail descends toward a prominent, forked ridge offering views northwest to the Big Sur watershed and Pacific. From this vantage point, you can see most of the remaining 3 miles of the Black Cone Trail as it winds past the western flanks of Black Cone before dropping into Strawberry Valley.

The trail dips through a small canyon that channels a headwater of the North Fork Big Sur River, at 12.6 miles from the trailhead. Across the canyon, the trail ascends to Shotgun Ridge, which overlooks the dozens of creeks, creeklets, springs, ravines, gullies, and broad valleys of the Big Sur drainage below. The ridge was named for a rusty 20-gauge shotgun that was left in the brush with other debris by the crew that forged this trail in the 1960s.

Beyond the ridge, the mostly waterless route reaches another small seep trickling from the mountainside. Fifty yards farther, there is a 200-yard spur down to comfortable Black Cone Camp. A year-round spring issues from the hillside in camp, which can accommodate up to four tents with room to spare.

Beyond the spur, the trail leads 0.3 mile toward a large, reliable creek, another headwater of the North Fork Big Sur. The creek lies along the northeastern flanks of Black Cone, which dominates the eastern skyline less than a half mile

GET TICK SMART

Ticks typically come out following winter's first major rains, and they like to hide out in dense thickets of brush and trees until they spot a worthy patch of skin to latch onto. Usually taking an hour or more to burrow into your skin, these tiny hitchhikers often go unnoticed until they swell with blood. Avoid letting them get this far by wearing long, light-colored clothing (to make it easier to spot the little bloodsuckers), and do tick checks at camp each night. If you find one, use tweezers to grip the tick as close to the skin as possible, and pull it straight out. A tick must be attached for at least 24 hours to transmit Lyme disease, which is very treatable if diagnosed early. If you develop a bull's-eye rash, pain, fever, headache, or muscle ache after a tick bite, see your doctor immediately.

from the trail. From here, contour past three minor ridges to the divide between Strawberry Creek, the Salinas River headwaters, and the North Fork Big Sur. The trail gradually descends an old bulldozed firebreak. Although the trail widens, poison oak returns along the remaining 0.8 mile to Strawberry Camp.

As you descend into Strawberry Valley, cross two small, seasonal creeklets (usually dry by midsummer), following the second creeklet 0.1 mile to Strawberry Camp. Though perched in a small valley, the camp, which can accommodate up to four tents in the shade of a sprawling oak, lies on sloping ground. While the creek may run dry by late summer, a 0.3-mile jaunt downslope to the Marble Peak Trail junction leads to water.

After traversing some of Ventana's highest ridges and mountains, connecting the trails of the Arroyo Seco drainage with the trails of the Big Sur River and Carmel River drainages, the Black Cone Trail ends here, at the South Fork Trail junction, 15.1 miles from the trailhead.

Retrace your steps to return to the trailhead.

BUILD-UP AND WIND-DOWN TIPS ·

When most people think of Big Sur hot springs, they think of Sykes Hot Springs. Few think of the **Tassajara Hot Springs**, located 4 miles south of China Camp on Tassajara Road. These hot springs, while less crowded than Sykes, are only accessible from late April to early September, when the Tassajara Zen Mountain Center is open. The springs are nestled in rugged, mineral rich Tassajara Creek canyon. Humans have used these healing grounds for centuries. The native Esselen people used the hot springs as traditional ceremonial grounds. Today, the springs are only open to guests with reservations at the Tassajara Zen Mountain Center from late April to early September. For reservations, call 831-659-2229 or 415-865-1899; for more information, see www.sfzc.org.

Along Tassajara Road, there are two small Forest Service campgrounds nearby: **White Oaks Campground** (7.9 miles south along Tassajara Road) and **China Camp** (10.7 miles south along Tassajara Road). Both campgrounds are open year-round on a first-come, first-served basis for $5 per night (seven and six sites, respectively). Facilities include vault toilets, fire rings, and picnic tables. For more information, see www.fs.fed.us/r5/lospadres, or call Los Padres National Forest Headquarters at 805-968-6640.

16

CONE PEAK TRAIL

Analise Elliot Heid

MILES: 10.2
RECOMMENDED DAYS: 2
ELEVATION GAIN/LOSS: 3110´/3110´
TYPE OF TRIP: Out-and-back
DIFFICULTY: Moderate
SOLITUDE: Moderate solitude
LOCATION: Ventana Wilderness
MAPS: USGS 7.5-min. *Cone Peak;*
      Big Sur and Ventana Wilderness by Wilderness Press
BEST SEASONS: Spring and fall

PERMITS

No wilderness permits are required in Ventana Wilderness. However, if you plan to use an open flame (campfire or cooking stove), you need a free fire permit. Campfires are permitted from late November through April (fire season is posted at the trailhead).

South of Nacimiento-Fergusson Road, get your fire permit at Pacific Valley Ranger Station (805-927-4211) on the east side of Highway 1, a mile north of the Sand Dollar Beach Day-Use Area, 30 miles north of Hearst Castle, and 60 miles south of Carmel. It is open daily, 8 AM to 5 PM.

Photo: Cone Peak dominates the skyline at 5155 feet, just 3 miles from the Pacific.

North of Nacimiento-Fergusson Road, get your permit at Big Sur Station (831-667-2315), located a half mile south of the park entrance on Highway 1. From Memorial Day through Labor Day, it is open daily from 8 AM to 6 PM; the rest of the year, it is open daily from 8 AM to 4:30 PM.

For more information, visit www.parks. ca.gov or www.fs.fed.us/r5/lospadres.

CHALLENGES ● ● ● ● ● ● ● ● ● ● ● ● ● ● ● ● ● ● ●

If you're bound for this summit when Cone Peak Road is closed (November through May), tack on the additional 5.2 miles each way between the trailhead and junction with Nacimiento-Fergusson Road.

HOW TO GET THERE ● ● ● ● ● ● ● ● ● ● ● ● ●

From Highway 1: Take Highway 1 54 miles south of Carmel or 44 miles north of Cambria to the Nacimiento-Fergusson Road junction, on the east side of the highway. Head east on Nacimiento-Fergusson Road and climb 7.3 very windy miles to the signed junction with Central Coast Ridge Road (better known as Cone Peak Road). Turn left on Cone Peak Road.

From Highway 101: From Highway 101, take the Jolon Road exit, 10 miles south of Greenfield and a mile north of the Salinas River crossing. Follow Jolon Road (County Road G14) 17.8 miles south to Mission Road. Proceed west onto Mission Road, and drive 0.2 mile to the Hunter Liggett Military Reservation gate (expect to show your driver's license and vehicle registration to enter). In 2.9 miles, turn left onto paved Nacimiento-Fergusson Road, which winds 17.9 miles to the signed junction with Central Coast Ridge Road (Cone Peak Road), 300 yards past the Forest Service's Nacimiento Station. Turn right on Cone Peak Road.

From Cone Peak Road: Drive north on Cone Peak Road for 5.2 miles to the signed trailhead on the west side of the road,

TAKE THIS TRIP

This is the shortest trail to one of the highest peaks in the Santa Lucia Range, 5155-foot Cone Peak. Trails to 5862-foot Junipero Serra, 4727-foot Ventana Double Cone, and 4417-foot Mt. Carmel require significantly more elevation gain and mileage to summit. Lording over the southern Ventana Wilderness, Cone Peak offers boundless views along the rugged flanks of the Santa Lucias to the rocky Pacific. The hike is best enjoyed in spring and fall, when fog banks roll well offshore. In winter, snow may fall on the summit, and temperatures can drop below freezing. Bring plenty of water and extra clothing along this exposed trail, and be prepared for rapidly changing conditions.

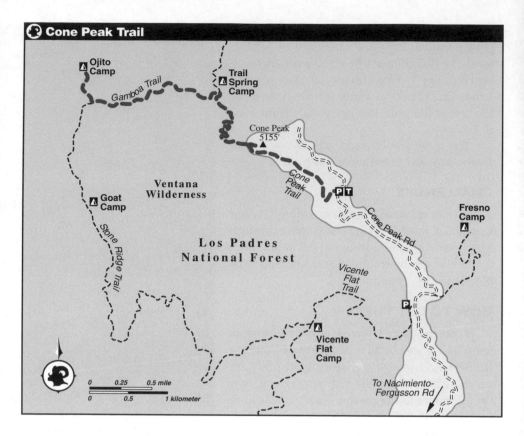

Cone Peak Trail

Ojito Camp

Gamboa Trail

Trail Spring Camp

Cone Peak 5155'

Cone Peak Trail

Ventana Wilderness

Goat Camp

Stone Ridge Trail

Fresno Camp

Los Padres National Forest

Cone Peak Rd

Vicente Flat Trail

Vicente Flat Camp

To Nacimiento-Fergusson Rd

0   0.25   0.5 mile
0   0.5   1 kilometer

beside a small turnout for up to four cars. There are no facilities or water at the trailhead.

Cone Peak Road is closed from roughly November through May (specific dates vary depending on weather and road conditions). Contact Los Padres National Forest Headquarters at 805-968-6790 or Big Sur Station at 831-667-2315 for details.

TRIP DESCRIPTION

From the signed trailhead on the west side of Cone Peak Road, head west to climb past dense thickets of manzanita, wartleaf, and tree poppies, which bloom brilliant yellow by late spring. These fire-adapted species are thriving in the wake of the 1999 Kirk Complex Fires, California's tenth largest recorded wildfire, which scorched more than 90,000 acres of wilderness.

At the top of a nearby saddle, gaze south for a stunning view of the southern Santa Lucia Range. Approaching a ridge, turn north to a second saddle, a half mile from the trailhead. As the trail steepens, the views encourage you onward. Watch your footing as you pass two rubble-lined gullies that continually erode onto the trail.

Skirting past a downed tree, you may notice the first appearance of encroaching poison oak, a rarity at this altitude. Although the trail was cleared in 2003,

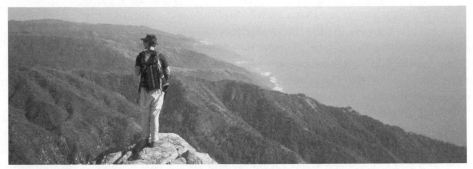

Peace and solitude can be found atop Cone Peak.

aggressive brush makes steady inroads. Dedicated Ventana hikers and wilderness advocates bring pruning sheers and machetes with them to keep the brush in check.

Reach an unmarked junction at 1.2 miles, where a spur on the left leads 100 feet south along the ridge for encompassing views of the Santa Lucias. To the right, the main route switchbacks down a ridge with scattered views through the remains of charred trees. The trail veers northwest to the Cone Peak Summit Trail junction, atop a narrow ridge 2 miles from the trailhead.

Turn east on the Cone Peak Summit Trail, which climbs the remaining 325 feet in 0.3 mile. Start out southeast, past drought-tolerant scrub oaks, manzanitas,

PRODIGIOUS CONE PEAK

Remarkable in many aspects, Cone Peak has intrigued people for millennia with its varied topography, geology, botany, and cultural history. Its western slopes form the steepest coastal grade in the continental U.S. Its bedrock comprises metamorphic rocks of the Salinian block, among the oldest rocks in the Santa Lucia Range. Its spectacular cliffs boast marble from an ancient seafloor that was transported here from Mexico along northwest-trending faults.

In the late 1800s, entrepreneurs found an overwhelmingly rugged peak that sheltered a wealth of natural resources. They would extract lumber, lime, tanbark, and even gold from these slopes and clefts. One company erected four enormous kilns along Limekiln Creek to purify some of the largest limestone deposits along the central California coast. The kilns still stand amid the redwoods at Limekiln State Park, along Cone Peak's western flanks.

Intrigued by the abrupt, distinct climatic zones from sea level to 5155 feet, botanists came in search of new plant species. Habitats vary from cool, damp redwood forests to rolling oak savannas and sun-scorched chaparral, each zone hosting dramatically different flora and fauna. In the 1830s, botanists first described the area's Coulter and sugar pines and Santa Lucia firs. The latter form an extensive stand on the peak's northwest slopes. Isolated from Sierra Nevada stands, secluded stands of sugar pines are limited to the highest peaks of the Santa Lucias.

sticky monkeyflowers, and yuccas, which shoot forth stalks of densely clustered, edible white flowers. As the trail switchbacks to cooler, north-facing slopes, the vegetation shifts to a cluster of endemic Santa Lucia firs and an isolated stand of sugar pines. The switchbacks soon lead to a dramatic ledge above a sheer rock face inhabited by cliff swallows, which dart skyward in search of tasty insects.

From the ledge, a final series of short switchbacks leads to the summit, at 5155 feet in elevation. Climb the lookout tower for more encompassing views: Clockwise from the north are the barren peaks of 4853-foot Ventana Double Cone and 3709-foot Pico Blanco. To the northeast rises 5862-foot Junipero Serra, the highest peak in the Santa Lucia Range. The ancient oak savannas of the San Antonio and Nacimiento valleys stretch south and southeast. From the summit, a 3.2-mile ridge drops west to the Pacific, comprising the steepest coastal slope in the continental U.S.—it's even steeper than the drop from 14,494-foot Mt. Whitney to Owens Valley. On the clearest days, often after winter storms, you can see the Sierra Nevada peaks east across the Salinas and San Joaquin valleys.

Retracing your steps back to the Cone Peak Trail junction, the trail turns right and leads northwest along a series of switchbacks to Trail Spring Camp. Trail Spring Camp offers one small site on sloping ground beside the unreliable headwaters of South Fork Devils Creek. To find water in dry months, anticipate a steep 300-foot descent 0.3 mile along the boulder wash. More adventurous hikers could check out Ojito Camp. The unmarked Ojito Camp Trail junction is 1.6 miles farther along the Gamboa Trail, which follows an ancient Native American trading route past Coulter pines and Douglas and Santa Lucia firs. Filtered views overlook the South Fork's remote swimming holes and the glistening Pacific beyond.

From the Ojito Camp Trail junction, turn right and head north, plunging 600 feet in the next 0.6 mile to Devils Canyon. Encroaching brush and large fallen snags obstruct portions of the route. Once at the banks of the South Fork Devils Creek, a faint overgrown trail leads 200 yards downstream along the swift creek to Ojito Camp, which has room for two tents. Those willing to venture cross-country will find myriad beautiful pools and cascades.

BUILD-UP AND WIND-DOWN TIPS

Assuming you are taking the more scenic route home along Highway 1, don't miss the chance to stop at **Nepenthe Restaurant** (Nepenthe, Highway 1, Big Sur 93920, 831-667-2345), a rustic yet elegant restaurant overlooking 40 miles of scenic coastline where condors soar directly above and golden eagles nest below. It's a great stop for coffee, pie, and epic views of Cone Peak.

The closest campground to the trailhead is **Kirk Creek Campground** (33 sites at $18 per night), on the west side of Highway 1, 0.1 mile north of the Nacimiento-Fergusson Road junction. Sites are first-come, first-served, and facilities include water and toilets. For more information, contact the Forest Service's Monterey District Headquarters at 831-385-5434.

17

POVERTY FLAT AND LOS CRUZEROS LOOP

Jean Rusmore

MILES: 13.9 (via Jackass Peak Road);
13.6 (via Middle Fork and the Narrows); add 4.6 for a side trip to Lost Spring and Mahoney Meadows
RECOMMENDED DAYS: 2–3
ELEVATION GAIN/LOSS: 2160´/2160´
TYPE OF TRIP: Loop
DIFFICULTY: Moderate
SOLITUDE: Moderate solitude on outgoing leg, Moderately populated to crowded on return leg on Manzanita Point Rd.
LOCATION: Henry W. Coe State Park
MAPS: USGS 7.5-min. *Mt. Sizer* and *Mississippi Creek*;
Pine Ridge Association's *Henry W. Coe State Park*
BEST SEASONS: Spring and fall (depending on water)

PERMITS •

There is a park fee and campsite reservations are required. Contact Henry W. Coe State Park, Box 846, Morgan Hill, CA 94038, 408-779-2728, or visit their website at www.coepark.org. Be sure to register with the park staff before starting your trip.

Photo: China Hole

95

TAKE THIS TRIP

This trip takes you around
the western area of Henry
W. Coe State Park—sam-
pling high ridges, dense
manzanita forests, oak savannas, and campsites be-
side two forks of Coyote
Creek. You will climb two
of the main ridges that run
northwest-southeast and
descend to historic Native
American and Spanish
explorer sites. In years
of plentiful rain, frocks of
spring wildflowers clothe
the hillsides and swimming
holes tempt hot hikers. By
skipping the Los Cruzeros
night and the exploratory
side trips, you could do
this trip as an overnight.

CHALLENGES

When you make your campsite reservation, inquire about the availability of water in
the creeks, and be sure to carry a water puri-
fier. Due to the heat and exposure, it's best to
get an early morning start up Middle Ridge,
and carry plenty of water. While no open
fires are allowed, you can use a backpacking
stove.

HOW TO GET THERE

From Highway 101 east of Morgan Hill
take East Dunne Avenue 13 miles east, climbing via innumerable switchbacks, to park
headquarters.

TRIP DESCRIPTION

Start your trip on the Corral Trail, beginning just across the road from park headquarters near the stop sign. This trail goes left
(downhill) into a little gully below the barn
and heads toward Manzanita Point. In and
out of oak-wooded ravines, the trail gently
contours along the hillside where chaparral
grows on the drier, south-facing slopes. In
less than a half mile you reach a tree-studded
grassland, an oak savanna. The large black
oaks growing on the north-facing slopes have
shiny, deeply lobed, 6-inch-long leaves with
sharp points. The new leaves, fuzzy and reddish in spring, become deep green in summer.
By fall—especially in colder locations—they
turn yellow tinged with red.

When the Corral Trail meets the Springs
Trail at 0.6 mile, you veer left (north) to cross
the wide Manzanita Point Road to a well-
marked trail junction. You take the Fish Trail
heading north, pass the Flat Frog Trail on
the left, and note the Forest Trail taking off
for Manzanita Point on your right. The latter
would be a fine route on your return to headquarters. Heading north you may see uphill
to the right (east) the fences of a corral that
Sada Coe built when she managed Pine Ridge

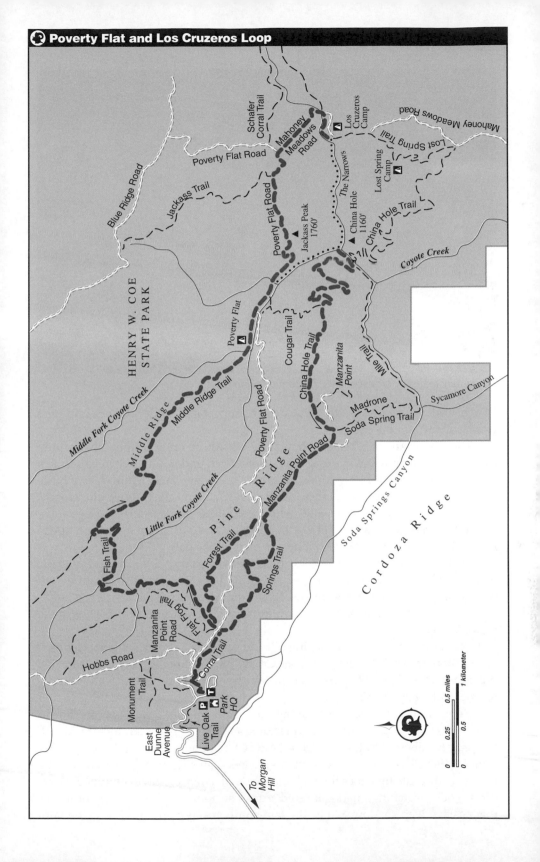

Poverty Flat and Los Cruzeros Loop

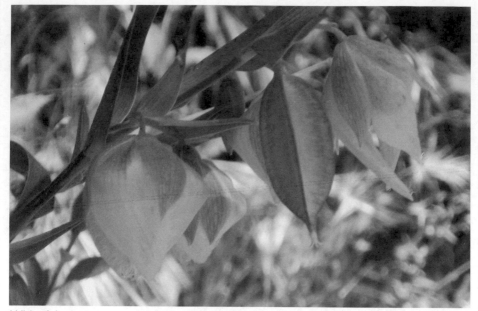

White fairy lanterns, or globe lilies, grace woodland trails.

Ranch. Today a backpack site, Old Corral Camp, stands under the oak and pine trees just north of the corral.

The Fish Trail then bends around the hillside to enter a tight, shady little canyon. On a hot day this is a welcome, cool stretch under dark bay trees beside a watercourse that is dry by summer, as are several other small tributaries of Little Fork Coyote Creek that you cross. After a few switchbacks through the woods, you arrive at an open, grassy valley where deep-blue heads of tall brodiaea wave above the emerging oats in spring. In summer and fall, the magnificent specimens of valley oak here stand out darkly against the pale gold grass.

In the fall you might watch for holes in the ground the size of a quarter, where the hairy-bodied, long-legged tarantula lines its little underground well with a silky web that catches the insects it eats. Also in Coe Park lives the tarantula hawk, an insect that stings the tarantula, paralyzes it, and lays its eggs in the victim's body.

Contouring along the east-facing hillside you make a quick switchback down to boulder-strewn Little Fork Coyote Creek. Now you climb 0.6 mile through mixed woodland and chaparral on the south-facing slope to reach the Middle Ridge Trail junction at 2.8 miles.

Here, from your 2480-foot vantage point on Middle Ridge you see northeast to 3000-foot Blue Ridge, which cuts diagonally northwest-southeast through the park for about 7 miles. The Middle Ridge Trail, for hikers and (except after rain) for bicyclists—horses are prohibited—lies on the sloping plateau of Middle Ridge. Your route first goes through the shade of a dense growth of huge manzanitas. Their glistening, mahogany-red trunks support a broad canopy of leaves that casts a deep shadow. On a still, late-summer day you might hear the faint rustle of papery curls of bark peeling from the trunks and falling to carpet the ground.

Then the path emerges onto grasslands, which soon widen, and you walk through a magnificent, broad, undulating savanna with immense, widely spaced valley and blue oaks. The trail slopes down on the south side of the broad ridge past a few old oaks riddled with woodpecker holes. As you descend, your view south over the canyon of the Little Fork is of Pine Ridge. You can pick out the Poverty Flat ranch road winding up through rugged woodlands of the ridge's north-facing slope, where this route will eventually take you.

About a mile from the Fish Trail junction, the trail turns northeast, crosses the ridge, dips into a few ravines, and then drops down the north side. Here the forest deepens, and trees of many species crowd the steep slopes—madrones, tall ponderosa pines, gray pines, and blue and black oaks interspersed with a few canyon oaks. Toyon, manzanita, and poison oak fill the understory and hardy, native bunchgrass flourishes on this hillside. You feel truly remote from civilization here—privileged humans in this wilderness. Often the only noises are the calls of many birds and the splashing of the creek in the canyon below.

On many switchbacks you continue southeast and down the steep slope for more than a mile. Arriving at the confluence of the Little and Middle Forks of Coyote Creek, you are on a narrow peninsula between them at 5.0 miles. Sunlight filters through the trees, and patterns of light dance on the waters of grass-edged pools.

The first Poverty Flat backpack camp is just across the Middle Fork on a broad flat under great oaks. Hop across on the rocks—there's no bridge here. Four other campsites are downstream beyond the ford where the Poverty Flat Road crosses. These campsites now are served by a very modern outhouse, something an early, unnamed homesteader did not have. The story goes that this settler held out for years against Henry Coe, who wanted to purchase this pleasant site—thus the name Poverty Flat. Here, also, was one of the park's largest Native American settlements, with abundant fish and game, and berries and other fruit nearby.

On your second day out, heading for Los Cruzeros Camp, you have two options—one cross-country, the other a road. The first is the shortest and entails less uphill but can be difficult, depending on the season and the depth of water in the Middle Fork. It requires more than a mile of scrambling downstream over rocks and boulders in the narrow confines of the creek's passage between the two promontories of Jackass Peak and Manzanita Point to reach China Hole. (This shortcut is not shown on the park map.) If the weather is warm, you might try a dip in one of the deep pools at the confluence of the Middle and East forks there. From China Hole it is another mile of off-trail rock hopping or walking over the gravelly streambed (if the water is low) along the Narrows of East Fork Coyote Creek to reach Los Cruzeros at 6.6 miles. When the water is high, neither of these interesting scrambles should be attempted.

The second option requires a stiff 0.8-mile pull up Poverty Flat Road as it switchbacks up the north side of 1760-foot Jackass Peak. Do this climb in the early part of a hot day to take advantage of the intermittent shade of overhanging valley oaks and occasional blue oaks. Coe Park's wide patrol roads can be hot in midday, so carry plenty of water. At the road's highest point there is an informal trail heading (right) for the tree-topped summit of Jackass Peak, but this trip continues on the main road, passes the Jackass Trail coming down from Blue Ridge on the left, and then reaches the junction with the Mahoney Meadows Road. Here the Poverty Flat Road veers left, but you bear right on the Mahoney Meadows Road at 6.5 miles.

Descending rapidly through rolling grasslands, you see northeast to Willow Ridge and the ragged Eagle Pines atop it, and south to the long Mahoney Meadows ridgelands. In spring the hillsides are gloriously strewn with an array of yellow, blue, and orange wildflowers. The meadows to the northeast, known for their brilliant spring flower displays, are called Miller Field, named for former land baron Henry Miller, who grazed great herds of cattle here.

In less than a half mile Mahoney Meadows Road crosses the East Fork Coyote Creek and heads uphill, but you can follow a narrow trail south along the east bank of the creek to its confluence with Kelly Cabin Creek. Situated on broad flats above the East Fork and shaded by sizable valley oaks are the three Los Cruzeros campsites at 6.9 miles.

When the explorer Juan Bautista de Anza and his men came through here from the San Antonio Valley, they named this place Arroyo del Coyote. The Spanish word *cruzeros*, meaning "cross" or "creek," might be the basis for its present name—Los Cruzeros. Maybe it was named for the creek crossing, or perhaps the small band of explorers set up a cross for prayer here before continuing on their journey. Today's travelers will find the site of their second night's stay a peaceful place, where several white-trunked sycamores survive and three beautiful valley oaks flourish on a gravel bar in the middle of the creekbed. The presumed Anza campsite at Los Cruzeros is now quite eroded by the floods of recent years, but the other campsites are fine.

Since the trip to Los Cruzeros from Poverty Flat is short, you may want to leave your pack and camping gear here, explore upstream along the East Fork's gravelly creekbed, and join the Schafer Corral Trail at the base of Miller Field. Or you could visit the Lost Spring campsite on the flanks of Mahoney Meadows.

SIDE TRIP: LOST SPRING

If you choose the latter, continue uphill (south) for 0.4 mile on Mahoney Meadows Road, past the original Los Cruzeros campsite, and then veer right (southwest) on the Lost Spring Trail, zigzagging uphill through light shade. The campsite at Lost Spring, just 0.7 mile from Los Cruzeros, is in a shady, black-oak woodland with a picnic table and fairly reliable year-round water.

If you feel like continuing farther, follow the well-graded trail 0.6 mile up to the junction of the main Mahoney Meadows Road and the China Hole Trail. Here on the wide, rolling grasslands are 360-degree views—ridge after ridge of mountains—and on either side the canyons of Coyote and Kelly Cabin creeks. In spring the grasslands are ablaze with color—blue lupines contrasting with yellow Johnny-jump-ups. In fall, too, there is brilliant color—poison oak turned red, pink, and orange and the gray-leaved, scarlet California fuchsia.

You could return to your Los Cruzeros campsite from the Mahoney Meadows Trail junction by way of the 2.2-mile China Hole Trail and the Narrows (if the water is low enough), descending on switchbacks through a cover of bay trees, with occasional black oaks towering overhead. At the base of the trail you come out on the east side of Coyote Creek and bear right (north), upstream to the deep pools and rocky beaches of China Hole, which invite you to stop for a swim or a snack. At the confluence of Middle and East Coyote creeks you bear right (due east) for 1 mile through the Narrows to reach Los Cruzeros—a 4.6-mile side trip.

To return to Coe Park headquarters after your stay at Los Cruzeros, take the Narrows route to China Hole (unless high water forces you to return via Poverty Flat and the 0.7-mile Cougar Trail along the north side of Manzanita Point). Then proceed downstream over and around rocks and under willows, alders, and young sycamores for 0.1 mile on the west side of Coyote Creek at 8.0 miles. Pick up the well-graded China Hole Trail and zigzag up the south-facing, grassy hillside, shaded by great oaks. In spring blue-flowered iris bloom beside the trail; in fall the small purple-flowered aster brightens the trailside. Then you walk into a 1994 prescribed-burn area now regrown with chaparral plants—chamise, ceanothus, and mountain mahogany, surmounted by skeletons of tall, dead manzanita.

Beyond the burn you step back into a mature manzanita forest of deep mahogany-red trunks and gray-green leaves, where occasional madrone and black oak trees pierce the manzanita canopy. At 10.6 miles you pass the Cougar Trail coming in on your right, and continue on the China Hole Trail 0.8 mile to reach Manzanita Point Camp 7 at 11.4 miles. Take the wide, unpaved Manzanita Point Road back toward headquarters. At the junction of Poverty Flat and Manzanita Point roads at 12.3 miles you can turn right (northeast) on the shady 1.1-mile Forest Trail—your best trail for a hot day—or take the 1.0-mile Springs Trail on the left (southwest side of ridge). Each trail contours gently back to its junction with the 0.6-mile Corral Trail, on which you continue to headquarters at 13.9 or 14.0 miles, depending on your route.

18

REDFERN POND LOOP

Jean Rusmore

MILES: 11.0
RECOMMENDED DAYS: 2
ELEVATION GAIN/LOSS: 1352´/1352´
TYPE OF TRIP: Loop
DIFFICULTY: Moderate
SOLITUDE: Moderate solitude to campsite,
       Solitude on trip to Vasquez Peak
LOCATION: Henry W. Coe State Park
MAP: USGS 7.5-min. *Gilroy Hot Springs*;
     Pine Ridge Association's *Henry W. Coe State Park*
BEST SEASONS: Spring and fall

PERMITS

There is a park fee and self-permits are required; complete and pay by check at the Hunting Hollow parking lot. You can find out more at www.coepark.org.

CHALLENGES

Be sure to treat pond water before drinking it, and use a stove instead of a campfire for cooking.

Photo: A mature madrone

HOW TO GET THERE • • • • • • • • • • • •

From U.S. Highway 101 on the north side of Gilroy, take Leavesley Road east about 1 mile to New Road and turn left (north). Turn right (east) onto Roop Road, which then becomes Gilroy Hot Springs Road, and continue east beside Coyote Creek, passing Coyote Creek County Park Road on the left. After 9 miles you reach the large Hunting Hollow parking lot on your right. Here you pay a state park fee at the kiosk and register for overnight camping, which you should have already reserved.

TRIP DESCRIPTION • • • • • • • • • • • • • • •

This trip begins through the gate at the southeast end of the Hunting Hollow parking lot. The first half mile along one of the tributaries of Coyote Creek is along a dirt road, through a wide valley with magnificent sycamores growing in the creekbed and huge bay trees nearby. In the fall ground squirrels busy themselves gathering winter supplies in the meadow near the creek. The trail crosses back and forth over the creek four times in the first half mile. In a wet spring you might get your shoes wet; carrying a hiking stick can help you across to dry ground.

After 0.5 mile you reach the junction of Lyman Willson Ridge Trail on the left—actually a wide trail that was once a ranch road. If you hear a squeaking noise here, it will not be a worried animal but a windmill, pumping water into a nearby horse trough. Beyond the junction under a large oak, a small fenced camping spot complete with picnic table, cupboard, and barbecue makes a good starting place for an equestrian trip.

Following the Lyman Willson Ridge Trail through a gate, past a corral shaded by walnut trees, your route heads east steeply uphill. You are now in oak woodland with typical Henry Coe open grassland visible on Middle Steer Ridge left across the canyon. In spring

TAKE THIS TRIP

In the more recently opened southwestern corner of Henry W. Coe State Park, this trip takes the backpacker up high, steep-sided ridges above tree-shaded canyons, and through remote grasslands dotted with oaks and punctuated by rocky outcrops. This area is also used by equestrians, as it has easy access for horse trailers, but its beauty deserves much wider acquaintance. Numerous small ponds are remnants of the cattle-grazing era, and this trip's overnight destination of Redfern Pond is one of the park's most attractive.

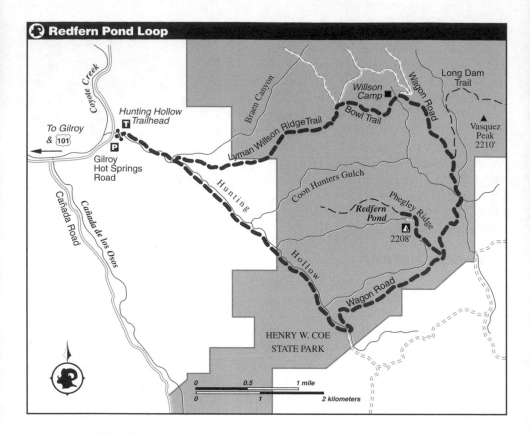

iris, brodiaea, and buttercups are everywhere; in fall the smell of tarweed permeates the air. As you ascend the ridge you see to the south the tree-covered slope of the next canyon, part of Phegley Ridge, and at an open spot catch a glimpse of distant Pacheco Peak and Lovers Leap near the Pacheco Pass Highway. If you look down-canyon west across the Santa Clara Valley, you can see Loma Prieta, the highest peak in the Santa Cruz Mountains.

After an uphill mile some rocks in the shade of blue oaks provide a convenient rest stop. Then comes a long stretch of open grassland before the trail contours right into the shade of some black oaks. As you climb, scan the trail for tracks of deer, coyote, fox, and bobcat, plus an occasional horse or human.

After 1.5 miles the trail levels out a little and crests a knoll on the ridge, where there are wide views east, south, and west. While Vasquez Peak to the east is the highest nearby point at 2210 feet, from here it's a rounded grassy knob. The trail crosses open grasslands for another mile to the junction with the Bowl Trail at 2.6 miles. As of this writing there is no sign, but it is easy to identify using your map. The Lyman Willson Trail continues straight uphill; the northward branch of the Bowl Trail, apparently little used, contours left. Your route follows the eastward-trending branch of the Bowl Trail right. Yellow tarweed smells very strong in the fall. You see two dammed cattle ponds, one below right, one immediately left. Grazing is no longer permitted in this part of the park, but wild animals also appreciate getting a drink.

Increasing numbers of rocky outcrops—a part of the Franciscan Formation composed of blue schist—add interest to the scene. Oaks grow picturesquely around these rocks. After passing a small nearby spring and attaining the trip's highest elevation at 2208 feet, the trail—now a rough road—begins to drop down to Willson Camp, the former cattle ranch of Lyman Willson at 3.5 miles. Nestled in the shade of a huge live-oak tree, the old house looks south across grasslands and canyons toward Pacheco Peak. It takes about 2½ hours to reach this place, whose remains include an old cowshed, two derelict house trailers, various shacks, and remnants of waterlines.

Lyman Willson was the son of an early Gilroy pioneer, Horace Willson, who emigrated from New Hampshire in 1853 to what was then known as San Ysidro. Horace accumulated large landholdings by homesteading and purchase in the Diablo Range east of Gilroy. His sons Edwin and Lyman ranched property of their own near Gilroy Hot Springs. While bringing a deer down Middle Ridge to Hunting Hollow from the family hunting camp in 1915, Lyman was thrown from his horse and killed. Edwin lived until 1937, but the ranch was sold eight years earlier. (The peak named for the Willson family and their ranch location is spelled with only one "l" on the USGS 7.5-minute *Gilroy Hot Springs* quad.)

From Willson Camp continue a short distance southeast to a trail junction with Wagon Road, a graded dirt road that follows Steer Ridge. As you head right (south) along the ridge, note the sign at the junction that says it is 6.9 miles north to Pacheco Camp and 1.8 miles north and then east to Vasquez Peak. Great views east, south, and west stretch before you. Looking below the trail at another stock pond you may catch a glimpse of a wild pig and piglets quenching their thirst. These descendants of escaped domestic pigs crossed with wild European boars have proliferated in the Diablo Range; you frequently see their rootings in the ground. Their tracks are similar to those of deer. Do not approach too closely because boars can be aggressive, as can a sow with piglets.

At another trail junction at 4.6 miles, the Long Dam Trail leads north and then east toward Vasquez Peak. But you continue south alternately descending steeply to cross three creeks and then again struggling steeply uphill. At 5.8 miles an unsigned track cuts off right toward the Redfern Pond Trail. In some seasons this may be hard to find, so continue on Wagon Road to the main junction at 6.0 miles. Here, next to a small stock pond, the Redfern Pond Trail heads right (north), rising gently uphill across the open grasslands of Phegley Ridge.

When you crest the ridge, about 0.5 mile farther, you reach a 2200-foot vantage point. Below you lies a large linear pond about 1.5 acres in size, partly encircled by tall reeds. The small dam is at the far end, and the pond drains to the west. Songs of red-winged blackbirds rise from the inviting bowl, and you may hear the cry of a red-tailed hawk cruising high above. Blue- and live-oak trees dot the grassy knolls above the pond, providing many inviting campsites. The state park map suggests a campsite above the pond to the right and another beyond the pond left of the trail.

You have the option of camping here two nights and taking a 5.2-mile round-trip dayhike east to Vasquez Peak, partly on roads and partly on a trail. To take this hike, return north on Wagon Road 1.4 miles and turn right on the Long Dam Trail. Curving around past a stock pond (Long Dam Pond), the trail climbs past Edith Pond and, 1.2 miles from Wagon Road, reaches Vasquez Road near Vasquez Peak.

When you continue your loop trip the next day, return from Redfern Pond to Wagon Road, which the route follows all the way to Hunting Hollow. First the road climbs steeply uphill, with very little shade until the ridgetop. Here you feel on top of the world (or at least Henry Coe Park), before making your final descent south to the tributary of Coyote Creek along which you began your hike.

The final 3 miles of this hike are along the valley of Hunting Hollow, with numerous creek crossings as you head northwest. Here again are the ground squirrels and brush rabbits that like meadows and bushes. In the fall tarantulas emerge from their holes looking for mates; they aren't dangerous but give them room to escape your tread. Among other tracks in the dust are linear grooves; these are made by snakes—occasionally rattlers—so watch your step.

At 10.5 miles you have completed the loop to the junction with the Lyman Willson Trail. Retracing your steps another half mile gets you to the trailhead parking. While this entire loop trip can take 6–8 hours and be done by strong hikers in a day, it makes a relaxing weekend getaway to a little-visited part of the Bay Area wildlands.

19

THE OHLONE WILDERNESS TRAIL

Matt Heid

MILES: 19.5
RECOMMENDED DAYS: 3
ELEVATION GAIN/LOSS: 6500´/6150´
TYPE OF TRIP: Point-to-point
DIFFICULTY: Moderately strenuous
SOLITUDE: Moderate solitude
LOCATION: Sunol Regional Wilderness, Ohlone Regional Wilderness, Del Valle Regional Park
MAPS: *Ohlone Wilderness Regional Trail Permit and Map*, *Sunol Regional Wilderness* and *Del Valle Regional Park* maps; USGS 7.5-min. *La Costa Valley* and *Mendenhall Springs*
BEST SEASONS: Spring and fall

PERMITS

A trail hiking permit/map is required to use the Ohlone Trail and is available at Sunol and Del Valle parks for $2; online at www.ebparks.org/parks/ohlone; or through the mail by sending your name, address, phone number, and a check for $2.50 to Ohlone Wilderness Trail, East Bay Regional Parks District, 2950 Peralta Oaks Court, P.O. Box 5381, Oakland, CA 94605-0381. Reservations are required for the five backcountry trail camps; contact the East Bay Regional

Photo: Hikers head out on the Ohlone Wilderness Trail, Sunol Regional Wilderness.

Park District reservation office (888-327-2757, 8:30 AM–4 PM Monday–Friday; $5 per person per night, plus a one-time reservation fee of $8). Dogs and campfires are prohibited.

CHALLENGES

The summer can be intense, with miles of exposed trail. Water can be scarce but is usually available at the five designated trail camps.

HOW TO GET THERE

The Sunol (starting) trailhead: Take Interstate 680 east of Fremont to the Calaveras Road exit and proceed 4.3 miles south on Calaveras Road to Geary Road. Turn left on Geary Road, reaching the entrance kiosk in 1.8 miles. The trailhead is located just past the visitor center.

The Del Valle (ending) trailhead: Take the North Livermore Avenue exit from Interstate 580. North Livermore Avenue becomes South Livermore Avenue as you follow it south. Turn right on Mines Road 1.5 miles south of town, go about 3.5 miles, and continue straight on Del Valle Road (Mines Road turns left) for 3.5 miles to the park entrance. Continue 0.8 mile past the entrance, and turn right toward the Lichen Bark Picnic Area and Ohlone Trail Parking Area.

TRIP DESCRIPTION

The Ohlone Trail is a route comprised of many different trails. Many junctions (but not all) will be posted to indicate the direction of the Ohlone Trail; most are numbered to correspond with the Ohlone Trail permit and map. Camping is permitted only at the five designated backcountry camps: Sunol Backpack Area, Doe Canyon Horse Camp, Maggie's Half Acre, Stewart's Camp, and Boyd Camp. Obtain water at the trailhead; none is available until the Sunol Backpack Area.

Register at the Ohlone Trail sign-in board and head across Geary Road to the wooden bridge over Alameda Creek. The mottled,

TAKE THIS TRIP

The Ohlone Trail journeys through some of the Bay Area's most remote terrain, a point-to-point adventure remarkable for its far-reaching views, majestic oak woodlands, and profuse spring wildflowers. This adventure connects Sunol Regional Wilderness with Del Valle Regional Park via Ohlone Regional Wilderness, a hidden, high-elevation wonderland accessible only by trail. Five designated backcountry camping areas provide a variety of overnight options.

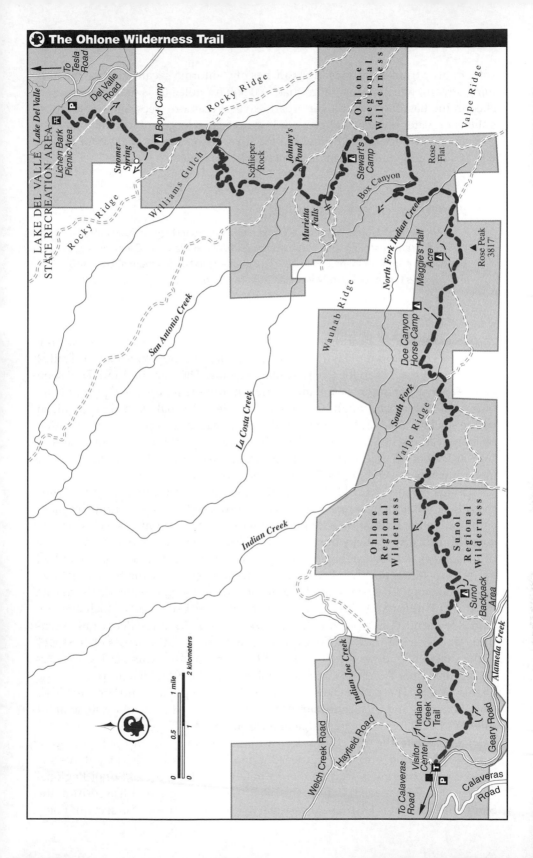

The Ohlone Wilderness Trail

LAKE DEL VALLE STATE RECREATION AREA

Lake Del Valle

To Tesla Road

Del Valle Road

Lichen Bark Picnic Area

Stromer Spring

Boyd Camp

Rocky Ridge

Rocky Ridge

Williams Gulch

Schlieper Rock

Johnny's Pond

Murietta Falls

North Fork Indian Creek

Ohlone Regional Wilderness

Stewart's Camp

Box Canyon

Rose Flat

Valpe Ridge

Rose Peak 3817

Maggie's Half Acre

Wauhab Ridge

San Antonio Creek

La Costa Creek

Doe Canyon Horse Camp

South Fork

Valpe Ridge

Indian Creek

Ohlone Regional Wilderness

Sunol Regional Wilderness

Sunol Backpack Area

Alameda Creek

Indian Joe Creek

Welch Creek Road

Hayfield Road

Indian Joe Creek Trail

Visitor Center

To Calaveras Road

Geary Road

Calaveras Road

0.5   1 mile
0   1   2 kilometers

smooth gray trunks and twisting branches of California sycamores line the gurgling stream, which drains more than 700 square miles (it is the largest watershed in the East Bay). With their broad leaves, sycamore trees can lose up to 50 gallons of water per day and grow only where such large volumes of water are available; watch for them throughout the hike. Also keep an eye out for poison oak and stinging nettle, common nemeses on this hike.

ALAMEDA CREEK ALLIANCE

Alameda Creek Alliance is a community watershed group dedicated to preserving and restoring the natural ecosystems of the Alameda Creek drainage basin. You can write them at Box 192, Sunol, CA 94516, call them at 510-845-4675, or visit them online at www.alamedacreek.org.

Cross the bridge, bear right, and continue straight on the Canyon View Trail as it passes junctions for Hayfield Road at 0.1 mile, the Indian Joe Nature Trail at 0.2 mile, and the Indian Joe Creek Trail at 0.3 mile. The Canyon View Trail soon climbs away from the creek and into a drier environment populated primarily by blue oaks. The most drought-tolerant oak species, blue oak is easily recognized by the shallow lobes and smooth margins of its leaves. You pass though the first of many cattle gates to come and reach a four-way intersection with the McCorkle Trail at 0.8 mile at 700 feet in elevation. Cows are still permitted to graze along much of the Ohlone Trail and are commonly seen in this area.

Go left on the McCorkle Trail, a more overgrown path that steadily climbs the ridgeline before turning east to traverse through chaparral, a shrubbier plant community that flourishes in more arid environments. Common species include coyote brush, toyon, sticky monkeyflower, bracken fern, coffeeberry, and plenty of poison oak. Valley oak begins to appear along this section as well, identified by its 2- to 4-inch deeply lobed leaves. You pass beneath some huge coast live oaks—look for their spiny, curled-under leaves—and then reach wide Cerro Este Road at 1.7 miles and 1180 feet. Bear left on Cerro Este Road, which steadily climbs to the next junction with the McCorkle Trail at 2.1 miles. Bear right to continue on the single-track McCorkle Trail, traversing steadily across open slopes with outstanding views west of Mission Peak and south toward Calaveras Reservoir, the upper Alameda Creek watershed, and the more distant peaks of the Diablo Range. The path makes a steep switchbacking drop into the "W" Tree Rock Scramble and then continues its traverse to reach the Backpack Road at 3.4 miles and 1150 feet and gated edge of the Sunol Backpack Area.

Past the gate, the trail climbs steeply up the hillside past spur paths to campsites 3–7, reaching sites 1 and 2 near the top. (Water is located just above site 3.) The route continues above, where a gate marks the edge of Sunol Regional Wilderness. For the next 2 miles, the hike passes through land leased from the San Francisco Water District—please stay on the trail during this section. Enjoy far-reaching views as you undulate through open grasslands dotted with rock outcrops and multitudes of spring wildflowers and then wind above the distinctive promontory of Goat Rock and turn uphill. Bear left at the first unposted junction with Goat Rock Road at 5.3 miles and 2170 feet and right at the second junction at 5.5 miles to continue west on Mid Road.

You quickly pass through another gate and enter Ohlone Regional Wilderness just before reaching a four-way junction with Billy Goat Road at 5.8 miles. Continue straight on Mid Road as it begins rising slowly toward the ridgeline above. The cities of the South Bay begin to appear in the distance, while intermittent views of distant South San Francisco can be spotted northwest. The route turns left on Bluff Road at 7.1 miles and then climbs to the ridgeline to meet Valpe Ridge Road at 7.4 miles and 2840 feet. Go right on Valpe Ridge Road, through another gate, and proceed along the airy slopes. The trail curves left where it meets Portuguese Point Road at 7.7 miles, dropping into the headwaters of Indian Creek, a tributary of Alameda Creek.

After crossing the creek, you resume climbing and soon crest 3000 feet for the first time. Views north open up; the massif of Mt. Diablo (3849 feet) is easily spotted more than 25 miles away. Black oaks also appear for the first time. A common denizen of higher elevations around the state, black oak is relatively uncommon in the Bay Area and found only at higher elevations in the Diablo Range and Santa Cruz Mountains. Recognize it by the large lobed leaves and pointy bristles at the leaf points. In spring its new leaves emerge a brilliant red.

You next pass the junction for Doe Canyon Horse Camp at 8.9 miles and 3380 feet, where a short side trip 200 feet down leads to the campsites' large clearing, water source, and outhouse. The continuing hike next reaches another junction with Portuguese Point Road at 9.3 miles; proceed straight to quickly reach a spur trail on the left for Maggie's Half Acre at 9.5 miles, located a quarter mile down the forested north slopes of Rose Peak.

The trail to Maggie's Half Acre rejoins the main route 0.6 mile past the campsites, but bypasses Rose Peak summit (3817 feet), a side trip not to be missed. The hike's highest point, Rose Peak is only 32 feet lower than Mt. Diablo and offers an exceptional 360-degree view. On a clear day you can peer from San Francisco to the Sierra Nevada. To tag the summit, remain on the Ohlone Trail, which passes just below the oak-studded high point.

Past Rose Peak, the trail passes the far junction for Maggie's Half Acre at 10.2 miles and 3590 feet and then briefly parallels the fenced park boundary. A private road splits right at 10.5 miles, but the route curves left to begin its northern journey toward Del Valle Regional Park. You next plummet more than 400 feet and cross the shady North Fork of Indian Creek. As you climb the opposite slopes, look down the Indian Creek drainage to spot the diminutive Coyote Hills on the edge of the Bay. Alameda Creek flows into the Bay immediately to their north.

The route passes Wauhab Ridge Road at 11.5 miles on the left and then cuts back to attain the ridgetop before dipping into Box Canyon. The trail passes a small cattle pond, climbs along the park boundary, turns left on Rose Flat Road at 12.4 miles, and then gently undulates north to reach the junction with the Greenside Trail at 12.9 miles. To reach Stewart's Camp, turn left on the Greenside Trail and descend 0.6 mile. Those staying overnight can rejoin the Ohlone Trail by continuing on the Greenside Trail and bearing right on Springboard Road to reach Johnny's Pond.

Continuing hikers should remain on the Ohlone Trail as it proceeds across the open meadows of Shafer Flat to reach the Jackson Grade Trail at 13.3 miles and 3460 feet. Head left (northwest) along the ridgeline that hems in the valley of upper La Costa Creek, where gigantic blue and black oaks punctuate fields flush with wildflowers. You encounter Johnny's Pond at a four-way intersection with Springboard Road at 14.0 miles, where distant views reach north to Mt. Tamalpais, the Golden Gate, and Mt. Diablo.

At this point, consider making the detour to nearby Murietta Falls (2990 feet), a thin rivulet dropping 60 feet over a cliff face. Though the waterfall is seldom more than a trickle, the rocky outcrops and required scramble are still exciting. The falls are located along the Greenside Trail, a half mile west of Stewart's Camp and a mile from Johnny's Pond via Springboard Road and the Greenside

Oak woodland, Ohlone Regional Wilderness

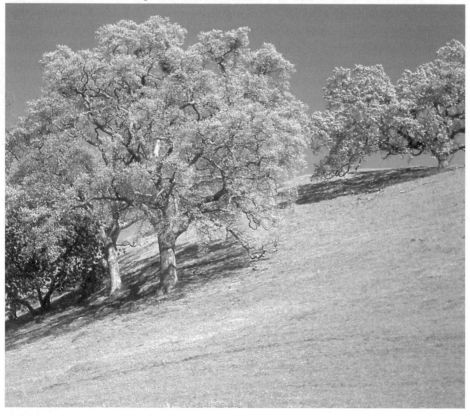

Trail. To find the cascade, head downstream along La Costa Creek from its inter-section with the Greenside Trail.

From Johnny's Pond, the Ohlone Trail continues straight on the Jackson Grade Trail and offers ever-vaster views of San Francisco, the East Bay Hills, Mission Peak, and north to your final destination, Lake Del Valle. Enjoy these final high-elevation views—the junction for the Big Burn is just ahead at 14.6 miles. Turn right and immediately begin the plummeting descent down the sin-gle-track trail.

On this north-facing slope, dense vegetation encroaches on the path in places and poison oak once again rears its ugly leaves. Dropping endlessly on numer-ous switchbacks, the trail loses 1400 feet of elevation in 1.7 miles before finally reaching the bottom of Williams Gulch at 16.3 miles. Here you pass beneath syca-mores and alders and cross the ephemeral creek. The trail gradually widens as it switchbacks steeply out of Williams Gulch, passes through fields of blue oak, and reaches the Rocky Ridge Trail at 17.0 miles.

Continue straight and resume the steep drop, quickly reaching Boyd Camp in 0.2 mile in a shrubby forest. From here the trail takes a direct, knee-jarring line downward, soon passing the junction for water on the Stromer Spring Trail at 17.6 miles and 1940 feet. Coyote brush becomes increasingly common, and man-zanita appears for the first time as the descent approaches its end.

Take time to sign the logbook at the Ohlone Trail sign-in panel by the Valleci-tos Trail at 18.5 miles and 1190 feet, which heads right down a creek gully toward the campground. The Ohlone Trail continues straight on a steadily descending traverse to finally reach trail's end at Lichen Bark Picnic Area at an elevation of 750 feet.

BUILD-UP AND WIND-DOWN TIPS ·

Tequila's Taqueria at 160 South Livermore Avenue in downtown Livermore has hearty portions and a jukebox. Plus it's near a **Peet's** coffee shop if you're craving some caffeine for the trip home.

20

PESCADERO CREEK LOOP

Michel Digonnet

MILES: 28.0

RECOMMENDED DAYS: 3

ELEVATION GAIN/LOSS: 5750´/5750´

TYPE OF TRIP: Loop

DIFFICULTY: Moderate

SOLITUDE: Solitude

LOCATION: Sam McDonald County Park, Pescadero Creek County Park, and Portola Redwoods State Park

MAPS: USGS 7.5-min. *Mindego Hill*, *La Honda*, *Franklin Point*, and *Big Basin*

BEST SEASON: Year-round

PERMITS

A permit is required for camping, on a first-come, first-served basis (i.e., you may be given a permit yet get there and find the first campground full and have to hike another 3 miles or so to the second campground); contact Big Basin's headquarters at 831-338-8861 or 831-338-6132 or 21600 Big Basin Way, Boulder Creek, CA 95006.

Photo: Pescadero Creek County Park

HOW TO GET THERE · · · · · · · · · · · · ·

The trailhead is in Sam McDonald County Park, a small redwood preserve that borders Pescadero Creek County Park. Take the Sand Hill Road exit on Interstate 280, and head west about 2.1 miles to Portola Road, which is on the right at the bottom of a grade. At the Y-junction 0.2 mile farther make a left, then continue 0.6 mile to a stop sign. Make the sharp left onto La Honda Road (Highway 84), which climbs the Santa Cruz Mountains 3.4 curvy miles to Skyline Boulevard at the crest. Cross Skyline Boulevard and continue 6.7 miles down Highway 84, a little past the sleepy town of La Honda, to Pescadero Road on the left. After 1.1 miles, in the sharp right hairpin bend at the junction with Alpine Road, stay right with the main road. Go another 0.6 mile to the inconspicuous entrance to Sam McDonald County Park on the right (announced by a small sign just before you reach it). Proceed up to the large paved area at the ranger station (usually closed) and park.

CHALLENGES ·

You will follow well-marked trails the whole way, so with a park map it would take special skills to get lost. Watch for poison oak on narrow trails, as it is quite common. Check yourself for ticks regularly. Make campfires only in the fire rings at the camps. Smoking is not allowed on the trails. The camps have no drinking water; bring your own, or purify or filter the creek water, which is otherwise a biological hazard. Come prepared for possible heavy rains in winter.

TRIP DESCRIPTION · · · · · · · · · · · · · · · · · ·

At Sam McDonald County Park the trail starts on the south side of the parking area, across from the ranger station, and ends shortly at the road on which you drove in. Cross the road and continue on the old logging road directly across it, which is Towne Trail. In the

TAKE THIS TRIP

The Pescadero Creek watershed is prime redwood country, part of a pristine system of forested ridges, hillsides, and valleys that stretches all the way to the Pacific Ocean. From the high rim of the creek's remote canyon, you wind down on steep lonesome trails through oak stands and ancient Douglas-fir forests, in a blissful mixture of sun and shade, until you reach the magnificent grove of giant redwoods by the edge of the creek.

The nearby campground is sheltered under old-growth redwoods high above the creek, peaceful and secluded. The next day, you carry a light pack on the long loop trail to remote Butano Ridge, a no-man's-land suffused with palpable solitude. On the final day, you return along a network of beautifully wooded trails that will take you past a derelict mill, an awe-inspiring giant redwood, a curious creek where crude oil naturally oozes into the stream, and impressive groves of ancient trees. So much beauty so close to one of the continent's largest metropolises is a miracle.

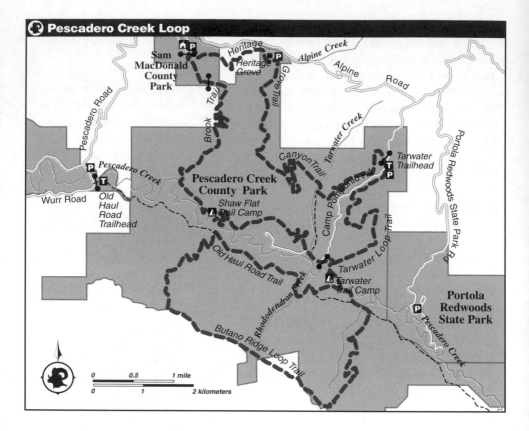

next 0.4 mile the trail climbs 350 feet through a dark old-growth forest of large trees. At the road junction, make a left and then a right shortly after, leaving the horse camp to your left. Continue up through a rolling meadow 0.3 mile to a foot trail on the right that cuts through a low grassy pass. After 150 yards, the trail splits at a spacious viewpoint overlooking the beautiful long forested canyon you are about to enter. The high ridge on its far side is Butano Ridge, your far-thest destination. At the bottom of this lush valley, hidden from view, flows the mastermind of this grand scenery—Pescadero Creek.

Take Brook Trail, the one on the right. It descends 750 feet in long switch-backs through a mixed forest of live oak, tanoak, bay laurel, and occasional madrone, with a mixed understory of huckleberry, blackberry, and poison oak. Year-round you are likely to see wildflowers here, as elsewhere on this trip, in-cluding hound's tongue, forget-me-nots, irises, and sticky monkeyflowers. After 1.6 miles Brook Trail crosses the wooden bridge over Towne Creek, at the end of a dim narrow canyon lined with giant redwoods. In the fall, the creek of-ten shrivels to a string of disconnected pools, but most winters it is a vigorous stream, sometimes with devastating force, as the enormous heap of torn trunks and limbs downstream from the bridge bears witness.

The trail ends shortly in the sharp curve of an abandoned logging road. Make a right, and look for a connecting trail on the left side 125 yards farther. Follow it 100 yards to the Pomponio Trail and make a left. For a short distance, these two trails overlook Jones Gulch, here a narrow channel winding between low sandstone walls, its rims covered with moss, its bottom coursed by a creek cloaked in perpetual darkness. Where it joins Towne Creek, the creek gives rise to a crystalline waterfall. Just past it, a narrow bridge swings high above Towne Creek. Drop your pack and take the small overgrown track that heads away from the creek on the far side of the bridge. It ends shortly at a barren slope that drops to the creek. Follow the slippery creek downstream back to the foot of the waterfall, along bedrock gauged with impressively deep cauldrons. On a warm day, this is a delightful spot to rest and cool off a little, deep beneath moss- and fern-covered cliffs.

The Shaw Flat Trail Camp, 0.7 mile east on Pomponio Trail, is one of the best backcountry camps on the peninsula. Located on a wide shelf high above Pescadero Creek, seemingly days from civilization and usually empty in spite of its proximity to one of America's largest urban areas, it is amazingly peaceful. Most of its eight sites are spacious and secluded. There are stumps to sit on, a fire ring with a grill, free firewood by the chemical toilet, and nonpotable water to put out your fire.

Do not miss the short walk to Pescadero Creek. Just continue east through the camp until the road becomes a single-track trail and curves tightly down to a majestic grove that holds some of the largest and most impressive redwoods in the park. The mighty little river is just below it, lined with an inviting sand beach. A roaring torrent of mud in winter, a bubbling brook of limpid water in summer and fall, Pescadero Creek is always faithfully there, snaking between the abrupt forested walls of its narrow canyon. This is a wonderfully serene spot for a picnic by the water's edge. Look for large crayfish crawling along the pebbly bottom and steelhead trout floating in the water. Even in summer the pool by the beach is deep enough to take a dip.

The next day, hike east on Pomponio Trail, a beautiful redwood trail smothered in a darkness that intimates silence. At midday the light has the magical reddish hue of *sempervirens* forests, dim yet strangely vivid, as if the forest was glowing from within. Stay on this trail 1.75 miles to the paved Camp Pomponio Road. This is the access road to a low-security county jail, so *do not go right* or you will be searched and questioned. Turn left instead, cross the steel bridge, and take the wide dirt road on the right 100 yards beyond it (Bridge Trail). In 0.4 mile it reaches a four-way junction. Make a right and head down 200 yards to Tarwater Trail Camp, where you can set up camp for the second night. Although overgrown and not as charming as Shaw Flat, it is just as desolate and quiet. For water access, walk back to the four-way junction and take Bridge Trail to the old steel bridge over Pescadero Creek, where a narrow trail drops to the stream.

To hike the Butano Ridge Loop Trail (10.7 miles from the camp and back), continue past the bridge up to the Old Haul Road Trail, turn left and walk 0.15 mile to the signed trail on the right. This one is steep: in 2.9 miles it ascends 1670 feet to Butano Ridge, the top half a succession of tight switchbacks. If you are in shape, it takes about an hour of vigorous cardiovascular exercise. The trail is under the cover of second-growth forest, and near the summit it passes a curious ledge of overhanging sandstone sculpted by erosion. The trail ends on an old logging road. Turn right and follow it 2 miles along Butano Ridge's undulating crest. Up there the air is cooler, and the walking, mostly downhill save for a few short climbs, is much easier. A short distance down the road grow a healthy stand of scraggly knobcone pines, one of only a few in the area. Much of the ridge is lined with groves of mature Douglas fir and redwoods. Through the stately trees you can catch glimpses of the rarely visited Butano Creek watershed to the north, one of the largest remaining swaths of unprotected land on the peninsula. Nature lovers will enjoy the majesty of the trees, the frequent switches from sun to shade, and the exhilarating sense of isolation.

The loop's downhill trail segment is marked by a small sign on the right. It snakes down 2.1 miles through a second-growth forest that gets darker along the way, to end at the Old Haul Road Trail. If you want to cool off, take the short Shaw Flat Trail across the road down to Pescadero Creek. To return, take the Old Haul Road Trail back up. The scenery alternates between densely packed spindly trees and old-growth stands bathed in sunlight. The horizontal slots cut in some of the stumps were made over a century ago to hold the springboards on which loggers stood to slowly saw the enormous trunks. After 2 miles, watch for the signed Snag Trail on the left, a scenic 0.4-mile shortcut that passes one enormous snag deprived of its bark on its way to Bridge Trail and ends a short distance from Tarwater Trail Camp.

The return on the last day starts on the Tarwater Loop Trail, perhaps the park's most diverse and scenic trail. At the four-road junction, turn left (north) and look for the trail sign on the right 0.1 mile farther. This leg of the trail climbs to a high point on Camp Pomponio Road (2.8 miles). It traverses several fern-lined old-growth stands, especially in its lower reaches, interspaced with mixed hardwood. In the late 19th century, a mill was operated along this trail about 0.3 mile in. It produced shingles instead of boards, which were easier to haul out from such remote locations. Look carefully for its long boiler and hefty support timbers hidden in the woods on the left. This trail's highlight is the gargantuan redwood a little past the midpoint. Shaped like a candelabra, crowned with massive vertical limbs thicker than most of the park's trees, it is one of the biggest on the peninsula. As you climb, the forest gradually changes to oak, madrone, and fir. At the top, cross Camp Pomponio Road, and start the second leg (1.5 miles) on the gated dirt road. Make a left on the foot trail 0.25 mile down. It descends gently through a series of bucolic meadows to a decaying barn under looming eucalyptus trees and an abandoned orchard below it. These are the remains of Tie Camp, a small dairy farm that once supplied milk products to local residents. The trail then enters the forest cover, crosses a narrow stream entrenched in dark-gray clay, and ends a little farther at a dirt road lined with giant redwoods.

Turn right on Canyon Trail. The narrow stream the trail crosses 200 yards away is Tarwater Creek. It is the site of a rare natural phenomenon: Crude oil oozes out of the creek bed in slender, sticky threads that often gather into thick black coatings. Farther on, you first follow a dark creek lined with major trees, then climb on tight switchbacks about 0.7 mile to Bear Ridge Trail and turn right. At one point this narrow path contours a deep precipitous slope covered with towering giants, offering an unusual perspective from the treetops *down* their massive trunks. When you first reach the ridge, look for a bench under a venerable Douglas fir, then a picnic table, just right of the trail. They both command grand views of the canyon you just explored.

About a half mile from the overlook, on the edge of an open meadow, a sign points you north to Heritage Grove Trail, a majestic path and befitting end to this trip. First it descends into the Alpine Creek watershed, then forks left and winds another mile at approximately constant elevation through a dark majestic forest. You will be walking under looming redwoods and firs with tall straight trunks more than 6 feet across. In summer, you might find orchids blooming by the side of the trail.

BUILD-UP AND WIND-DOWN TIPS

On the way out, I like to stock up on carbs and proteins with a hearty ranch-style breakfast at **Alice's Restaurant**, a local landmark lost on Skyline Boulevard at the intersection with Highway 84. The waiters are friendly, the burger menu innovative, and the back patio beautifully landscaped and restful. In the warmer months you can eat outside at picnic tables, and in the winter you can warm up your bones in the cabin-style dining area.

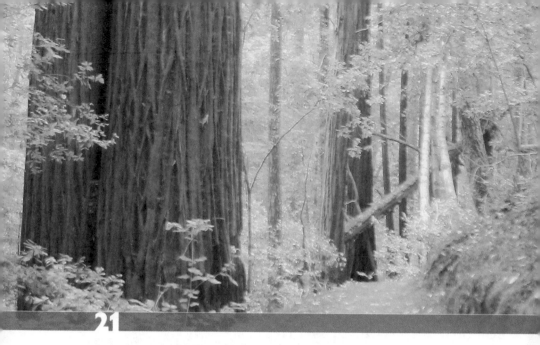

21

SKYLINE TO BIG BASIN

Michel Digonnet

MILES: 26.5

RECOMMENDED DAYS: 4

ELEVATION GAIN/LOSS: 3550′ / 5150′

TYPE OF TRIP: Point-to-point

DIFFICULTY: Moderate

SOLITUDE: Solitude

LOCATION: Long Ridge Open Space Preserve, Portola Redwoods State Park, Pescadero Creek County Park, Redtree Properties L. P., and Big Basin Redwoods State Park

MAPS: USGS 7.5-min. maps *Mindego Hill* and *Big Basin*

BEST SEASON: Year-round

PERMITS

A permit is required for camping, on a first-come, first-served basis (i.e., you may be given a permit yet get there and find the first campground full and have to hike several more miles to another one); contact Big Basin's headquarters at 831-338-8861 or 831-338-6132 or 21600 Big Basin Way, Boulder Creek, CA 95006. Slate Creek Camp is usually closed December through April—double check its availability during this period before planning your trip.

Photo: *Redwoods along the Skyline-to-the-Sea Trail*

HOW TO GET THERE • • • • • • • • • • • • •

On Interstate 280 in Palo Alto, take the Page Mill Road exit. Drive Page Mill Road about 10 miles south to Skyline Boulevard at the crest of the Santa Cruz Mountains. Turn left and follow Skyline Boulevard 4.9 miles to the signed entrance to the Long Ridge Open Space Preserve, on the west side. If you are coming in from the south, from Saratoga take Highway 9 up to Skyline Boulevard at Saratoga Gap, then Skyline Boulevard north 1.5 miles to the same spot. Parking overnight at or near this location is prohibited, so arrange to be dropped off.

To be picked up in Big Basin Redwoods State Park, from Saratoga Gap drive southwest on Highway 9 a distance of 6.1 miles to its junction with Highway 236, then take this narrow, very windy road 8.1 miles to the park headquarters.

CHALLENGES •

All trails are well marked, so route-finding is easy. Watch for poison oak on narrow trails, as it is quite common. Check yourself for ticks regularly. Campfires are not allowed at either campground. Smoking is not allowed on the trails. The camps have no drinking water. Bring your own, or purify or filter the creek water. Come prepared for possible heavy rains in winter.

TRIP DESCRIPTION • • • • • • • • • • • • • • • •

From Skyline Boulevard, first head down Hickory Oaks Trail. This old ranch road crosses a pastoral landscape of grass-covered hills studded with the venerably old oak trees after which it is named. Some very large specimens thrive on these cooler heights, their wide crown supported by tangles of misshapen limbs. This is a striking example of the oak woodlands for which California is famous, its grassland bright gold in the long dry season, tender green in winter. This area commands

TAKE THIS TRIP

This is, without a doubt, the most scenic and off-beat wilderness route across the Santa Cruz Mountains. From the crest of the range you will descend across typical California rolling grassland studded with ancient oaks to the densely forested canyon of Pescadero Creek, then climb on the far side to the lofty summit of Butano Ridge, and finally drop along restful Opal Creek to the redwood heart of Big Basin. The side trip into the Peters Creek watershed, home of the peninsula's tallest tree, is unparalleled in the entire range for its seclusion and outstanding groves of towering redwoods.

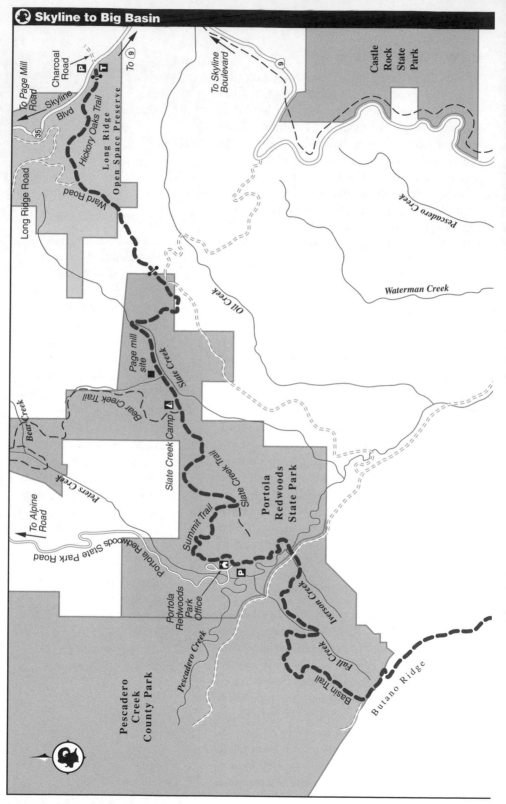

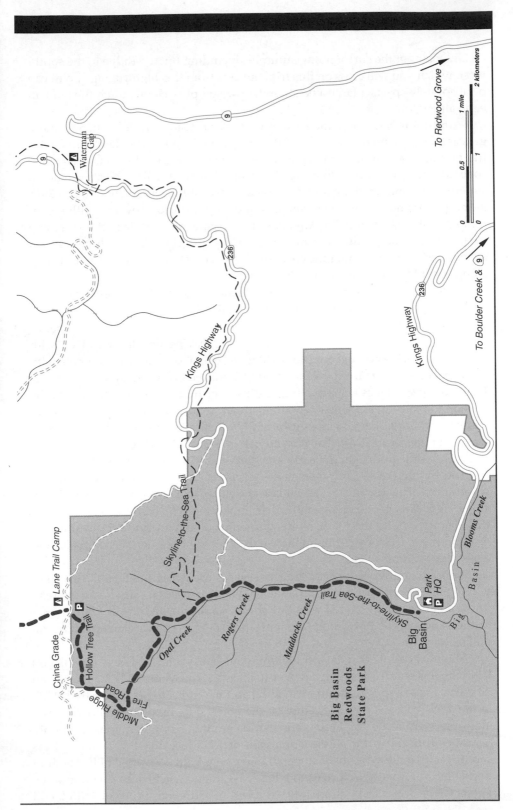

distant vistas of the surrounding summits, including Butano Ridge to the southwest, which you will cross on this trip. Sunsets from this high vantage point can be absolutely spectacular, especially when wispy pink clouds torch the land an eerie alpenglow.

After 1.1 miles, where the trail ends at Ward Road, turn left. There is more grassland for a while, then the road ducks into a mixed forest of laurel and oaks, fragrant after a rain. It opens up again as it drops steeply along an open slope covered with low shrubs typical of California chaparral. This open stretch offers superb views into the long and deep watersheds of Pescadero and Oil creeks, a grand panorama of unspoiled canyons and ridges thickly covered with a continuous mat of tall evergreen. After passing the gate into Portola Redwoods State Park, the road begins its descent along a steep ridgeline. You will pass by an abandoned farm, then enter the cover of an oak and Douglas-fir forest, dropping along abrupt inclines interspaced by short terraces.

About 0.8 mile into the park, the steel gate of the Redtree Properties blocks farther progress. Just before it, a small sign on the right directs you to Slate Creek Trail. You enter a forest of redwood and fir, its understory here a lush cover of fern and blackberry, there a brown carpet of decaying needles sprinkled with starflower. Dark second-growth areas logged several decades ago alternate with small pockets of mature trees that seeded hundreds of years ago. After about 1 mile the trail makes a sharp left and dips over human-made stairs cut in the hillside to Slate Creek. This lively little stream is usually not very deep, but in winter, you might have to cross it carefully on slippery rocks and providential logs and hope to stay dry. The next stretch is beautiful and serene. The canyon brightens as the tree cover thins to a long grove of well-spaced ancient redwoods coursed by the creek. The steep slopes disappear under green carpets of redwood sorrel. This idyllic passage ends at the site of Page Mill, marked by a large, aging sign. This is one of two mills that lumberman William Page operated in this vicinity around the 1860s. Nothing remains of this historic venture, but this is a great spot to sit by the bubbling creek, soak your feet in its cool pools, and enjoy the soothing silence.

Another quarter mile up the trail, past steep road-cuts and fallen trees, takes you to Slate Creek Camp, on the left at a major crossroad. Its six sites are spread down a gentle slope covered with low shrub, under the high roof of tall fir, madrones, and spindly redwoods. Privacy is limited—but chances are high that you will be on your own.

The next day, take a day off lugging your backpack and take a dayhike on Bear Creek Trail. After hiking all over the Santa Cruz Mountains for more than 20 years, I yet have to find a more magical and magnificent place. The trail starts at the crossroad just past the camp, on the north side. Ignore the unnecessarily alarming sign at the trailhead—this loop is anything but strenuous. It is only 6.5 miles round-trip for an elevation gain of 1550 feet, most of it gradual except for a 0.4-mile very steep slope a ranger once called Cardiac Hill. The trail first climbs gradually as a road to a low pass, then switchbacks down into the Peters Creek watershed, all in a mixed forest of redwood, fir, oaks, laurel, and madrones. The road then turns into a foot trail, drops along Cardiac Hill, and reaches Bear Creek.

Words fail to describe the beauty, seclusion, and haunting silence that permeate the confluence of Bear and Peters creeks, along the last 1.5 miles. The low banks along Peters Creek are home to one of the largest concentrations of giant redwoods in these mountains. You will be walking in awe through a high-vaulted cathedral supported by the massive straight trunks of immense trees, craning your neck to gaze up at the dark-green canopy tens of feet higher up. Where the trail reaches Bear Creek, amble a short distance up the shallow stream. Funneled between steep, closely spaced canyon slopes, its limpid water gathers in deep holes, spreads over shallow gravel beds, then tumbles over small cascades. Submerged rocks are petrified—coated with a veneer of limestone deposited by the calcareous water. Fallen tree trunks span the narrow gulch. Just a little farther, the trail reaches the start of the loop. Head north, on a broad bank covered with fern, within sight of the gurgling waters of Peters Creek. The next crossing, at the north end of the loop, is a great place to take a rest and have lunch, at the foot of mighty trees. The tallest redwood on the peninsula grows in this vicinity but enormous trees are so numerous that it is impossible to pick it out.

The rest of the loop is equally impressive. It climbs to, then follows a wide bench 50 to 100 feet above the creek, from which you are treated to awesome plunging views of the deeply furrowed, elephantine trunks of the local giants. The last crossing of Peters Creek is the hardest because the creek is wider and rocks are fewer and slippery, but in the right season it is fun to get wet.

On the third day, take gently sloped Slate Creek Trail 1.1 miles to Summit Trail, under the cover of a redwood forest lined with thickets of huckleberry and wax myrtle. Then head down Summit Trail's long switchbacks 0.8 mile to a paved service road at the bottom of Portola Redwoods State Park. If you want to refill with city water, turn right on this road and walk 0.5 mile to the fountain outside the ranger station. Otherwise turn left on the service road, cross Pescadero Creek (the bridge was washed out in the winter of 2008, so you might need to get your feet wet), and climb the steep grade to Long Haul Road Trail.

Portola Trail starts right across the old haul road, by the park board. From here to Basin Trail just below the crest, it is a hefty 1590-foot climb in 2.8 miles. Portola Trail is comparatively gentle and suffused with a restful mood. It follows Fall Creek for a while, which always has a good flow. At one place the stream leaps into a narrow cleft and gives birth to a singing waterfall. The enormous dam of fallen trees just above it is a silent reminder of the phenomenal forces such meek streams can develop when swollen by heavy rainstorms. At the first junction, make a left on Ridge Trail. Much steeper, it shoots up the side of a sloppy ridge, culminating in a few dozen short, heart-pumping switchbacks—a satisfying grind and the only physically demanding part of this trip.

At the next junction, make a left on the signed Basin Trail. Although all of it is on high ground, this trail is mostly under tree cover and offers surprisingly few good views. The exception is the scenic overlook 0.4 mile out: It commands glorious vistas of sprawling ridges to the northeast, a brilliant patchwork of grass meadows and dark-green forests. Look carefully for the hollow tree that grows in this vicinity, along the left side of the trail. It is a rare natural occurrence: You can step into it and look straight up its trunk, which a fire cored out all the way through to the top long ago—and the tree is still alive. After 0.8 mile, the trail enters an easement on Redtree Properties land. Stay on it 1.3 miles as it gently undulates on or near a ridge covered with mixed hardwoods. It ends at China Grade Road, at the northern boundary of Big Basin Redwoods State Park.

Lane Trail Camp is 0.2 mile down the trail that starts across the road. It has six sites defined by logs, in a dimly lit setting of skinny madrones and oaks. This is not the most scenic camp around, but it is peaceful and far away from everything.

The last segment first heads down Hollow Tree Trail, then south on Skyline-to-the-Sea Trail. This well-signed route, about 7.1 miles long, crosses the northern corner of Big Basin Redwoods State Park, created in 1901 to preserve what was still then a little-known natural wonder—extensive groves of exceptionally large trees. Thanks to this early preservation, this beautiful area was spared from almost any logging, and today it is host to an unusually high density of virgin redwood stands. Hollow Tree Trail has its share of majestic trees. Gentle and downhill the whole way, it is a tranquil finale to a memorable trip. Most of it follows Opal Creek, a quiet little stream that tumbles lazily through a mixed woodland at first, then through increasingly finer and more impressive redwood as the elevation drops. Along the way, look for the trail's namesake, a hollow tree near the top of the trail, shortly after a creek crossing. Silt particles in suspension in the water makes the creek reflect light from within like an opal. This peculiar iridescence is especially striking in the creek's lower reaches along Skyline-to-the-Sea Trail. Some of the redwoods along the final mile or so are simply gigantic.

BUILD-UP AND WIND-DOWN TIPS

At the end of your trip, do not miss the unforgettable **Redwood Trail**. It begins just across the road from the park headquarters. In a half mile, this easy loop packs in one of densest collections of colossal redwoods on the peninsula, including the Mother and Father of the Forest. Drive Highway 236 east a few miles to the town of **Boulder Creek** for a wide selection of restaurants to recharge your batteries in a quaint setting.

22

SKYLINE-TO-THE-SEA TRAIL

Matt Heid

MILES: 29.3

RECOMMENDED DAYS: 3

ELEVATION GAIN/LOSS: 2500´/5100´

TYPE OF TRIP: Point-to-point

DIFFICULTY: Moderate

SOLITUDE: Moderately populated

LOCATION: Castle Rock State Park, Big Basin Redwoods State Park

MAPS: USGS 7.5-min. *Mindego Hill, Cupertino, Castle Rock Ridge, Big Basin, Franklin Point*, and *Point Año Nuevo; Castle Rock State Park Map; Big Basin Redwoods State Park Map; Trail Map of the Santa Cruz Mountains 1 & 2*

BEST SEASONS: Spring and fall

PERMITS

Advance reservations are required for the backcountry trail camps and can be made up to two months in advance by calling 831-338-8861, daily 10 AM–5 PM. Sites cost $10 per night (maximum 6 people per site), and there is a $5 nonrefundable reservation fee that must be mailed to the following address to secure the site: Big Basin Redwoods State Park, Trail Camp Reservations, 21600 Big Basin Way, Boulder Creek, CA 95006. Pay your camping fees at the self-service station

Photo: Old-growth redwoods on the Skyline-to-the-Sea Trail

TAKE THIS TRIP

From the ridgeline spine of the Santa Cruz Mountains, the Skyline-to-the-Sea Trail descends through lush woodlands, passes sweeping vistas, lines crystalline streams, explores old-growth redwood forest, visits beautiful waterfalls, and then reaches the Pacific Ocean at Waddell Beach. It may be the best-known backpacking trip in the Bay Area, but the scenery and adventure are irresistibly epic.

at the Castle Rock trailhead (exact change required) or Big Basin headquarters. For more information, visit www.bigbasin.org.

CHALLENGES

Securing a campsite at popular Sunset Trail Camp in Big Basin Redwoods State Park can be challenging on the weekends. In winter, rains can be heavy and the shady forest is an extremely damp environment.

HOW TO GET THERE

Trailhead at Castle Rock State Park: Take State Highway 35 south of the State Highway 9 junction for 2.5 miles; the posted entrance is located on the west side of the road.

Trailhead at Waddell Beach: Take State Highway 1 to Waddell Beach, located 4.0 miles north of Davenport. Turn inland at the closed (but unlocked) gate north of Waddell Creek and follow the road 0.5 mile to the Waddell Creek Ranger Station and parking lot. Public transportation is available daily to Waddell Beach from the Metro Center in downtown Santa Cruz on Santa Cruz Metro Route 40 (www.scmtd.com, 831-425-8600).

TRIP DESCRIPTION

Seven trail camps are available for year-round overnight use. Water is available at some locations, campfires are not allowed (Castle Rock is an exception), and pets are prohibited everywhere. Castle Rock Trail Camp is the largest and offers 20 sites. Campfires are permitted outside of fire season (typically December through May). Waterman Gap Trail Camp has six sites in a young forest near State Highways 9 and 236. The sound of traffic on the nearby roads is intrusively audible. Water is usually available. Lane Trail Camp is accessible via a 4.2-mile detour from the main route. Six lightly used sites are available, but no water is available. Jay Trail Camp nestles in the main visitor complex surrounding Big

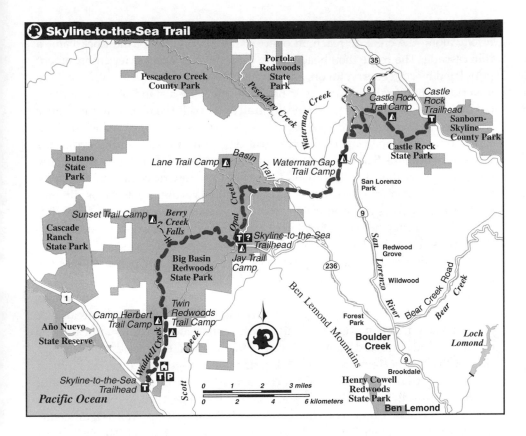

Skyline-to-the-Sea Trail

Portola Redwoods State Park

Pescadero Creek County Park

Pescadero Creek

35

9

Castle Rock Trail Camp

Castle Rock Trailhead

Sanborn-Skyline County Park

Waterman Creek

Butano State Park

Lane Trail Camp

Basin Trail

Waterman Gap Trail Camp

Castle Rock State Park

San Lorenzo Park

9

Cascade Ranch State Park

Sunset Trail Camp

Berry Creek Falls

Opal Creek

Skyline-to-the-Sea Trailhead

Redwood Grove

San Lorenzo River

Bear Creek Road

Bear Creek

Big Basin Redwoods State Park

Jay Trail Camp

236

Wildwood

1

Twin Redwoods Trail Camp

Ben Lemond Mountains

Forest Park

Loch Lomond

Camp Herbert Trail Camp

Waddell Creek

Scott Creek

Boulder Creek

Año Nuevo State Reserve

9

Brookdale

Skyline-to-the-Sea Trailhead

Scott Creek

0   1   2   3 miles

0   2   4   6 kilometers

Henry Cowell Redwoods State Park

Pacific Ocean

Ben Lemond

Basin headquarters and is adjacent to Highway 236. Amenities include water, hot showers in adjacent Blooms Creek Campground, and the small general store near headquarters. Sunset Trail Camp features 10 sites and is accessed via the fairy-tale-perfect Berry Creek Falls Trail, a 1.2-mile detour off the main route. Berry Creek is a third of a mile away and provides water. Camp Herbert shelters in a grove of redwoods and bay trees by mellifluous Waddell Creek and provides six lightly used sites. Twin Redwoods Trail Camp sits in a shady copse of giant bay trees adjacent to Waddell Creek. Given the discrepancies between the trail mileages listed in park literature, on trail signs, and as measured on topographic maps, the distances included below have been made as accurate as possible.

From the Castle Rock parking area, head past the small forest of signs that marks the trailhead at 3070 feet in elevation and proceed straight on the Saratoga Gap Trail. A mixed-evergreen forest of Douglas fir, tanoak, and madrone shades the path as you begin the descent into the Kings Creek drainage, one of the uppermost headwaters of the San Lorenzo River. The trail drops into a dry gully and quickly passes a trail to Castle Rock on the left at 0.1 mile, a worthwhile and short side trip to some wild sandstone formations. Sword ferns and bigleaf maples appear as the trail continues downward, crosses the creek, and passes the Ridge Trail on the right at 0.5 mile.

A few young redwoods can be spotted as the Saratoga Gap Trail continues briefly along the creek to reach an overlook at 0.7 mile for Castle Rock Falls, a thin cascade. The route then heads away from the creek to a drier environment populated by coffeeberry, toyon, and fragrant California bay. The path traverses a world of chaparral and sandstone boulders, entering a stand of rustling black oaks shortly before reaching a connector trail on the right that leads to the nearby Ridge Trail at 1.5 miles and 2560 feet. Excellent views soon open up as you continue on the Saratoga Gap Trail. On a clear day, you can peer south beyond the vast drainage of the San Lorenzo River and across Monterey Bay to the Monterey peninsula, more than 40 miles away. To the west, the low ridge that separates the San Lorenzo River and Pescadero Creek watersheds is apparent; the Skyline-to-the-Sea Trail follows this divide en route to Big Basin Redwoods State Park. Tall Bonny Doon Ridge hems the San Lorenzo River to the southwest, while Butano Ridge rises above the deep canyon of Pescadero Creek to the west.

Gradually descending, you pass thick coyote brush and poison oak as the narrow trail winds along sheer slopes. A sharp bend to the right then leads you through a thick forest of tanoak and madrone to the Ridge Trail on the right at 2.5 miles. To reach the trail camp, bear left and then left again on the wide fire road to reach the main area at 2.7 miles. Knobcone pines abruptly appear, their twisted architecture and namesake cones making them easy to identify. The 15 sites of the Main Camp area are nearby off the Saratoga Gap Trail, while the 5 sites of more-removed Frog Flat Camp are a quarter mile downhill on the Service Road Trail, just below the intersection with the Frog Flat Trail.

From the Main Camp, continue on the wide Saratoga Gap Trail as it descends and passes the Frog Flat Trail on the left at 3.0 miles and 2240 feet. The trail drops into the moist gully of Craig Springs Creek, crosses the small stream, and then curves left to reach the Travertine Springs Trail on the left at 3.4 miles. Follow the Travertine Springs Trail as it initially parallels the stream and then banks right to begin a 2-mile undulating traverse, dropping to cross the San Lorenzo River on a wooden bridge at 4.4 miles and 1680 feet. You next encounter the trail's namesake, Travertine Springs at 5.2 miles, surrounded by massive bay trees, a protective wooden fence, and a few ramshackle structures in the area. Past the spring, the Travertine Springs Trail crosses a small bridge and ends at the Saratoga Toll Road Trail at 5.5 miles.

Turn left to descend and pass a culvert, a dam, and then an old bridge. The route curves south past Tin Can Creek and reaches Beckhuis Road on the right at 6.3 miles. Follow Beckhuis Road as it climbs to the ridge, reached either via the main road or the cutoff trail that splits left along the way. Upon reaching the ridge at 6.7 miles, turn left to descend close to Highway 9 and cross several more fire roads. Redwoods and buckeye trees appear in damp, shady spots along this section, while a scrubby chaparral community of coyote brush, manzanita, chamise, and sticky monkeyflower grows on the drier west-facing slopes. The trail eventually curves away from Highway 9 to reach Waterman Gap Trail Camp at 9.6 miles.

From this camp, the trail narrows and briefly climbs before descending to cross Highway 9 and Mill Road. Past Mill Road, the trail crosses Highway 236, parallels it briefly, and passes the Saratoga Toll Road Trail on the left at 10.2 miles. You then recross Highway 236 and follow it for several undulating miles through dense second-growth redwood forest, crossing several private roads en route. After crossing Highway 236 once again at 13.5 miles, the hike finally curves away from the road.

The boundary of Big Basin Redwoods State Park is not marked, but the transition is readily apparent as several old-growth trees appear along the trail. The trail leads past the East Ridge Trail on the left by trickling Boulder Creek and then turns uphill to cross Highway 236 yet again. You climb out of the San Lorenzo River watershed and cross paved China Grade Road at 14.8 miles, where the flora abruptly changes to dry chaparral marked by the presence of coyote brush, toyon, yerba santa, buck brush, and canyon live oaks. You have excellent views toward the southwest, including the deep drainage of Waddell Creek and the still-distant Pacific Ocean. Past the road, the trail quickly encounters the Basin Trail on the right at 14.9 miles and 1980 feet.

SIDE TRIP: LANE TRAIL CAMP

Lane Trail Camp offers six campsites in a dense forest of tanoak in one of Big Basin's least visited areas. A 6-mile loop follows the Basin Trail to the campsites and then returns to the main route via the Hollow Tree Trail. Rejoining the Skyline-to-the-Sea Trail 1.8 miles past the Basin Trail junction, this variation adds 4.2 miles and 700 feet of elevation gain and loss to the overall journey. The last reliable water source is at Waterman Gap Trail Camp, though a few ephemeral trickles can be found along Basin Trail during wet periods.

From the Basin Trail junction, the Skyline-to-the-Sea Trail continues through dense chaparral punctuated by spindly knobcone pines—enjoy the hike's final views as you traverse the slopes. The route then turns downhill, curves right to reenter lush redwood forest, and crosses two small headwater trickles of Opal Creek shortly before the Hollow Tree Trail enters from the right at 16.7 miles and 1270 feet.

For the next 8 miles, the hike remains entirely within magnificent old-growth redwood forest. You cross Opal Creek on a wooden walkway and follow the burbling stream past large chain ferns and humongous redwoods. You next reach paved North Escape Road near an informative kiosk. Cross Opal Creek on the paved bridge and then immediately bear right to return to the trail, which briefly parallels the road, momentarily rejoins it, and then passes the Meteor Trail on the right. The route touches the road again at another bridge crossing at 17.7 miles and 1040 feet. The Sequoia Trail continues on the opposite side, but the Skyline-to-the-Sea Trail leaves the road at this point to remain on the right (west) side of Opal Creek.

Cruising close to the water past the fluted trunks of giant redwoods, the trail next reaches Maddocks Creek, where an interpretive placard tells the story of an early settler who built an entire cabin from a single redwood tree. Look for the soft leaves of hazel bushes as you continue on the muddy trail, pass the Creeping Forest Trail and Gazos Creek Road, and then reach the Dool Trail on the right at 18.8 miles and 960 feet, which is named for the third park warden of Big Basin Redwoods State Park. Continue straight to quickly reach the junction for the Big Basin headquarters area on the left at 19.2 miles. To reach Jay Trail Camp and the park visitor center and small general store, turn left here to cross Opal Creek. The camp is a quarter mile south of park headquarters on the north side of the highway.

PHOTOGRAPHY TIPS

Photographing old-growth redwood forest is notoriously challenging; achieving a sense of scale is difficult. Try to place a known object (person, backpack, etc.) in the frame to provide a reference point. And for the best results, shoot on overcast or foggy days. The even lighting eliminates the contrast issues that arise from more sun-dappled conditions.

The continuing hike quickly passes the Hammond Connector on the left and begins a steady climb out of the East Waddell Creek drainage. After several switchbacks, the trail crests into the West Waddell Creek drainage at the junction with the Howard King Trail.

Continuing straight, you pass a connector to the Sunset Trail on the right at 20.3 miles and rapidly descend though spectacular old-growth redwood forest—dozens of perfect trees fill the forest in every direction. A bridge soon leads across Kelly Creek, where an alternate route splits right and runs along the stream before rejoining the main trail 0.4 mile later. Past the Timms Creek Trail at 21.6 miles and 530 feet, the canyon narrows and becomes rockier. The trail drops to cross West Waddell Creek, briefly climbs to a tantalizing view of Berry Creek Falls, and then descends to reach the Berry Creek Falls Trail at the confluence of the two creeks.

Even if you're not staying at Sunset Trail Camp, drop your pack here and make the brief side trip to Berry Creek Falls. The Berry Creek Falls Trail immediately leads to a large viewing platform for the waterfall, a misty cascade that nourishes lush surrounding greenery. Thimbleberry and sword fern coat the damp ground below, tanoak and redwoods rise above, and five-finger ferns wave from the surrounding steep, mossy slopes. The continuing trail climbs steeply above the falls and crosses Berry Creek, staying close to the water in a fairy-tale world of giant trees. The muddy path next reaches Silver Falls, climbing above it via a steep cable-protected section to reach Golden Falls, a series of cascades that slide over brilliant orange sandstone. The trail then curves right to climb out of the narrow creek canyon and reach the Sunset Trail. To reach Sunset

Trail Camp, turn left and ascend the narrow trail to Anderson Landing Road in 0.2 mile. Six sites are available directly across the road (follow the signs); four more are 0.1 mile and 70 feet lower around a large turnout.

From the Berry Creek Falls Trail, the Skyline-to-the-Sea Trail descends to cross rushing West Waddell Creek on a seasonal bridge. Arcing bigleaf maples overhead provide ideal hunting grounds for spiders. Dozens of perfect webs are everywhere, their strands glistening with the moisture of fog and rain. Past this point, the trail widens to become a fire road and the forest immediately transforms into denser, younger second-growth. The route follows the wide and level fire road for the remainder of the hike.

The trail passes the Howard King Trail on the left at 23.3 miles and 350 feet and then recrosses the creek and encounters a bike rack for ocean-bound pedalers. Crossing the stream one last time, the trail passes a few old-growth trees, momentarily narrows to avoid a large washout, and reaches the Henry Creek Trail on the right. The canyon broadens and members of the approaching coastal scrub community start to appear: ceanothus, sticky monkeyflower, coyote brush, coffeeberry, blackberry tangles, poison oak, and stinging nettle. The trail slowly descends to the McCrary Ridge Trail on the left at 26.2 miles and 100 feet, crosses East Waddell Creek on a metal bridge, and reaches Camp Herbert.

Past Camp Herbert, the trail runs along the boundary between parkland and gated private property. Redwoods become increasingly scarce and poison oak explodes in abundance. Soon the large, two-headed redwood tree appears that gives Twin Redwoods Trail Camp its name. Continuing, the Skyline-to-the-Sea Trail quickly passes the Clark Connection Trail on the right, which leads to an alternate, hikers-only route back to Waddell Creek Ranger Station. To take this narrower, less-traveled trail, bear right to cross Waddell Creek and then turn left downstream (the Clark Connection Trail continues upslope). The path climbs briefly and contours along the slopes, crossing several small creeks. Enjoy a few intermittent views of the area—including a glimpse of the Pacific Ocean—before descending to reach Waddell Creek Ranger Station.

If you remain on the easier road, you quickly reach closed Alder Camp on the right at 24.6 miles and then pass through the hike's final redwood grove. Here lurks a huge and gnarled specimen known as the Eagle Tree, spared the logging ax due to its contorted shape. The broad trail widens as it passes a gated private road on the left, crosses Waddell Creek one last time, and passes through a section of private property—please stay on the road. You pass another private road shortly before reaching Horse Camp and the Waddell Creek Ranger Station at 28.8 miles. The hike's final journey to the beach follows the paved road from the parking area to the unlocked gate by Highway 1. Cross the busy road to reach the sandy expanse of Waddell Beach and journey's end.

BUILD-UP AND WIND-DOWN TIPS ·

To refuel after your hike, hit up the **La Cabana Taqueria** in Davenport for reasonably priced—and exceptionally good—burritos and Mexican food. They're located right by Highway 1, and you can call them at 831-425-7742.

23

COAST TRAIL

Matt Heid

MILES: 14.6

RECOMMENDED DAYS: 2

ELEVATION GAIN/LOSS: 2150´/1900´

TYPE OF TRIP: Point-to-point

DIFFICULTY: Moderate

SOLITUDE: Crowded

LOCATION: Point Reyes National Seashore

MAPS: USGS 7.5-min. *Inverness* and *Double Point*; *Point Reyes National Seashore and West Marin Parklands* by Wilderness Press; Tom Harrison's *Point Reyes National Seashore*

BEST SEASONS: Spring and fall

PERMITS

Camping is permitted only at Coast and Wildcat Camps, 1.5 and 9.1 miles from the trailhead, respectively. Campsites can be reserved up to three months in advance by calling 415-663-8054, 9 AM–2 PM Monday through Friday. Reservations can be made in person at the Bear Valley Visitor Center anytime during open hours. You can also make a reservation by fax; download the appropriate form at www.nps.gov/pore/activ_camp_fax.htm and send it to 415-464-5149. Most campsites have a maximum capacity of six, but several larger group sites

Photo: The south end of Double Point from Pelican Hill

are also available. Campsites cost $15 per night for 1–6 people, $30 per night for 7–14 people, and $40 per night for 15–25 people. Payment by Visa or Mastercard is due at the time telephone reservations are made and reservations are nonrefundable. *Permits must be obtained from the Bear Valley Visitor Center prior to your trip.* After-hours pick-up is allowed—permits are placed in a wooden box by the information board in front of the visitor center. If sites are available, walk-in registration is possible for same-day departures.

CHALLENGES

Point Reyes is an extremely popular destination; most trail camps fill up months in advance for Friday and Saturday nights. This hike also requires a car shuttle; the two trailheads are 60 to 90 minutes apart by road.

HOW TO GET THERE

Palomarin (ending) Trailhead: Head west from Highway 1 on unposted Olema-Bolinas Road, located immediately north of Bolinas Lagoon. In 1.2 miles, the road reaches a T-junction—go left and continue on Olema-Bolinas Rd. for 0.5 mile. Turn right on Mesa Road and follow it 4.6 miles to the large parking lot at road's end, passing a Coast Guard radar station and the Point Reyes Bird Observatory along the way. The last 1.3 miles are unpaved.

Bear Valley Visitor Center: To pick up your backcountry permit, head north on Highway 1 from its intersection with Sir Francis Drake Boulevard in Olema and immediately turn left on Bear Valley Road. In 0.5 mile, turn left again to reach the visitor center.

Northern (starting) trailhead: Take Bear Valley Road 1.5 miles north of the Bear Valley Visitor Center, turn left on Limantour Road, and follow it west for 7 miles. Turn left immediately prior to the main Limantour Beach parking lot, and proceed 0.4 mile to the southernmost parking area.

TAKE THIS TRIP

This hike travels the length of Point Reyes' Philip Burton Wilderness on the Coast Trail, a point-to-point journey that never leaves the oceanside as it cruises by secluded beaches, exceptional views, a beautiful waterfall, and two coastside camping areas. Gentle trails and ready access from the Bay Area further highlight this trip.

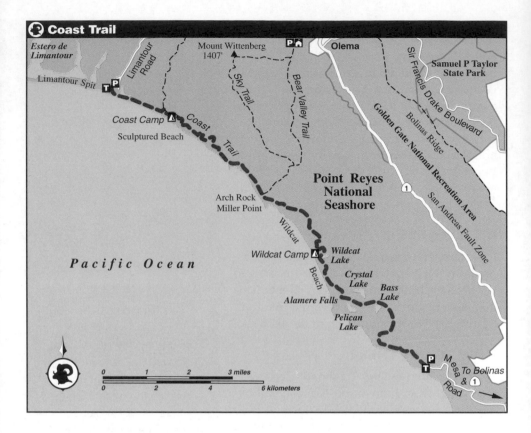

TRIP DESCRIPTION

Head toward the water from the trailhead, following the obvious path past common members of the coastal scrub plant community: coyote brush, coffeeberry, blackberry, lupine, yarrow, ceanothus, cow parsnip, and a few creekside alders. On clear days, Chimney Rock is visible to the west across Drakes Bay, marking the east end of the Point Reyes Headlands. To the south, a large eucalyptus tree indicates the location of Coast Camp.

Head down the beach, keeping an eye out for harbor seals in the surf and herons, ducks, and shorebirds in the nearby marshy wetlands. You can follow the beach all the way to Coast Camp, though the loose sand makes for strenuous going at times. The Coast Trail offers easier walking and can be accessed just past the marsh where a lone bishop pine rises from the sandy dunes, about halfway to Coast Camp.

From Coast Camp at 1.5 miles and 50 feet in elevation, continue south on the broad Coast Trail as it climbs above the small valley and attains the blufftop. For the next 4 miles, the Coast Trail travels atop the headlands; cliffs and steep drainages hem the coastline below. The trail curves around Santa Maria Creek, the first of several creek gullies, and passes the Woodward Valley Trail on the left at 2.1 miles.

The Coast Trail next encounters a wide junction at 2.3 miles that provides access to a small cove at the south end of Sculptured Beach, a worthwhile side trip. Follow the narrow path and stairway down to the ocean, where outcrops of Monterey Shale are dramatically overtopped by the loosely consolidated Drakes Bay Formation. (A sequence of sedimentary layers up to 8000 feet thick, the Monterey Shale formation was deposited on the granite bedrock of Point Reyes National Seashore over the past 20 million years.) At low tide, it is possible to travel from here to Coast Camp past the many formations of Sculptured Beach. Extreme caution is in order—there is no exit from the beach to escape encroaching waves.

DRAMATIC WEATHER CHANGES

From April through October, thick fog blankets Point Reyes' low-lying coastal region and strong onshore winds are common. The fog encounters a formidable obstacle at Inverness Ridge, however, and is often unable to overcome the thousand-foot rise in elevation, leaving eastern regions to bask in more frequent sunshine. On any given day in summer, it may by sunny, calm, and more than 80 degrees at Bear Valley but foggy, breezy, and in the low 50s just a few miles east. Be sure to wear layers.

Continuing south on the Coast Trail, the route loops around a small creek and passes through an area affected by the 1995 Vision Fire, which burned more than 12,000 acres in the central wilderness area; blackened snags jut from the coastal scrub. Hardy coyote brush and bush lupine predominate in the regenerating landscape, joined intermittently by sage and morning glory. The trail curves around several more small drainages and then gradually descends to reach an enormous eucalyptus by another creek. A remnant of U Ranch, this arboreal gargantua marks the access point for Kelham Beach at 4.9 miles, a remote and cliffy strand. From the beach, you get views south toward the sea stacks offshore from nearby Arch Rock and beyond to distant Double Point.

Continuing south on the Coast Trail, you pass the Sky Trail on the left at 5.1 miles shortly before reaching the Bear Valley Trail near Arch Rock. Take the time to visit this distinctive landmark, readily accessed by the many paths that crisscross the area. The view from its open blufftop is excellent, stretching north along adjacent Kelham Beach to Point Resistance and beyond. On the south side of Arch Rock, a well-worn but precarious path descends into the mini-gorge of Coast Creek. At low tide, you can walk through the Arch to access Kelham Beach to the north. To the south, a small pocket beach stretches a short distance to Millers Point.

The southbound Coast Trail next crosses Coast Creek and attains an open ridgeline. Expansive views open up as the trail climbs to 300 feet in elevation and encounters a path on the right, where a short 20-yard detour leads to a small knoll and gravestone marker for Clem Miller, a local congressman who fiercely advocated for the creation of the National Seashore. Miller Point below is named in his honor. The views become ever more thrilling as you continue the ridgeline ascent. Your climb eventually levels out at one of the best vistas in the entire seashore.

Looking north, the long curving arc of Limantour Beach and Drakes Beach terminates in the prominent mass of Point Reyes itself. On clear days, the sharp points of the Farallon Islands are visible to the southwest. On days of exceptional visibility, you can spot the three lumpy rocks of the seldom-seen North Farallones to the west-southwest. To the south, Wildcat Beach and its southern terminus at Double Point are visible. A short distance farther, you encounter the North Spur Trail.

Remain on the Coast Trail as it leaves the vistas behind and enters a dense world of coastal scrub. The trail parallels the headwaters of a deep creek drainage and then gently ascends to the South Spur Trail on the left at 8.0 miles and 840 feet. Bear right to continue on the Coast Trail, which turns south to offer additional ocean views before curving east above the deep valley of Wildcat Creek; Wildcat Camp is located at its mouth. Look for Wildcat Lake and Pelican Hill to the south as you traverse down to meet the broad Stewart Trail entering from the left at 8.4 miles. Turn right and follow the Coast Trail—now a wide fire road—as it winds through a forest of bay and Douglas firs, switchbacks steeply down, and arrives at the open blufftop of Wildcat Camp.

POINT REYES DAIRY RANCHES

In the latter half of the 19th century, a series of dairy ranches were established throughout the Point Reyes peninsula. Famed for their high-quality butter, these ranches were named by the letters of the alphabet; starting with A Ranch by the lighthouse, the ranches progressed clockwise around the peninsula to Z Ranch on Mount Wittenberg.

From here, it is possible to hike 1.3 miles south along the sands of Wildcat Beach to reach Alamere Falls, a unique beach backpacking experience and a more direct and level route to your next destination. Note, however, that sections of the beach can be impassable during high tides and heavy surf, and that there is no exit between Wildcat Camp and Alamere Falls. To continue inland instead, follow the Coast Trail as it climbs through a thick corridor of willow and vetch to reach the Ocean Lake Loop at 9.3 miles and 220 feet.

Bear right on this more scenic alternative that rejoins the Coast Trail in 1.1 miles. The narrower path ascends past brush-lined and inaccessible Wildcat Lake, reaches a bench with views north to Wildcat Beach, and then drops to bank around marshy Ocean Lake. A gentle rise returns you to the Coast Trail. Bear

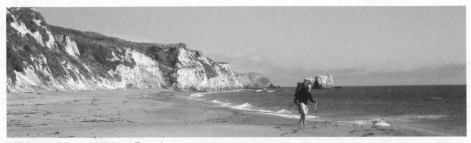
Hiking north on Wildcat Beach

right on the Coast Trail and descend into the Alamere Creek drainage, where alder, elderberry, and thimbleberry thrive in a moister environment.

The route curves around the stream valley, begins climbing, and reaches an unposted spur trail on the right at 10.9 miles. This overgrown and brushy path leads 0.3 mile down to Alamere Falls, unseen until the very end; scrambling is required to reach the stream and its series of cascades, which end as a sheet of water tumbling directly onto the beach below. A rocky chute leads down to the ocean, but requires some difficult scrambling. The bluffs are impressive, and the tilted exposed layers of Monterey shale are spectacular south of the falls.

Return to the Coast Trail and continue south, immediately reaching another unposted spur trail on the right. The small trail climbs 0.3 mile to the top of Pelican Hill (480 feet) and the north end of Double Point, another recommended side trip. Far-reaching views look south and north from the summit. An inaccessible cove beach below is often filled with hundreds of hauled-out seals. In the region around Double Point, Monterey Shale has become involved in a huge landslide nearly 4 miles long and at least 1 mile wide. As this huge block of land slips slowly toward the sea, depressions are formed that fill with freshwater lakes such as Pelican and Bass lakes.

From here, the Coast Trail makes a rising traverse above beautiful Pelican Lake and passes a junction for unexciting Crystal Lake on the left at 11.6 miles. Next up is larger Bass Lake, which provides the hike's best freshwater swimming opportunity and is popular with nudists; a short spur path leads to an open area on its north shore. Continuing, the Coast Trail gradually rises above the lake and then winds through a dense forest of Douglas fir punctuated by several swampy ponds. You pass the Lake Ranch Trail on the left at 12.4 miles, drop over a small divide, and curve around a creek gully choked with willows, horsetail, watercress, and bracken ferns. Several more small creeks follow as the trail winds near the open blufftops. Good views south open up as you proceed. Just before reaching the trailhead, the trail enters a thick eucalyptus grove where a few enormous trees hulk; one huge Hydralike specimen watches your final steps home.

BUILD-UP AND WIND-DOWN TIPS ·

The **Olema Inn and Restaurant** opened on July 4, 1876, and was one of the few buildings in the area to survive the 1906 earthquake. Fully restored in 1998, it makes for a pleasant and historic visit or very gourmet post-hike dinner.

24

BEAR VALLEY LOOP

Matt Heid

MILES: 15.8
RECOMMENDED DAYS: 2–3
ELEVATION GAIN/LOSS: 2000´/2000´
TYPE OF TRIP: Loop
DIFFICULTY: Moderate
SOLITUDE: Crowded
LOCATION: Philip Burton Wilderness, Point Reyes National Seashore
MAPS: USGS 7.5-min. *Double Point*,
       Tom Harrison's *Point Reyes National Seashore*
BEST SEASONS: Spring and fall

PERMITS ●

Camping is permitted only at Sky and Glen Camps, 2.9 and 11.2 miles from the trailhead, respectively. Campsites can be reserved up to three months in advance by calling 415-663-8054, 9 AM–2 PM Monday through Friday. Reservations can be made in person at the Bear Valley Visitor Center anytime during open hours. You can also make a reservation by fax; download the appropriate form at www.nps.gov/pore/activ_camp_fax.htm and send it to 415-464-5149. Most campsites have a capacity of only 6 people, but several larger group sites are also available. Campsites cost $15 per night for 1–6 people, $30 per night for 7–14

Photo: Looking north from the Coast Trail across Drakes Bay people, and $40 per night for 15–25 people. Payment by Visa or Mastercard is due at the time telephone reservations are made and reservations are nonrefundable. *Permits must be obtained from the Bear Valley Visitor Center prior to your trip.* After-hours pick-up is allowed—permits are placed in a wooden box by the information board in front of the visitor center. If sites are available, walk-in registration is possible for same-day departures.

CHALLENGES

Point Reyes is an extremely popular destination; most trail camps fill up months in advance for Friday and Saturday nights.

HOW TO GET THERE

Head west on Bear Valley Road; the turn-off is located immediately north of the intersection of Highway 1 and Sir Francis Drake Boulevard in Olema. In 0.5 mile, turn left to reach the Bear Valley Visitor Center and trailhead parking.

West Marin Stagecoach Route 68 makes 4–5 runs daily from Monday through Saturday from San Rafael to Inverness, stopping at Bear Valley Visitor Center along the way (415-499-6099; www.marintransit.org).

TRIP DESCRIPTION

From the Bear Valley Trailhead at 80 feet in elevation, head north on the Morgan Trail, which runs parallel to the fenced margin of Morgan Horse Farm and quickly passes the Woodpecker Trail on the left at 0.1 mile and 170 feet. Established to breed and train horses for national parks around the country, Morgan Horse Farm once had a herd of nearly 80 animals. Today individual parks maintain their own stables, and Morgan Horse Farm keeps only a few horses for trail patrol and maintenance in the seashore.

The trail soon enters a mixed-evergreen forest of Douglas fir, tanoak, and bay, and

TAKE THIS TRIP

Explore the full spectrum of Point Reyes National Seashore on this loop hike, which tours the lush forest atop the peninsula's highest ridgelines, descends past far-reaching views, and then explores the salt-swept coastline before returning inland via Bear Valley. Pitch a tent at Sky Camp and Glen Camp for a relaxing two-night journey; for an overnight trip, Glen Camp is near the midpoint of the hike.

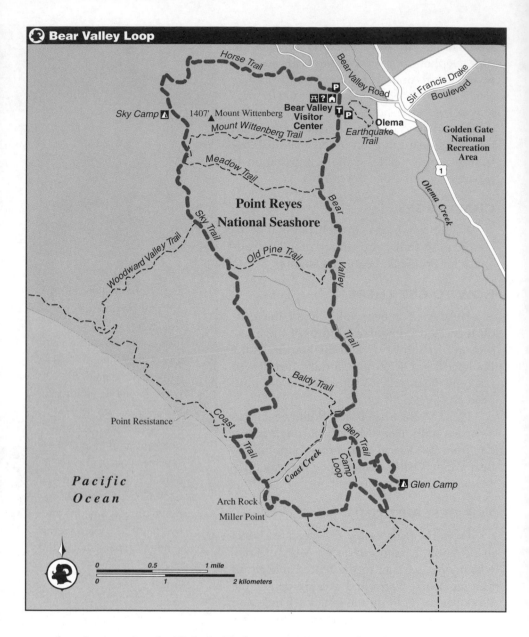

Bear Valley Loop

Horse Trail

Bear Valley Road

Sir Francis Drake Boulevard

Sky Camp ▲   1407'▲ Mount Wittenberg   **Bear Valley Visitor Center**

Mount Wittenberg Trail

Olema

Earthquake Trail

Golden Gate National Recreation Area

Meadow Trail

Olema Creek

Point Reyes National Seashore

1

Bear

Sky Trail

Old Pine Trail

Valley

Woodward Valley Trail

Trail

Baldy Trail

Point Resistance

Coast

Glen Trail

Trail

Camp Loop

Pacific Ocean

Coast Creek

▲ Glen Camp

Arch Rock

Miller Point

0   0.5   1 mile

0   1   2 kilometers

reaches the junction for Kule Loklo by a massive tanoak at 0.4 mile. (The short side trip to Kule Loklo leads to a reconstructed village of the Miwok Indians, the area's prior inhabitants.) Continue on the Morgan Trail, which gently descends to the Horse Trail by a wooden bridge at 0.6 mile. Turn left on the Horse Trail and prepare to ascend!

As you start the climb, look for the sinuous limbs of coast live oaks twining among the drooping branches of bay trees and stout trunks of Douglas firs. Stinging nettle, fuzzy-leaved hazel bushes, blackberry tangles, soft thimbleberry leaves, and wood and sword ferns fill the understory. Wreaths of poison oak climb the trees. The single-track trail becomes steep and rutted as it steadily climbs to 900 feet, where it briefly levels out. Granite rocks, part of Point Reyes' bedrock core, can be found here in the trail.

A MIGRANT PIECE OF LAND

The deepest bedrock of Point Reyes is granite, formed in the region of Southern California approximately 85 million years ago. When the San Andreas Fault became active 28 million years ago, land west of the emergent fault began to slowly migrate north at the rate of 2–3 centimeters per year, traveling hundreds of miles over the ensuing millennia. Point Reyes was one of these; it continues its northward march today.

After a final ascent, the Horse Trail crests Inverness Ridge, contours south through a more open area, and passes the Z Ranch Trail on the left at 2.5 miles. You walk past some loose, layered outcrops of Monterey Shale, which caps the bedrock granite throughout most of the wilderness area. The Horse Trail ends at the wide fire road of the Sky Trail at 2.9 miles and 1050 feet. Turn left on the Sky Trail and cruise into Sky Camp at 3.4 miles.

Continue south past Sky Camp on the easy-cruising Sky Trail, which passes the Mount Wittenberg and Meadow trails on the left at 4.0 miles and enters a section of mature mixed-evergreen forest. Douglas firs tower overhead and strain moisture from the fog, keeping the environment lush and green year-round. Moss-bearded branches and tree-bound ferns droop above abundant elderberry, huckleberry, blackberry tangles, and sword ferns. In September, the huckleberry bushes dangle with abundant—and deliciously edible—blue-black berries.

The Sky Trail next passes the Woodward Valley Trail on the right and climbs briefly to reach the Old Pine Trail on the left at 5.0 miles. Remain on the Sky Trail as it gently descends and then crests a small rise where the surrounding environment transitions to low-lying coastal scrub. Here the Baldy Trail splits right at 6.4 miles to drop into Bear Valley, but you remain on the Sky Trail and descend toward the increasingly visible ocean. The route passes a few burnt snags—remnants of the 1995 Vision Fire, which burned 12,000 acres of the seashore—and reaches a small saddle cloaked with coyote brush. The descent continues, becoming steeper near the end as it makes a final drop via two switchbacks to reach the Coast Trail at 7.9 miles and 130 feet.

The continuing hikes bears left on the wide and sandy Coast Trail south, which quickly leads to the Bear Valley Trail and nearby promontory of Arch Rock at 8.4 miles. (A right turn on the Coast Trail leads in 0.2 mile to an enormous eucalyptus situated by a small creek, which marks the access point for Kelham Beach, a remote strand of cliffs and sandy solitude.) Take the time to visit the open blufftop of Arch Rock, readily accessed by the many paths that crisscross the area. The view is excellent, stretching north along adjacent Kelham Beach to Point Resistance and beyond. On the south side of Arch Rock, a well-worn but precarious path descends into the mini-gorge of Coast Creek. At low tide, you can walk north through the Arch to access Kelham Beach. To the south, a small pocket beach stretches a short distance to Miller Point.

Heading south on the Coast Trail, your continuing route crosses Coast Creek and then climbs to the open ridgeline. Expansive views open up as the trail climbs to 300 feet and encounters a path on the right, where a short 20-yard detour leads to a small knoll and gravestone marker for Clem Miller, a local congressman who advocated fiercely for the creation of this national seashore. Miller Point below is named in his honor. The Coast Trail continues its ascent along the ridgeline and the views become ever more thrilling. Your climb eventually levels out at one of the best views in the seashore.

DEER IN POINT REYES

A dozen native marine mammals, 37 land mammals, and 45 percent of all bird species in North America have been sighted within Point Reyes National Seashore. Native black-tailed deer are common, and two introduced deer species also live here: axis deer, native to India and identified by their reddish-brown coat with white spots, and fallow deer, native to Europe and easily distinguished by their large mooselike antlers.

Looking north, the long curving arc of Limantour Beach and Drakes Beach terminates in the prominent mass of Point Reyes itself. On clear days, the sharp points of the Farallon Islands are visible to the southwest. When the weather provides exceptional visibility, you can spot the three lumpy rocks of the seldom-seen North Farallones to the west-southwest. Wildcat Beach and its southern terminus at Double Point are visible to the south.

Just past the viewpoint, you encounter the North Spur Trail at 9.8 miles and 760 feet. Turn left, take the North Spur Trail inland to the Glen Trail in 0.2 mile, bear right, and proceed on the level Glen Trail to the Glen Camp Loop Trail on the left at 10.4 miles. Follow the Glen Camp Loop Trail past the Greenpicker Trail on the right and slowly descend through a young forest. Glen Camp becomes visible below shortly before the trail banks right and drops steeply into camp at 11.2 miles.

From Glen Camp, your journey continues on the Glen Camp Loop Trail, which narrows to single-track as it rises briefly past eucalyptus and huckleberry bushes and then traverses above a deep gully. The trail skirts a clearing, crosses a small stream, and meets the Glen Trail at 12.1 miles and 460 feet. Turn right and follow the Glen Trail, which briefly runs level with a glimpse of the ocean and then descends through mixed-evergreen woods to emerge in a clearing of coastal scrub and coast live oak. The trail curves right, drops parallel to Coast

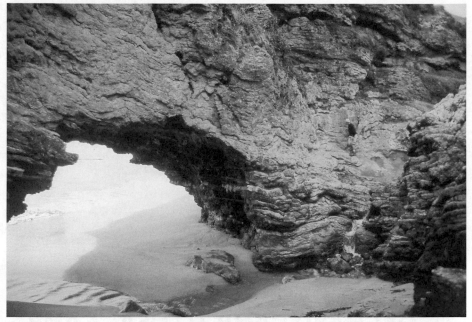

Arch Rock—notice the hiker descending the rocks.

Creek into a lush riparian world, and reaches the Bear Valley Trail by a bike rack at 12.7 miles and 170 feet.

Turn right on the broad trail and head inland alongside alder-choked Coast Creek. The arching branches of massive bay trees shade your journey to Divide Meadow at 14.2 miles and 320 feet, a pleasant rest stop. Ringed by coast live oaks, the meadow sits on the divide between the Olema Valley and Coast Creek watersheds and is the only low-elevation gap through Inverness Ridge. A hunting lodge owned by the Pacific Union Hunting Club of San Francisco once sat in the northwest corner, a backcountry base for pursuing bears and mountain lions from the 1890s until the Great Depression. The lodge has long since been removed; two huge introduced Monterey pines and a few patches of exotic pink flowers are all that remain.

Continue on the Bear Valley Trail and enter one of the seashore's most majestic forests. California bay, alders, and tanoak thrive. Mighty Douglas firs rise above, each unique in form and character. Bracken ferns, thimbleberry, blackberry tangles, sword ferns, elderberry, five-finger ferns, and gooseberry grow abundantly beneath their crooked branches. On your way out, you pass the Meadow Trail at 15.0 miles and Mount Wittenberg Trail at 15.6 miles on the left and then emerge into a more open landscape. Bear Valley Trailhead is just ahead.

BUILD-UP AND WIND-DOWN TIPS ·

The **Olema Inn and Restaurant** opened on July 4, 1876, and was one of the few buildings in the area to survive the 1906 earthquake. Fully restored in 1998, it makes for a pleasant and historic visit or very gourmet post-hike dinner.

25

LOST COAST TRAIL: ORCHARD CAMP TO USAL CAMP

Matt Heid

MILES: 16.7
RECOMMENDED DAYS: 3
ELEVATION GAIN/LOSS: 3800´/3800´
TYPE OF TRIP: Point-to-point
DIFFICULTY: Moderately strenuous
SOLITUDE: Moderate solitude
LOCATION: Sinkyone Wilderness State Park
MAPS: USGS 7.5-min. *Hales Grove*, *Mistake Point*, and *Bear Harbor*; *California's Lost Coast* by Wilderness Press
BEST SEASONS: Spring and fall

PERMITS

Backcountry camping is allowed only at three designated trail camps: Wheeler, Little Jackass, and Anderson Gulch. There is a fee of $3 per person per night for the trail camps, payable outside the Needle Rock Visitor Center or at the Usal Camp fee station. There is no trail quota.

Photo: Above the Lost Coast

CHALLENGES ·

The two ends of the Lost Coast Trail are far apart by road (2–3 hours' driving time) and a car shuttle is required to complete the hike. The weather can be fickle. Fog blankets the region from June through mid-September, interspersed with clear days and strong northwest winds. Heavy rains usually strike by late October and can inundate the coast well into April. If you're planning a winter visit, call the park in the days just before your trip to verify access; flooding and slides can close the roads for weeks at a time.

HOW TO GET THERE · · · · · · · · · · · · · · ·

Orchard Camp (starting) Trailhead: Take the Highway 101 exit for Redway and Shelter Cove. From Redway, follow Briceland Thorn Road toward Shelter Cove 16.5 miles to Chemise Mountain Road and turn left (south). The road rapidly turns to dirt, reaching a four-way junction in 6.3 miles—turn right onto the least significant road. The descent from here is steep, narrow, and not passable for trailers or RVs. While four-wheel-drive vehicles will have an easier time, low-clearance cars can make a slow descent. The Needle Rock Visitor Center is 3.2 miles from the junction; the trailhead is 2.4 miles farther south at the road's end. The road is closed beyond the visitor center during the rainy season, making it necessary to walk this final stretch.

Usal Beach (ending) Trailhead: Take Mendocino County (Usal) Rd. 431 north from Highway 1 at milepost 90.88. The unmarked and easily missed turnoff is 13.9 miles west of the Highway 1 junction with Highway 101 and approximately 3 miles north of Rockport. The one-lane dirt road is impassable for trailers and RVs but easily handled by all other vehicles. In 5.4 miles you reach the area's first campsites, located in a large grassy field. Trailhead parking is 0.3 mile farther on the left.

TAKE THIS TRIP

Dark cliffs tower more than 1000 feet above the crashing sea. Small creeks carve deep gullies between the bluffs, providing access to unusual black sand beaches and remote camping areas. The Lost Coast Trail tours it all on a point-to-point journey remarkable for its scenery, wildlife, and strenuous hiking.

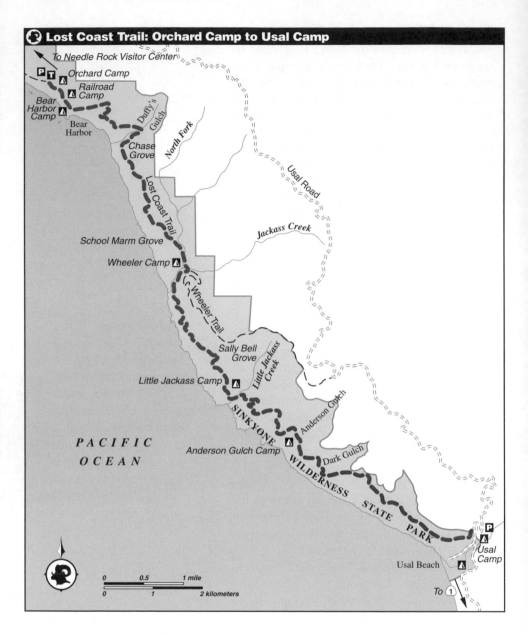

Lost Coast Trail: Orchard Camp to Usal Camp

To Needle Rock Visitor Center

Orchard Camp

Railroad
Camp

Bear
Harbor
Camp

Bear
Harbor

Duffy's Gulch

Chase
Grove

North Fork

Usal Road

Jackass Creek

School Marm Grove

Lost Coast Trail

Wheeler Camp

Wheeler Trail

Sally Bell
Grove

Little Jackass Camp

Little Jackass Creek

SINKYONE

Anderson Gulch

Anderson Gulch Camp

Dark Gulch

WILDERNESS

PACIFIC
OCEAN

STATE

PARK

Usal
Camp

Usal Beach

To 1

0   0.5   1 mile
0   1   2 kilometers

TRIP DESCRIPTION

The hike follows the Lost Coast Trail between Orchard Camp and Usal Camp, a strenuous trek best done in three days. For being along the coast, there is virtually no level walking on this hike: the trail constantly encounters sheer creek canyons, descending quickly and ascending steeply hundreds of feet at a time. While the hike can be done in either direction, this description runs from north to south.

Soon after leaving the trailhead at Orchard Camp, the trail is joined by a spur trail from Railroad Camp. Then it winds down to the spectacular coastal vista at Bear Harbor at 0.4 mile, a doghole port established in the late 1800s to transport lumber from the area. Nothing remains of prior development but pleasant campsites tucked away from the ocean. Next comes a general introduction to the Lost Coast Trail experience of repeated ascent and descent. Climbing a steep and narrow stream gully, the trail passes through luscious greenery. Large sword ferns splay everywhere, moss covers the thick trunks of alder and California bay, the large leaves of blue elderberry line the stream bank, and every possible nook and cranny bursts with life. You have time to enjoy all this because the trail is remarkably steep. After you attain the ridge, the trail traverses around Duffy's Gulch and through the first grove of old-growth redwoods before gently climbing along the blufftop. Views into the sheer gulch of Jackass Creek open up where the trail makes its steep descent to Wheeler Camp at 4.7 miles, passing through another old-growth redwood grove just before the first campsites.

Wheeler Camp was the location of a wood processing facility from 1951 until 1960, run by the Wolf Creek Timber Company. The small company town included a store, bunkhouse, and school, but was deliberately burned for liability reasons in 1969. Remnants of the mill include knee-high periscopelike tubes protruding from the ground, which were used to test the underground flow of toxic diesel fuel that leaked from the facility. While no fuel is known to have reached Jackass Creek, to be safe obtain your water upstream from the site. If it's raining or windy, the campsites nearest the redwood grove are nicest. If it's sunny and clear, continue along the trail to uphill sites south of the beach.

On your way to the beach, a trail diverges left as you enter the more open meadow—continue straight, winding along the edge of the beach before climbing steeply to almost 1100 feet. Keep an eye out for the small trees lining the top of the cliff, some of which are as old as those in the surrounding forest, with remarkably stout trunks hidden beneath their twisted foliage. Shelter Cove can

Roosevelt elk

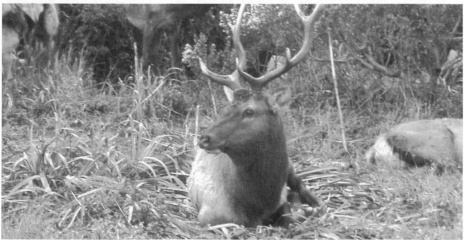

TREKKING POLES

Using trekking poles can help minimize knee impact on steep descents. On a 25-degree grade, poles reduce compressive forces on the knees by 12 to 25 percent. They also reduce knee strain on level ground, though by a lesser amount (approximately 5 percent). To set the pole height, hold the handle out in front of you with the tip on the ground and your arm at your side. For level or uneven terrain, your elbow should form a right angle when the pole is properly adjusted. For sustained downhill sections, lengthen the pole a few inches to compensate; for uphill miles, shorten it.

To use the straps properly, first insert your hand through the loop in an upward motion from underneath. Then grasp the handle, positioning the portion of the strap closest to the pole between thumb and index finger. Part of the strap should now lie between your hand and the grip, with the rest wrapping snugly around your wrist. Adjust the size of the loop to fit closely. With the straps properly fitted, you can much more effectively transfer energy between the ground and your upper body.

be spotted north from near the cliff top, before the trail plummets down through dense tanoak forest to Little Jackass Camp at 9.2 miles. Sites are fewer than at Wheeler Camp and farther from the wonderfully secluded beach.

The trail continues inland opposite the creek, quickly entering the Sally Bell Grove, an old-growth redwood stand named for a Sinkyone woman who fled here after an attack on her village at Needle Rock in May 1864 by Lieutenant William Frazier and the Battalion of Mountaineers. Passing many substantial redwoods, the trail makes a very steep ascent to 800 feet before immediately dropping to Anderson Gulch Camp at 11.7 miles at 250 feet. Here, the campsites are small and hidden among the trees. You pass the best sites shortly after crossing the creek.

Another brief up-and-down brings you to Dark Gulch at 12.3 miles, where the final and most arduous section of the hike begins. A prolonged stretch of climbing brings you to—at more than 1100 feet—the highest point on this hike, almost directly above the ocean. The thick forest of tanoak, bigleaf maple, and redwood opens into fields of low-lying coyote brush and blackberry tangles. South, the trail can be seen winding along the bare ridgetop. Ocean views are exceptional, Usal Beach is visible, and a keen eye can identify Highway 1, 7 miles south of here, twisting along the coast before turning inland. It's a gradual descent from here to Usal Beach, ending with several steep switchbacks that deposit you near some nice campsites.

BUILD-UP AND WIND-DOWN TIPS ·

Eighteen walk-in campsites ($15 per night) are scattered around the **Needle Rock** area, an option for a late-night arrival or superb base camp for exploring the surrounding area on dayhikes.

26

LOST COAST TRAIL: KING RANGE WILDERNESS LOOP

Matt Heid

MILES: 30.6
RECOMMENDED DAYS: 3–4
ELEVATION GAIN/LOSS: 5800´/5800´
TYPE OF TRIP: Loop
DIFFICULTY: Strenuous
SOLITUDE: Moderate solitude
LOCATION: King Range Wilderness and National Conservation Area
MAPS: USGS 7.5-min. *Shelter Cove, Shubrick Peak*, and *Honeydew*;
King Range National Conservation Area by the BLM
BEST SEASONS: Spring and fall

PERMITS

A backcountry permit is required, available at the trailhead or from the Bureau of Land Management King Range Office. A California Department of Forestry permit is required for campfires, which are permitted except when a fire closure is in effect (typically late June through late October).

Photo: Get lost.

TAKE THIS TRIP

Established in 2006 as one of the state's newest wilderness areas, the 42,585-acre King Range Wilderness encompasses the rugged and wild coastline of the northern Lost Coast. It includes the western flanks of the King Range, which lurch upward from the ocean to its high point atop 4088-foot King Peak, less than 3 miles from the coast. Small streams carve deep ravines through the coastal bluffs, providing water and oceanside campsites for beach-walking hikers, while rugged and seldom-traveled trails journey through the high, dry interior of the King Range. This loop hike tours it all.

CHALLENGES

A 4.5-mile section of beach is passable only at low tides; take note of when they occur (posted at the trailhead). Heavy rain can turn streams into dangerous torrents that may be difficult or impossible to cross; watch the weather. A 2003 wildfire burned much of the King Range, leaving an open charred landscape with lots of sun exposure. Bear canisters are mandatory (violators are subject to a $150 fine) and can be rented at the BLM King Range Office for $5 per trip with a credit card deposit.

HOW TO GET THERE

Take the U.S. Highway 101 exit for Redway and Shelter Cove. From Redway, take Briceland Thorn Road toward Shelter Cove. In 13.2 miles you'll pass the BLM King Range Office on the left (open year-round Monday–Friday 8 AM–4:30 PM; intermittently on summer weekends; 707-986-5400). Continue another 7.1 miles to Beach Road and turn right toward Black Sands Beach, reaching the Black Sands Beach Trailhead and parking area in 0.9 mile. Potable water is available. No camping is permitted from the parking area to Telegraph Creek, 0.2 mile north.

TRIP DESCRIPTION

A view north from the blufftop parking area reveals much of your approaching hike. The broad clearing of Big Flat, your northernmost beach destination, is discernible in the distance. Inland, Horse Mountain rises as the first prominent ridgeline, followed by Saddle Mountain, where a keen eye can spot a trail—your return route—descending its flanks. The small pyramid of King Peak peeks out beyond Saddle Mountain, crowning the top of Miller Ridge. Shubrick Peak and Lake Ridge loom beyond.

Follow the sidewalk down to the beach. Dark-colored greywacke and shale—loosely

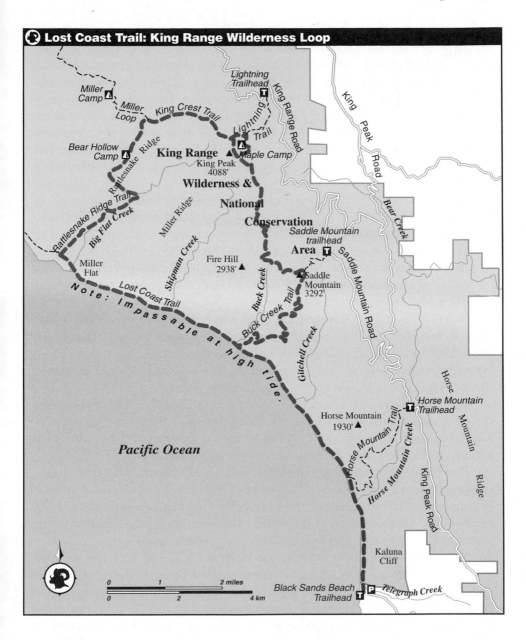

Miller Camp

Miller Loop

King Crest Trail

Lightning Trailhead

Lightning Trail

King Range Road

King Peak Road

Bear Hollow Camp

Rattlesnake Ridge

King Range
King Peak
4088'

Maple Camp

Wilderness &

Rattlesnake Ridge Trail

Big Flat Creek

National

Miller Ridge

Shipman Creek

Conservation

Saddle Mountain trailhead

Bear Creek

Area

Fire Hill
2938'

Buck Creek

▲Saddle Mountain
3292'

Saddle Mountain Road

Miller Flat

Lost Coast Trail

Buck Creek Trail

N o t e :   I m p a s s a b l e   a t   h i g h   t i d e .

Gitchell Creek

Horse Mountain
1930' ▲

Horse Mountain Trail

Horse Mountain Creek

Horse Mountain Trailhead

Horse Mountain Ridge

Pacific Ocean

King Peak Road

Kaluna Cliff

0   1   2 miles
0   2   4 km

Black Sands Beach Trailhead

Telegraph Creek

consolidated layers of sand and mud—compose much of the mountains here, eroding to form the beach's distinctive black sand and cobbles. You'll be walking on it for the next 8 miles, a fatiguing exercise in the loose terrain. The wet sand below high tide line usually offers the firmest footing.

Heading north, you soon pass Telegraph Creek on the right, followed by a rivulet emerging from below the Kaluna Cliffs. The beach narrows at this point and a giant house-sized boulder bulges from the shore. As you approach Horse

Mountain Creek at 1.6 miles, you encounter an elaborate driftwood shelter, the first of many to come. A nice tent site nestles north of the creek mouth.

Past Horse Mountain Creek, you soon pass the Horse Mountain Trail heading inland and then wander by low terraces hiding a few pleasant campsites. (Along most of the beach, anywhere that appears to have camping potential probably has an established site.) The beach narrows again and the first offshore rocks appear as you approach Gitchell Creek at 3.7 miles, which tumbles out of a 30-foot-wide gash in otherwise featureless cliffs. A huge driftwood shelter has been constructed on the north side of the stream; a nice tent site can be found on a small terrace a short distance north.

The next 4.5 miles of beach are impassable for several hours on either side of high tide (longer if there is significant swell). Time your passage appropriately and don't risk getting caught—there is no escape up the vertical cliffs. Past Gitchell Creek, the beach steepens and hems against sheer outcrops. Huge debris piles lie jumbled at the mouths of steep ravines. Big Flat briefly disappears from sight as you curve around a horseshoe of coastline and pass a pretty stream rushing out of a lush alder grove overhead.

You next reach Buck Creek at 5.2 miles, which pours into the surf by a wild wall of contorted rock layers. Numerous campsites perch just inland from the shore, many with ocean views (and exposure to wind). The Buck Creek Trail—your return route—heads uphill from here on its way toward Saddle Mountain, visible in the back of the valley.

Past Buck Creek, the beach narrows further and boulder fields extend into the tidal zone. Watch for seals hauled out on the rocks. Shipman Creek, a substantial stream that emerges from a broader valley, is next at 6.6 miles with a few inland sites in addition to the requisite driftwood shelter.

Past Ship Creek, the beach becomes rockier and strewn with cobblestones, creating the toughest walking conditions yet. Offshore wash rocks are abundant. You enter the 2003 burn area just prior to reaching Big Flat, where the cliffs shorten abruptly. Although there is no obvious path leading off the beach, take the first opportunity to scramble onto the easy-walking terrain above.

You emerge onto the broad outwash plain of Big Flat at 8.2 miles, an open grassland interspersed with boulder piles, stunted Douglas firs, and profuse wildflowers. Burnt trees lance the surrounding slopes, mute evidence of the 2003 wildfire. The trail passes several driftwood shelters. Level tenting areas are abundant by the shore; exploration inland reveals many more possibilities, though dense alder groves preclude camping directly along the creek. The beach is readily accessible, here a rough cobblestone strand of fist-sized stones.

As you continue north, increasingly deep views peer up the Big Flat Creek watershed. Rattlesnake Ridge rises above the drainage to the north, part of your continuing route. The trail next crosses Big Flat Creek at 8.5 miles, a substantial, but broad, waterway readily rock-hopped in most conditions. The volume of debris at its mouth, however, makes it easy to imagine the power of this river in flood, and the fury of the ocean during big surges.

TECTONIC ACTIVITY IN THE KING RANGE

The King Range is California's most seismically active area and tectonic forces push the range upward an average of 10–13 feet every 1000 years. In 1992, an earthquake lifted the entire range 3–4 feet in minutes.

The rock fields diminish north of the creek and an expansive meadow stretches toward the mountains, where a small parcel of private property—including a grass landing strip and two small houses—nestle in the grass and trees. You pass another large driftwood shelter as you walk north on the lupine-covered path. The coast curves here and you can once again see ridges in the distance, which diminish in size as they recede north; Oat Ridge is the farthest, Kinsey Ridge rises in front of it. Looking inland, you can spot King Peak at the head of the Big Flat Creek drainage, the tallest summit on the right. Adjacent to the left is Peak 3996; your continuing route to the summit wraps around its backside.

Your journey now turns right and heads inland along the edge of the private property. At a broad road at the end of the runway, bear right on an unsigned single-track trail that quickly enters the trees. The path quickly widens and returns to the burn area. Poison oak is everywhere. The flora rapidly shifts to a much drier chaparral community; coyote brush, ceanothus, and sticky monkeyflower increase in abundance.

At one point, the trail forks by a campsite. A right turn leads down to the water, but you take the more obvious path left to quickly reach a tributary in a lush ferny glade. The trail becomes rougher and winds along loose slopes above the stream. A recent landslide closed a portion of the trail here, and you must cross to the other side to avoid this impassable section. An exciting rock-hop leads to the opposite side, where you immediately recross the stream to reach a pleasant campsite on the far shore.

The trail then crosses the North Fork of Big Flat Creek at 10 miles, a sizable waterway of achingly clear pools, then curves back to cross the main creek. The gradient now increases, the creek rushes, and the path steeply climbs above a level campsite below. Switchbacks lead to a view of the watershed ahead; the trail winds around a narrow gorge, drops back into the lush creek corridor, and follows the jumbled streambed. You hop over two more tributaries and then descend to cross the main creek by another campsite. Fill up your water bottles; this is your last source for the next 3 miles.

Switchbacks lead you above an inaccessible grotto pool, where the real uphill grind begins. Over the next 2.9 miles, the trail climbs 2400 feet via 84 switchbacks to reach Bear Hollow Camp atop Rattlesnake Ridge. The well-graded trail steadily zigs and zags upward through a burned forest of Douglas fir snags, joined by an increasing number of living specimens as you crest 1000 feet. Around 1500 feet (switchback 45), you pass though a burned zone that offers views of Miller Ridge and King Peak through the trees. Chaparral slowly increases. At 1700 feet (switchback 50), Big Flat becomes visible below for the first time. The trail then makes a series of tight switchbacks near the ridgeline and briefly crests at 2000 feet (switchback 61), where you enjoy your first level moment since leaving Big Flat Creek.

Expansive views of Miller Ridge continue as you climb to the small knob and burnt manzanita atop Peak 2059. The route then resumes its switchback marathon, eventually cresting atop the ridge (switchback 74) to enjoy increasingly full views of the river mouth and central Big Flat area. The trail curves up the ridge, passes views of the dramatic slides in an adjacent drainage, and then finally reaches the posted spur to Bear Hollow Camp and Spring on the right at 13.4 miles and 2770 feet.

The spur drops 50 feet down to the campsite, which offers space for three tents in a shadeless, viewless glen of fire-killed madrone and Douglas firs. The nearby spring flows strongly. Past camp, the trail resumes a switchbacking ascent and winds through head-high thickets of regenerating chaparral to touch the ridgeline at 3000 feet. You soon crest the ridge and enjoy an astonishing view of the massive cliffs and slides of the upper North Fork headwaters. After a brief level section, surmount the final switchbacks and make a rising traverse to reach the King Crest Trail at 14.2 miles and 3440 feet.

SIDE TRIP: MILLER CAMP

To visit pleasant Miller Camp (2.8 miles round-trip with 1250 feet of elevation gain and loss), head north on the King Crest Trail. The trail quickly passes an established (but dry) campsite and then traverses the severe slopes along the north side of the ridge to reach an old metal sign posted for Miller Camp at 0.6 mile. Turn right and follow the faint trail on a long rocky traverse through a nice grove of living Douglas firs. The path steepens, encounters a posted and reliable "bonus spring" at 2830 feet, and switchbacks steadily downward. You pass a few isolated specimens of sugar pine at 2500 feet—look for the giant cones—before reaching a posted junction for the spring (left) and camp (right), located a short distance downhill. The spring is actually a flowing stream, which disappears beneath an enormous outwash of angular debris flushed down the mountain after the recent fire. A stand of old-growth Douglas firs protrude from the detritus, heavily charred but still very much alive.

Back at the junction with the King Crest Trail, head south and enjoy your first views east toward the Eel River watershed. Looking due east on a clear day, you might be able to spot Lassen Peak more than 120 miles away on the far side of the Central Valley. The trail traverses along the ridge's west slope and then summits Peak 3620. Views north encompass the rolling terrain of the Mattole River watershed. King Peak appears ahead beyond the pyramidal form of Peak 3996. A slow descent leads through more burn zone, where young manzanita grow among the skeletal fingers of their forbears. You pass through a corridor of head-high madrone and encounter a canyon live oak clinging steadfastly to the rocks at the ridge's narrowest point. Severe cliffs plummet away to the north; admire the tenacious trees that manage to survive in this rapidly eroding terrain.

The trail rises briefly, travels beneath some twisted live oaks, and then begins a level traverse on the north side of Peak 3996. The eastern flanks of the King Range escaped the flames for the most part, and you now enjoy an uncharred, shady forest of mature trees. At times, the trail skirts across some very loose slopes where the sheer terrain below drops 1000 feet in less than a half mile. This section is mildly unnerving—if you slipped, you might not stop. The trail eventually turns a corner and reenters the sun. After a brief drop, it climbs back to the ridgeline via a bouldery field of sandstone chunks. You momentarily ascend the ridgeline, bear left to return to the shady slopes, and reach the Lightning Trail at 16.4 miles and 3710 feet.

From here the recommended route is to head left on the Lightning Trail and obtain water (and spend the night) at Maple Camp, your only source for the next 9 miles. (Alternatively, you can drop your packs here, get water, and return to climb King Peak via the King Crest Trail. A roofed, three-sided shelter sits just below the summit.) Heading down the Lightning Trail, you enjoy another bout of switchbacks, which deposit you at the junction for Maple Camp. (The Lightning Trail continues downhill for another 1.9 miles and 31 switchbacks to reach the end of King Range Road, accessible only by high-clearance vehicles and closed during the rainy season—not a recommended entry or exit point.) Turn right and follow the trail toward Maple Camp, which soon offers views southeast toward the rolling hills. The rocky trail winds downward to meet a laughing brook in a stand of large, unblemished Douglas firs. A brief rise brings you to Maple Camp at 17.0 miles, where a half dozen tent sites dot the slopes like rocky nests. Bay trees and a few bigleaf maples shade the creek.

Continuing past camp, your route runs alongside the creekbed, which soon fills with water once again. The trail crosses the brook, makes a few switchbacks, and then traverses left to return to the sun-scoured world of burnt madrone and manzanita. Views open up to the northeast and then southeast, as you ascend the loose and rocky path through the scrub. Glimpses of nearby King Peak appear shortly before you rejoin the King Crest Trail.

To tag the summit (0.4 mile one-way with 260 feet of elevation gain), drop your pack and head north through a gravelly moonscape. The trail slowly rises on a steady traverse beneath the intermittent shade of scraggly canyon live oaks. About halfway up, the route returns to the ridgeline. Some final S-turns lead to the summit and the three-sided cement shelter that nestles just below it.

LOST COAST RAINFALL

The Lost Coast is California's wettest area, with the highest ridges averaging 200 inches per year; Shelter Cove averages 69 inches annually. Despite this moisture, coast redwoods are unable to grow along the King Range due to the lower incidence of fog. Cape Mendocino blocks the area from the predominant northwest winds—and the fog it pushes onshore.

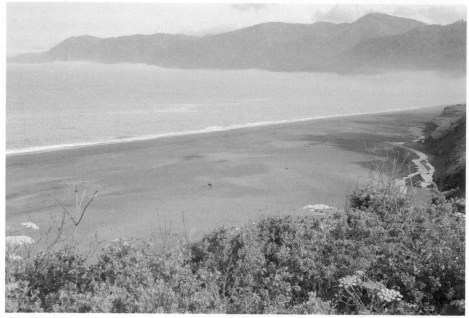

The King Range looms beyond Black Sands Beach.

The view is tremendous, a 360-degree sweep. The Big Flat Creek watershed pours into the ocean; Shubrick Peak guards its northern flanks. The King Range marches away in both directions, its spine traced by the King Crest Trail. Farther north, the Mattole River flows in the midst of rumpled topography. The deep drainage of Shipman Creek is next to the south, separated from Big Flat by Miller Ridge. The Buck Creek watershed is just beyond, separated from Shipman Creek by Fire Hill. In the southern distance you can make out the Kaluna Cliffs near Shelter Cove and the coastline of Sinkyone Wilderness on the farthest horizon. The high bumps of the Trinity Alps dimple the northeast horizon, and more than 10 ridges recede into the eastern distance.

Back at the earlier junction with the Maple Camp Trail at 17.5 miles, head south on the King Crest Trail. The Shipman Creek watershed appears below to the west as you travel along the ridgeline. Saddle Mountain looms ahead like a crouching lion. The route weaves on and off the ridgeline, descends a series of steep switchbacks, and makes a brief, but steep drop. The exposed roots of canyon live oaks and Douglas firs grip the eroding hillside nearby.

The trail then traverses steeply upward and widens to road width; it was used for access during the 2003 fire. You now cruise on the easy-walking trail, passing a few level campsites (dry) and restricted views into the Shipman Creek drainage. The route rises briefly and then slowly descends through a section of unburned forest to wind above the headwaters of Buck Creek. (You can spot the Buck Creek Trail—your route back to the ocean—on the ridgeline hemming Buck Creek in to the south.) Saddle Mountain soon appears ahead. You pass a large pullout and campsite (dry) and then make a steady sustained climb through mature Douglas fir forest as Buck Creek rushes audibly down below. The gradient eases shortly before you reach the Buck Creek Trail at 21.8 miles.

Turn right on the Buck Creek Trail, which immediately becomes single-track as it briefly rises and then begins its steady drop to the sea. Cruising along the south side of the ridge, it offers intermittent views south across the adjacent Gitchell Creek drainage. The route soon emerges on the open ridge, sticks close to the ridgeline, and then switchbacks right to make a long traverse. You momentarily regain the crest and then drop steeply to pass below Peak 2081; this section of trail was rerouted following the 2003 fire. A narrow traverse leads steadily down to a long shady cruise. After crossing the ridge, the trail steepens and descends into a lusher forest environment. Bay and sword ferns appear as the path traverses down. Eventually the route turns into the Buck Creek drainage and enters a cooler environment thriving with ferns, irises, and healthy fir trees. Alders, poison oak, and blackberry proliferate as well. The ocean becomes audible ahead as the trail descends through tall grass, emerges by Buck Creek's uppermost campsite, and leads down to the water at 25.4 miles. From here, retrace your earlier steps along the beach to the trailhead.

BUILD-UP AND WIND-DOWN TIPS

Be sure to acquire all necessary supplies before arriving in Shelter Cove. The town's small general grocery has limited merchandise and is expensive. **Redway** is your last best option on the way in, though **Ukiah** or **Willits** are your best bets for groceries.

KLAMATH MOUNTAINS

T he remote Klamath Mountains cover a large portion of northwestern California and southwestern Oregon, a region rich in diversity spanning the spectrum from coastal forests to alpine heights. Two of California's most pristine wilderness areas are found within the Klamath Mountains. The Trinity Alps Wilderness, northwest of Redding, contains 515,000 acres of rugged backcountry with more than 500 miles of trails. The Marble Mountain Wilderness, southwest of Yreka, contains 227,000 acres, about half the size of the Trinity Alps but with nearly the same trail mileage. Since these wilderness areas are well away from major population centers, they are not heavily visited. Some trails in the Klamath Mountains are more popular than others, but the opportunity for solitude is much higher here than in the Sierra Nevada, for instance. While you may not encounter many other people on the trail, you might see some cattle, as grazing is allowed during certain periods (check with the Forest Service for exact dates if you wish to avoid these bovine invasions). With a thousand miles of trail, the Klamath Mountains present a plethora of backpacking opportunities beyond the handful of trails described in this guide. Not many other areas in California present such geographic diversity within such close proximity, spanning the range from coastal forests to alpine heights. The region is more than worthy of consideration for backpacking adventures beyond the routes described here.

THE TRINITY ALPS

The Trinity Alps are characterized by rushing streams, high waterfalls, mountain lakes, granite peaks, and cool, deep forests. Set aside as a primitive area in the 1930s, the area was officially added to the wilderness system in 1984. Three national forests, Shasta-Trinity, Klamath, and Six Rivers, oversee the administration of the Trinity Alps. Four trips are described in this guide within the Trinity Alps. The trail to Canyon Creek Lakes is perhaps the most heavily used path in the otherwise lightly used wilderness, providing a suitable weekend trip (or longer) to a trio of scenic high lakes in the central Alps. A much longer journey follows the tumbling course of the North Fork Trinity River and Grizzly Creek to spectacular Grizzly Falls and picturesque Grizzly Lake, both in the shadow of Thompson Peak, at 9002 feet the highest summit in the wilderness. The third trip is located in the remote western part of the Trinity Alps, a semiloop journey at lower elevations that visits a slice of the historic mining district, where hundreds of people once worked the mines and lived in nearby towns from the 1880s to the 1920s. The fourth trip tours the northernmost Trinity Alps with a side trip to Mt. Eddy and its overwhelming view of Mt. Shasta. Although wilderness permits (and campfire permits) are required in the Trinity Alps, quotas do not exist and permits can easily be obtained by self-registration at any ranger station.

THE MARBLE MOUNTAINS

The Marble Mountains were set aside as a primitive area in the early 1930s, reclassified as wilderness in 1953, and then included in the original Wilderness Act of 1964. Klamath National Forest is solely responsible for administration of the Marble Mountains Wilderness. Rising in the heart of their namesake wilderness, the Marble Mountains, vertical cliffs of layered marble, plummet more than 1000 feet into the valleys below. Sky High Lakes basin lies nearby. Several bodies of water speckle the flat and idyllic basin, providing an ideal base camp for exploring the surrounding peaks and views. The other Marble Mountains trip in this guide is a loop that visits two of the more popular lakes in the area, as well as some of the least visited spots in the wilderness. Wilderness permits are not required in the Marble Mountains, although campfire permits (available at any ranger station) are required.

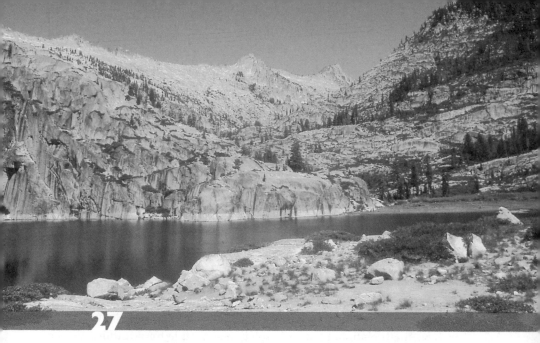

CANYON CREEK LAKES AND L LAKE

Mike White

MILES: 16.5
RECOMMENDED DAYS: 2
ELEVATION GAIN/LOSS: 4260´/4260´ to L Lake and back;
3325´/3325´ to Lower Canyon Creek Lake
and back
TYPE OF TRIP: Out-and-back
DIFFICULTY: Moderately strenuous
SOLITUDE: Moderately populated
LOCATION: Trinity Alps Wilderness
MAPS: USGS 7.5-min. *Mt. Hilton*;
U.S. Forest Service *A Guide to the Trinity Alps Wilderness*
BEST SEASON: Summer through early fall

PERMITS

A wilderness permit is required for all overnight trips in the Trinity Alps Wilderness, and a campfire permit is also required if you plan to have one. Both permits can be obtained by self-registration at the ranger station in Weaverville.

Photo: The Canyon Creek Lakes are some of the most scenic lakes in the Trinity Alps.

CHALLENGES •

Since this is perhaps the most popular trail in the Alps, get an early start on the weekend to secure the best campsites. Better yet, take this trip during the week to minimize the crowds. Campfires are prohibited in the upper Canyon Creek watershed, beginning 500 feet beyond the Boulder Lakes Trail junction.

HOW TO GET THERE •

From Weaverville, which is about 45 miles west of Redding, continue westbound on Highway 299 for 8 miles to the tiny town of Junction City, and turn right (north) onto Canyon Creek Road. Drive 13.8 miles on Canyon Creek Road to the large parking area at the road's end. The trailhead is equipped with a pit toilet and picnic table.

TRIP DESCRIPTION •

From the well-signed trailhead, the Canyon Creek Trail branches left from the Bear Creek Trail, as you head north on slightly rising tread. Soon leveling off, the trail then makes a moderate descent among bigleaf maple and dogwood to a boulder hop of Bear Creek. From the creek, the trail climbs around the shoulder into the main canyon, well above Canyon Creek. A long, steady ascent ensues, where you pass through the dry vegetation of an open, mixed forest of canyon and black oaks, incense cedars, Douglas firs, and ponderosa pines. The climb continues uninterrupted until you reach an informal junction with a use trail heading down 200 yards to a large flat and the relocated McKay Camp just below the Sinks, a large rockslide where the creek adopts a subterranean course. For interested backpackers, McKay Camp offers fine campsites and good fishing nearby.

TAKE THIS TRIP

A hiking companion posed this question on a recent trip, "What if you could hike in only one mountain range for the rest of your life, which one would it be?" After careful consideration, I responded firmly, "The Trinity Alps!" From dense, low-elevation coastal forests to glaciated granite peaks reaching 9000 feet and everything in-between, few other mountain ranges in California possess the wide range of diversity found within the Trinity Alps.

The Canyon Creek Trail takes backpackers into the best of the Alps: Sapphireblue lakes, tumbling creeks, dramatic waterfalls, abundant wildflowers, rugged granite peaks flanked by permanent snowfields, exquisite scenery, and splendid vistas are all here in abundance. Beyond the backpacking, peakbaggers, amateur naturalists, anglers, rock climbers, and cross-country enthusiasts will find diversions aplenty in the heart of the range. The Canyon Creek Trail is popular by Trinity Alps standards—for good reason—but perhaps is the best sampling of what makes this area so spectacular and unique.

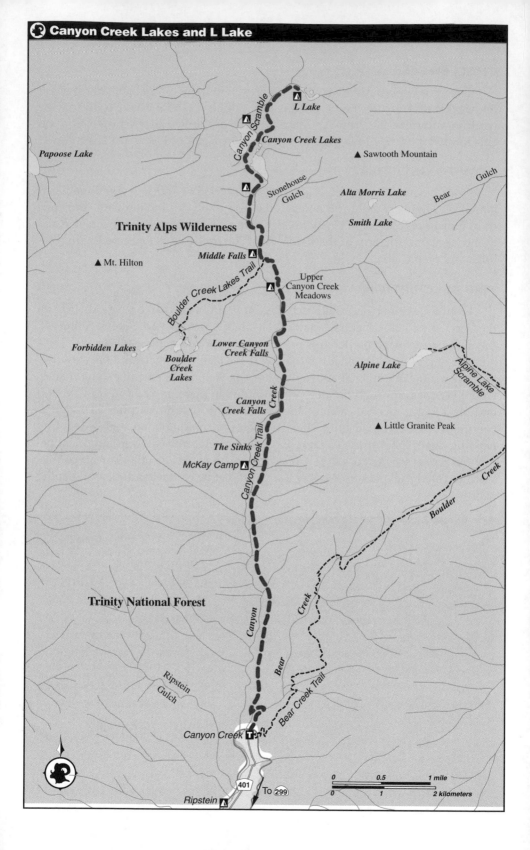

L Lake

Canyon Scramble

Canyon Creek Lakes

Papoose Lake

▲ Sawtooth Mountain

Stonehouse Gulch

Bear Gulch

Trinity Alps Wilderness

Alta Morris Lake

Smith Lake

Middle Falls

Boulder Creek Lakes Trail

▲ Mt. Hilton

Upper Canyon Creek Meadows

Forbidden Lakes

Lower Canyon Creek Falls

Boulder Creek Lakes

Alpine Lake Scramble

Alpine Lake

Canyon Creek Falls

Canyon Creek Trail

Creek

▲ Little Granite Peak

The Sinks

McKay Camp

Boulder Creek

Trinity National Forest

Canyon

Creek

Ripstein Gulch

Bear Creek Trail

Bear

Canyon Creek T

401

To 299

Ripstein

0	0.5	1 mile
0	1	2 kilometers

From the junction, a moderate climb leads to the first source of water since Bear Creek, where a pleasant little stream glides across the trail through a narrow swath of vegetation. As refreshing as this water may appear, you might want to hold off on acquiring any for a little while, as the trail soon crosses this stream two more times via a pair of switchbacks. Leaving the thrice-visited stream behind, continue the ascent up the east side of the canyon. The old trail used to follow the creek bottom past spectacular Canyon Creek Falls, but nowadays hikers must settle for the distant roar of the falls and perhaps an incomplete and unsatisfying cross-canyon glimpse through dense brush and moderate forest. Farther up the trail, you draw near to the creek and pass by Lower Canyon Creek Falls, a less prestigious fall but one with a wonderful swimming hole at the base, offering a great way to beat the heat on a hot afternoon.

Another stretch of climbing leads to a level stretch of trail with some pleasant, shaded campsites nearby. Just beyond the campsites, you stroll through waist-high ferns alongside the quiet surroundings of Upper Canyon Creek Meadows. In early season, the marshy meadows are carpeted with a wide array of flowers.

Lower Canyon Creek Lake beneath jagged Mt. Hilton

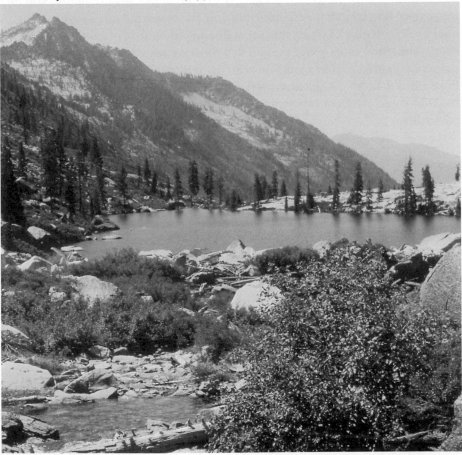

Early evening may provide a good chance to see some deer grazing on the lush foliage.

From the meadows, the moderate climb resumes through light to moderate forest cover, crossing some usually dry seasonal streams along the way. Near the 5-mile mark, you climb over granite ledges and soon reach a large forested flat, littered with boulders, where some decent campsites are not far from the creek. For the adventurous, a rugged and steep cross-country route leaves this flat and climbs the gulch to the east to Smith and Alta Morris lakes, a pair of beautiful subalpine lakes situated at the southeastern base of craggy Sawtooth Mountain. The beginning of the route is the most difficult section, as you must force your way through heavy brush at the base of the ridge. Once you get above this band of brush, the way is much easier but still requires a good dose of stamina, route-finding skill, and a bit of mountaineering ability. Although the total distance from the flat to Smith Lake is only 1.5 miles, plan to spend the better part of a morning or afternoon making the rugged, cross-country ascent.

At the far end of the flat, just before a steep ascent up a cliff, a faint use trail branches west through the trees for about 0.1 mile to the base of Middle Falls, a dramatic series of cascades tumbling over granite ledges and finally plunging into a deep bowl. From the use-trail junction, the main trail turns east and begins a series of switchbacks across the cliff, following the course of a little creek up the slope. The grade eases above the cliff in a forested azalea dell and then proceeds up gently graded trail to a junction with the Boulder Creek Trail, 5.7 miles from the trailhead. From the junction, a short, steep descent on the Boulder Creek Trail leads to some excellent campsites on forested flats alongside Canyon Creek at 6.75 miles.

SIDE TRIP: BOULDER CREEK LAKES

If the main trip isn't enough for you to get your fill of the Alps, you could climb 1.5 miles to a set of delightfully scenic lakes at the junction with the Boulder Creek Lakes Trail. Compared to Canyon Creek Lakes, the Boulder Creek Lakes see far fewer visitors, perhaps due to a section of trail that is among the steepest in the Alps and gains about 600 feet in a half mile. However, perseverance brings great reward, as the picturesque lakes and a host of smaller ponds fill glacier-scoured depressions in a nearly treeless granite basin, where vistas of rugged peaks and ridges abound. A side trip to the Boulder Creek Lakes adds a distance of 3 miles and an elevation gain/loss of 1650/200 feet to your trip.

Remaining on the Canyon Creek Trail, you near the creek again and pass some more good campsites before reaching the end of the azalea dell (and the easy walking) at the base of another set of switchbacks. Climb around the next falls on Canyon Creek, where there are some more campsites near the stream and scattered around the cliffs above the falls. Continue upstream to a crossing of Canyon Creek, which can be made either by fording the stream or by crossing a fallen log. Proceed through the trees to the base of another falls and the last

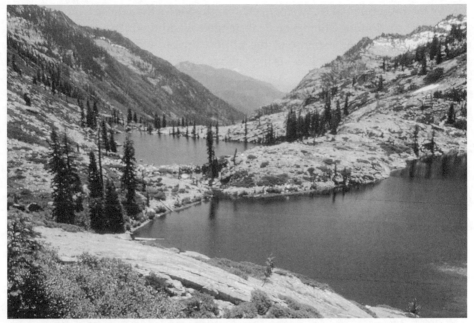

Canyon Creek Lakes from the scramble route to L Lake

campsite before the lakes. From there, a winding ascent over granite slabs leads to the shore of Lower Canyon Creek Lake.

The pristine waters of Lower Canyon Creek Lake fill a deep granite bowl sprinkled with a smattering of weeping spruces, red firs, and Jeffrey pines clinging to the limited pockets of soil scattered around the basin. The lack of a dense forest grants visitors the delight of widespread views in every direction. To the east, steep hillsides rise up toward the sky, culminating at the top of rugged Sawtooth Mountain. Lower cliffs on the west offer vistas of snowcapped Mt. Hilton, while to the north, filling a notch at the head of the canyon, is the jagged summit of 9002-foot Thompson Peak, highest peak in the Trinity Alps.

Although numerous campsites dot the shoreline, camping at Lower Canyon Creek Lake is not recommended, as most of the sites are way too close to the lake. The lack of deep soil for adequate waste decomposition combined with the lake's popularity creates a potentially serious environmental problem. The U.S. Forest Service is reluctant to institute an outright ban on camping at Lower Canyon Lake, so the proper response of earth-friendly backpackers would be to camp in the forest below and dayhike up to the lake.

If Upper Canyon Creek Lake or L Lake is your goal, turn northwest from the southern tip of the lower lake and climb toward the low ridge above. Many years ago, orange blazes were sprayed on the rock to help delineate the route, but most of these marks have fortunately faded away over time, replaced by a series of ducks. Follow this scramble trail, which eventually turns north and surmounts the cliffs high above the west side of the lake. Beyond the lake, the path rounds a rock rib, shortly ascends a gully, and then tops out on the dike between the lower and upper lakes, where even grander views than those from the lower lake greet you. Joining Thompson Peak, jagged Wedding Cake springs into view, along with the arcing expanse of the upper canyon, where myriad waterfalls, born from springs and snowfields high above, spill across the steep granite walls of the horseshoe-shaped basin. Above the east shore, you can catch a glimpse of the stream draining L Lake 800 vertical feet higher. At the far end of the upper lake, the inlet creek meanders through the pastoral scene of a deep-green, grassy delta. As at the lower lake, campsites along the water's edge should not be used. With a little effort, more appropriate sites can be found near the far edge of the delta, or sprinkled around the upper basin beyond the lake. The verdant delta was formerly submerged when miners built a wood-timbered dam, raising the level of the lake about 6 to 8 feet. Today the only evidence of the former dam is the white bathtub ring on the granite walls around the lakeshore. Despite the heavy traffic, fishing is still reported to be fairly good at Upper Canyon Creek Lake for fair-sized eastern brook and rainbow trout.

A defined path continues around the southeast shore to the outlet stream's exit from the lake. To get across the fast-moving creek, you will either have to make a knee- to waist-high ford or be very agile and quite bold as you jump the rocky gorge (if you choose the latter option, be very careful not to fall into the creek—such a fall could be disastrous). Beyond the creek a faint path continues a short distance and then dead-ends at a strip of beach below an illegally close

A picturesque fall adds scenic wonder to a campsite along Canyon Creek.

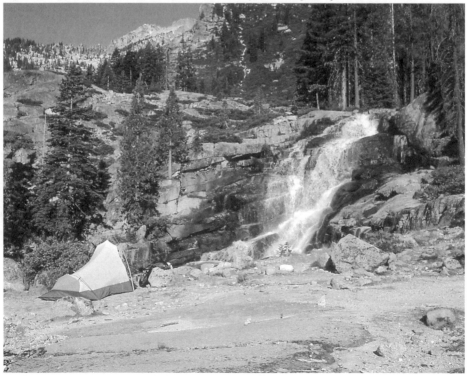

campsite. Just above this campsite, a use trail climbs steeply up the hillside, beginning the climb to L Lake.

Most backpackers are content to go no farther than Canyon Creek lakes, satisfied with the rewards that their moderate effort has reaped. The ascent to L Lake—at least while burdened with a backpack—is another story altogether. Although a path of sorts leads to the lake and the distance is less than a mile from Upper Canyon Creek Lake, the route can hardly be considered an improved trail and the elevation gain is nearly 1000 feet. Campsites at L Lake are limited as well, but the few and hardy souls willing to make the journey should have a good shot at solitude, at least after the last of the dayhikers have headed back to lower regions.

To reach L Lake, follow the use trail from the campsite near the strip of beach along the northeast shore of Upper Canyon Creek Lake up a steep gully for a short distance and then northeast, making an upward traverse across the top of the first granite knob. Continue to climb across open terrain on the east face of the canyon, following a ducked route over sloping granite ledges and through steep gullies, until you reach the outlet stream from L Lake, about a mile from the shore of Upper Canyon Creek Lake. Along the way you are blessed with splendid views of Canyon Creek Lakes, the Canyon Creek drainage, and Mt. Hilton dominating the western skyline. Turn east-northeast and climb along a ducked route up the outlet for about 0.4 mile to the lake. As you approach the lake, you enter light forest and pass a narrow strip of meadow alongside the creek.

Obviously the lake was named for its irregular shape, which roughly resembles the letter "L," although a small circular pond near the northeast shore must have at one time been part of the lake, when the shoreline didn't bear this resemblance. Shallow at the west end, L Lake gains some depth at the far end, providing a fine home for a healthy population of eastern brook trout. Mountain hemlocks, weeping spruce, and red fir grace the shoreline, adding a somewhat somber effect to the lake's ambiance. The 2-acre lake is jammed into the narrow cleft of a cirque, the deep chasm very nearly surrounded on all sides by steep rock walls. The southeast flank of the basin rises up sharply to culminate in the very summit of towering Sawtooth Mountain, 2350 feet above. Permanent snowfields below the peak give the area a decidedly alpine feel, even though the lake is only 6525 feet above sea level. The northern rim of the basin sharply divides the Canyon Creek drainage from that of the equally popular Stuart Fork.

Campsites near the lake are somewhat limited but seemingly sufficient for the low number of backpackers willing to lug their gear all the way up here. The best, forested spots occur near the meadows below the lake, while more exposed sites with grand views can be found on top of a rocky hill south of the outlet. Since mosquitoes can be a nuisance for a few weeks in midsummer, a campsite on top of the hill may offer the benefit of a breeze.

At 8.25 miles from the trailhead, a base camp at L Lake affords backpackers with an extra day or two many additional opportunities to further their adventures. For those with mountaineering skills, a climb of Sawtooth Mountain and the incomparable view from the summit can be quite rewarding. However, be aware that the final pitch requires Class 3–4 climbing skills, and possibly cram-pons, an ice axe, and a rope, depending upon the conditions. Cross-country en-thusiasts have the option of following a strenuous route north across a saddle in the ridge and down the other side to Mirror and Sapphire lakes. Even if you lack the skill or desire for such rigorous pursuits, L Lake can be a great spot for simply whiling away the hours in relaxation. At the conclusion of your stay, retrace your steps to the trailhead.

BUILD-UP AND WIND-DOWN TIPS

The quaint town of Weaverville offers a few decent options for grabbing a bite to eat before or after your trip. In the historic section of town, the **Garden Café** is a fine place to have breakfast, especially on their shaded patio; they're open for breakfast and lunch every day except Tuesday. Just up the street, the **La Grange Café**, which is open every day except Sunday, serves excellent meals for lunch and dinner. East of the historic section of town, try **Millers Drive-In** for an old fashioned hamburger (although a for sale sign was up during my most recent visit).

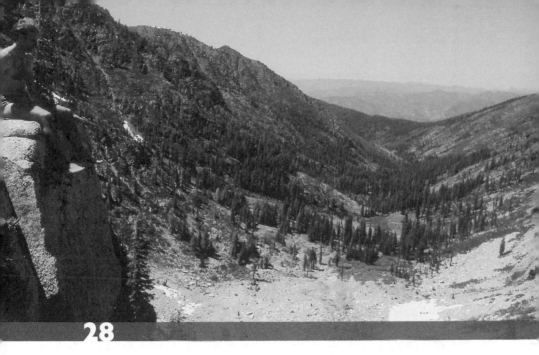

28

NORTH FORK TRINITY RIVER TO GRIZZLY LAKE

Mike White

MILES: 35.0
RECOMMENDED DAYS: 4–7
ELEVATION GAIN/LOSS: 6925′/1775′
TYPE OF TRIP: Out-and-back
DIFFICULTY: Moderately strenuous
SOLITUDE: Moderate solitude
LOCATION: Trinity Alps Wilderness
MAPS: USGS 7.5-min. *Thurston Peaks*, *Cecil Lake*, and *Thompson Peak*;
U.S. Forest Service *A Guide to the Trinity Alps Wilderness*
BEST SEASON: Summer through early fall

PERMITS

A wilderness permit is required for all overnight trips in the Trinity Alps Wilderness, and a campfire permit is also required if you plan to have one. Both permits can be obtained by self-registration at the ranger station in Weaverville.

Photo: At the brink of Grizzly Falls and outlet of Grizzly Lake

TAKE THIS TRIP

Starting at an elevation near 3000 feet, with the possibility of reaching 9002 feet on top of Thompson Peak, the Trinity Alps highest summit, this route exposes visitors to the diversity for which the area is renowned. For the first 10 miles the elevation gain is a paltry 1000 feet, as the trail follows the gentle route of the North Fork Trinity River and lower Grizzly Creek through a wide range of trees, ferns, and flowers. Along the way are a number of old cabins and plenty of leftover relics from the mining days. The last 7.5 miles gain nearly 6000 feet, passing through mixed conifer and red fir forests, and mountain meadows on the way to extraordinarily scenic, subalpine Grizzly Lake nestled into a granite cirque below jagged Thompson Peak. Immediately below the lake, spectacular Grizzly Falls shoots over the lip of the basin and plummets nearly 100 feet toward verdant Upper Grizzly Meadow at the head of a U-shaped canyon.

This is the long way to Grizzly Lake, as an incredibly steep but short route from the remote China Gulch Trailhead will get you there in a mere 7 miles. Consequently, this relatively short trail combined with the incredible scenery draws a high number of admirers; don't expect to be alone at the lake. However, you can reasonably expect a generous dose of solitude all the way from the trailhead to the China Gulch junction.

CHALLENGES

While camped at Grizzly Meadows, be sure to protect food from the critters—deer and marmots seem to be more of a problem here than bears. Since you will have to ford some significant streams along this route, pack along an extra pair of lightweight and quick-drying footwear.

HOW TO GET THERE

From Weaverville, which is about 45 miles west of Redding, continue westbound on Highway 299 for 15 miles to a bridge over North Fork Trinity River and a turnoff for Old Helena. North of the townsite, a narrow, paved road crosses the North Fork and then continues up the East Fork of the North Fork 2.7 miles to a junction with Hobo Gulch Road. Turn left and follow the narrow, very crooked, and sometimes steep gravel road on an 8-mile-plus climb to the top of a ridge between the North and East forks. From there, a steep downgrade leads 5 miles to the trailhead, 0.3 mile above the primitive Hobo Gulch Campground.

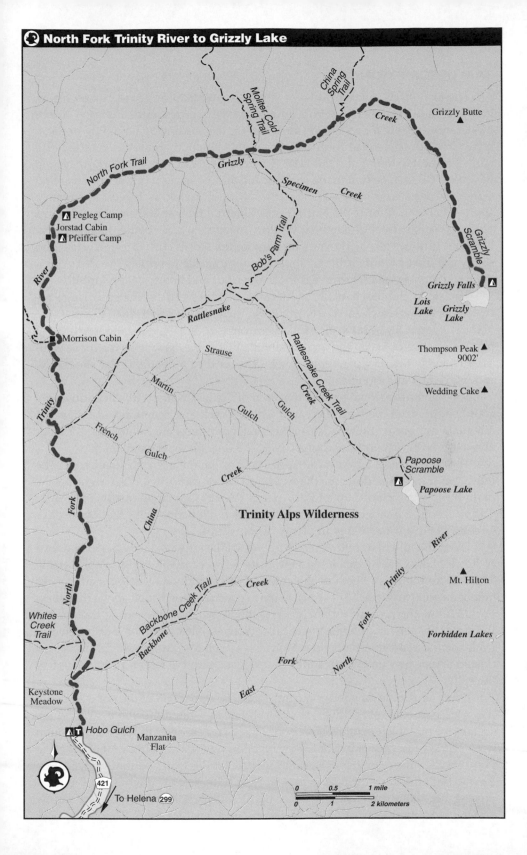

China Spring Trail

Molter Cold Spring Trail

Creek

Grizzly Butte ▲

North Fork Trail

Grizzly

Specimen

Creek

Grizzly Scramble

△ Pegleg Camp
Jorstad Cabin
■ △ Pfeiffer Camp

Bob's Farm Trail

Grizzly Falls △

River

Lois Lake

Grizzly Lake

Rattlesnake

Thompson Peak ▲
9002'

■ Morrison Cabin

Strause

Rattlesnake Creek Trail

Wedding Cake ▲

Martin

Gulch

Gulch

Creek

Trinity

French

Gulch

Gulch

Creek

Papoose Scramble

△

Papoose Lake

Trinity Alps Wilderness

China

Fork

River

Trinity

North

Backbone Creek Trail

Creek

Fork

Mt. Hilton ▲

Forbidden Lakes

Whites Creek Trail

Backbone

Fork

North

Keystone Meadow

East

△ T *Hobo Gulch*

Manzanita Flat

421

To Helena 299

| 0 | 0.5 | 1 mile |

| 0 | 1 | 2 kilometers |

TRIP DESCRIPTION ·

The trail starts out almost level from the trailhead in dense, mixed forest, leads 0.2 mile to a junction with a spur from the campground, and then climbs moderately steeply for a short distance before descending to a crossing of Backbone Creek. A somewhat confusing three-way junction greets you on the north bank. Farthest to the right, Trail 11W07, signed RUSSELL CABIN, heads northeast up Backbone Creek. The trail to the left, leading almost straight beside the river and signed PAPOOSE LAKE-LOW WATER TRAIL, BEAR WALLOW MEADOWS, travels upstream a short distance and fords the North Fork. The trail then splits: One branch turns west up Whites Creek and to Bear Wallow Meadows, and another faint low-water trail continues alongside the west bank of the North Fork through brush and soggy ground to a ford farther upstream. Your trail, signed solely PAPOOSE LAKE, is the middle path, which turns slightly to the right and heads steeply uphill.

The steep climb eventually moderates, as you head up the spur ridge between Backbone Creek and the North Fork, then travels north along the east side of the canyon. Climb above the canyon bottom through a pleasant, open forest of madrones, canyon oaks, and an occasional sugar pine, as well as the more common Douglas firs and ponderosa pines. Descend to a beautiful flat shaded by incense cedars and Douglas firs.

Soon you drop down to meet the trace of the low water trail. An entire army could set up camp between here and China Creek and seemingly still have an adequate supply of firewood. Another flat with excellent campsites is higher above the river just north of China Creek, 2.3 miles from the trailhead.

The trail divides again at the upper end of the flat above China Creek. The left-hand trail drops down to the river and more campsites. Veer right on the main trail, which climbs up and down and then passes the remnants of Strunce Cabin. About a quarter mile farther, you reach a junction with the Rattlesnake Creek Trail in a broad flat with plenty of campsites.

From the junction, follow the left-hand trail, signed GRIZZLY CREEK, to a ford of Rattlesnake Creek (difficult in high water) and campsites on the north bank. Then climb the ridge north of the creek in five, moderately steep switchbacks before curving around the nose of a ridge to continue north well above the North Fork. Follow the contour for a while and then a steeply descending traverse, as the trail cuts across an almost vertical rock face. After another level stretch of trail, you descend to a flat below Morrison Gulch and Morrison Cabin. A sign posted at a nearby junction reads RATTLESNAKE LAKE to the left and GRIZZLY LAKE to the right.

Veer right at the junction and climb from the upper end of the flat well up on the steep east bank of the river, as the trail makes a horseshoe bend around the spur ridge on which perches Morrison Cabin. The grade is almost level through deep woods until breaking out into the open again at Pfeiffer Flat, delivering you almost to the doorstep of Jorstad Cabin, 8.2 miles from the trailhead. George Jorstad built this cozy little cabin back in 1937, where he lived while hand-placer-mining his claim until passing away in 1989 (hand-placer mining is done by either gold panning or running water through a sluice box). The cabin, now under the care of the U.S. Forest Service, has so far escaped the two most common calamities of such structures—fire and vandalism. This idyllic site certainly deserves your utmost consideration and respect. Away from the cabin, an easy amble under towering ponderosa pines, incense cedars, and Douglas firs leads to Pegleg Camp at 8.7 miles near the confluence of Grizzly Creek and North Fork Trinity River, with plenty of firewood and room for a few tents.

Leaving the North Fork, the trail turns east from Pegleg Camp to follow the narrower canyon of Grizzly Creek on good tread, built up on the south slope since the canyon bottom is steep and choked with alders. After nearly a mile, a ford, without any log footbridges nearby, takes you to the north side of the canyon. From there, you climb moderately steeply above more alders and willows and then level off in a jumble of rock piles that marks the old mining site of China Gardens.

Beyond the diggings, climb steeply for 200 yards to an old ditch, walk along it for a quarter mile to a tributary stream and another steep pitch, and then ascend more gradually to Mill Gulch, 3 miles from Pegleg Camp.

Trail junctions are close together in Mill Gulch: At the creek, a seldom-used and never maintained trail, signed TRAIL 11W02, CECIL LAKE, climbs upstream. Just beyond the creek, another trail, signed PAPOOSE LAKE, SPECIMEN CREEK, NORTH FORK, HOBO CAMP, heads across Grizzly Creek and up Specimen Creek. Your trail, which continues upstream along Grizzly Creek, is clearly defined at all junctions with signs as well.

SIDE TRIP: PAPOOSE LAKE

If you have an extra day or two, you might as well visit lovely Papoose Lake, 8 miles up the Rattlesnake Creek Trail. If you choose to visit Papoose Lake after Grizzly Lake, avoid the temptation to take the shortcut from the Grizzly Lake Trail up the Specimen Creek Trail to Bob's Farm and then down the other side, as this is one of the steepest and roughest trails in the entire wilderness—you're better off going the full distance from Grizzly Lake back down Grizzly Creek and the North Fork Trinity River to the Rattlesnake Creek Trail junction.

From the junction, head northeast toward Papoose Lake on an old, level wagon road across the wide floor of lower Rattlesnake Creek canyon. Where the canyon narrows, follow single-track trail moderately up the southeast wall away from the old road. After a brief diversion into Martin's Gulch, the trail rejoins the road and continues to a series of log rounds that block further progress and diverts traffic to the left through rock debris to a ford of Rattlesnake Creek, 1.7 miles from the junction. A campsite is along the creek immediately past the ford.

From the ford, climb up to the old road again, now on the northwest side of the canyon, and then ascend moderately with a few steeper pitches through mixed forest to a junction with the brutally steep trail to Bob's Farm. Continue ahead (east) to a manzanita-filled clearing and then climb steeply and drop just as steeply to a crossing of Mill Creek, where a single campsite lies next to the creek.

Climb moderately away from Mill Creek on good tread for 0.5 mile to a crossing of Middle Fork Rattlesnake Creek, which usually combines a boulder hop and a logjam to complete successfully. Another 2 miles of stiffly ascending trail veers southeast to red-fir-shaded Enni Camp, located on a glacial moraine 6.3 miles from North Fork Trinity River.

The trail continues southeast up the canyon, climbing steeply east of the creek. About 0.75 mile from Enni Camp, you encounter large granite boulders and cross to the south bank, as the creek turns east. Discernible tread deteriorates and ducks show the way east across a sloping bench through ceanothus and manzanita and over more boulders. At the end of this bench, a steep climb leads along the top of a cliff above the creek. At the bottom of a vertical face of meta-morphic rock you follow the trail south and then double back to zigzag up a crack to a ledge above. Cross this ledge eastward, climbing over boulders, and look for ducks leading south to two less vertical faces with a ledge in between. Above the third rock face, continue south along the west edge of a deep gorge through which the outlet falls from the lake. Beyond a hump of solid granite, you overlook gorgeous, teardrop-shaped Papoose Lake. A number of campsites near the outlet are badly overused—look for excellent spots farther upslope in the rocks above the northwest shore.

The trail up Grizzly Creek gets steeper between the Specimen Creek junction and the China Spring junction, which is just beyond a clear, cold, little stream cascading down a gully to the north. From this junction, the China Spring Trail-head is a mere 2.5 miles north over the Salmon River Divide, 1350 feet up to the crest and 1600 feet down the other side. Continuing up the canyon, you begin to turn south in thick woods well away from the creek. At 1.3 miles from the junction, the trail climbs out of the trees and over a glaciated, metamorphic rock outcrop, offering you your first far-ranging views since you left the trailhead. The higher valley above reveals the typical U-shape left by glaciers, in contrast to the V-shape of the nonglaciated canyon below.

Proceed up the valley on traverses alternating with switchbacks that gain altitude across patches of brush and broken rock. From openings about 3 miles from the China Spring junction are the first glimpses of Thompson Peak and the permanent snowfields clinging to the northern flank. Small meadows, willow flats, and groves of red firs soon replace the brush on the more level floor of the upper valley, with good campsites above and below a spring flowing across the trail. Climb moderately steeply over exposed rock and through stands of firs to the north edge of Upper Grizzly Meadow. Directly ahead, beyond lush grasses and wildflowers, the outlet from Grizzly Lake leaps from a precipice to dissolve in cascades of white foam and mist in the tumbled blocks of granite below—one of the more dramatic sights you'll see in the Trinity Alps. Good to excellent campsites in shady groves of red fir are on the south and west sides of the meadow and between the trail and the creek below the meadow at 17 miles from the trailhead.

The route up to Grizzly Lake from the meadow has been designated as a "scramble" trail, the purpose of which is to define a single route up the very steep slope, but to discourage people from carrying backpacks up to camp at the lake. Only experienced hikers should attempt the steep and strenuous route. Above the lower talus at the head of the canyon, a virtual granite staircase has been constructed, marked by periodic cairns. Approximately halfway up the slope, a spring-fed stream flows down a rock channel, beyond which you can pick up a dirt trail that leads to a rock outcrop. Behind the outcrop, a steep path passes through a cleft leading along the upper channel of the stream and across a field of wildflowers. Cross another branch of the stream to where an easier trail, somewhat indistinct, passes over boulders, through lush vegetation, and across another watercourse, before following an angling traverse across the slope. The trail eventually becomes distinct again in an area of scattered conifers and leads to the north shoreline of spectacular Grizzly Lake.

Spectacular Grizzly Falls just below Grizzly Lake

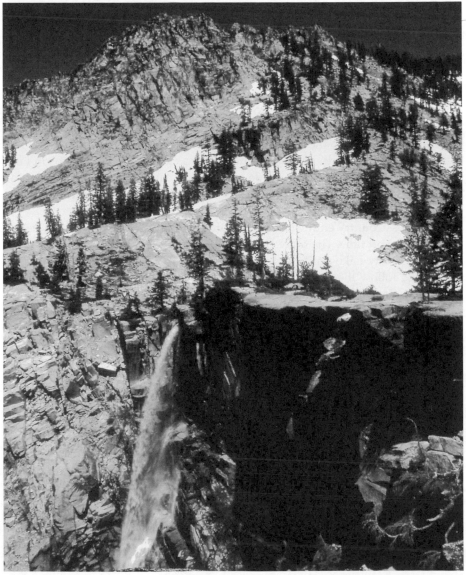

Here the full expanse of deep, blue, Grizzly Lake and its magnificent basin lies before you. Nearly level slabs of granite ease into the water west of the outlet, offering splendid opportunities for pondering the scene, sunbathing, or taking a quick dip into the chilly waters. Scattered mountain hemlocks, red firs, foxtail pines, and whitebark pines grow in cracks and pockets of soil around the granite basin. Lush gardens of wildflowers bloom in tiny pockets of meadow long after their lower counterparts have faded in the valley below. Above the cliffs to the southeast, a large, higher cirque and shelf on the north face of jagged, 9002-foot Thompson Peak hold perpetual snowfields.

For rugged backpackers willing to haul their packs up the steep scramble route, a handful of useable campsites at Grizzly Lake are found on rock slabs along the north shore and among trees on a ridge and peninsula above the northwest shore. Firewood is scarce and what little wood you might find should not be burned.

Rock climbers will find plenty of good vertical and overhanging rock both above and below the lake. For the more prosaic, who desire to reach the highest summit in the Alps, the route from Grizzly Lake is straightforward: From the north shore, work above the cliffs to the southwest, and then angle across granite slabs above, which may be snow-covered in early season, to the low point on the ridge leading up to the summit. Follow the backside of this ridge to the top, where views are superb. For those who desire a closer look at Thompson Peak but have neither the desire nor time to reach the summit, excellent views can be had at the top of the ridge above Lois Lake, including a panorama with Mt. Shasta to the east.

For cross-country enthusiasts, the route to diminutive Lois Lake can be traversed in a short time. The route climbs clefts in the ridge southwest of the north shore of Grizzly Lake until reaching the top of the ridge. From there, turn left (west) and follow the ridge to a saddle, where another ridge meets it from the northwest. Carefully drop down southwest from the ridge to where you can see Lois Lake below, sitting serenely in a small cirque, descending approximately 350 feet to the shore.

After a satisfying stay at Grizzly Lake, retrace your steps 17.5 miles to the trailhead.

BUILD-UP AND WIND-DOWN TIPS ·

The quaint town of Weaverville offers a few decent options for grabbing a bite to eat before or after your trip. In the historic section of town, the **Garden Café** is a fine place to have breakfast, especially on their shaded patio; they're open for breakfast and lunch every day except Tuesday. Just up the street, the **La Grange Café**, which is open every day except Sunday, serves excellent meals for lunch and dinner. East of the historic section of town, try **Millers Drive-In** for an old fashioned hamburger (although a for sale sign was up during my most recent visit).

29

NEW RIVER AND SLIDE CREEK TO HISTORIC MINING DISTRICT AND EAGLE CREEK

Mike White

MILES: 24.0
RECOMMENDED DAYS: 3–6
ELEVATION GAIN/LOSS: 6875´/6875´
TYPE OF TRIP: Semiloop
DIFFICULTY: Moderate
SOLITUDE: Solitude
LOCATION: Trinity Alps Wilderness
MAPS: USGS 7.5-min. *Jim Jam Ridge* and *Dees Peak*;
U.S. Forest Service *A Guide to the Trinity Alps Wilderness*
BEST SEASONS: Late spring and throughout fall

PERMITS

A wilderness permit is required for all overnight trips in the Trinity Alps Wilderness, and a campfire permit is also required if you plan to have one. Both permits can be obtained by self-registration at ranger stations in Weaverville, Big Bar, or Willow Creek.

Photo: *Much of the route to the Historic Mining District follows delightful streams.*

TAKE THIS TRIP

There's a good chance you might not see another soul on this 24-mile semiloop trip through the remote western Trinity Alps. However, solitude is not the only feature, as the trail takes you through the Historic Mining District, an area rich in history from the bygone days of mining activity during the late 1800s and early 1900s. Although it is hard to believe when you're standing on the site, at one time Old Denny had 500 residents. Along with the history, you will travel partway along the cascading waters and deep green pools of Slide and Eagle creeks.

CHALLENGES

Poison oak is found at the lower elevations along this route—know how to identify it and avoid it in the field. These trails may not be in the best shape from year to year, as the western part of the Alps is a little-used area of the wilderness. Stream crossings in spring may be dangerous during periods of high water—always check with the U.S. Forest Service for current conditions before heading out on the trail. Considering that the entire trip is below 5000 feet in elevation, summers can be exceedingly hot, making spring and fall the ideal times for a visit.

HOW TO GET THERE

Leave Highway 299 at Hawkins Bar, 46 miles west of Weaverville and 10 miles east of Willow Creek, and head toward Denny on County Road 402. Beyond a high bridge over the Trinity River, you go a quarter mile to an intersection, where you turn west and then north beside Hawkins Creek and proceed past several houses and a subdivision to another intersection. Turn right and begin the long, twisting climb headed generally east up Trinity River canyon.

At 6.3 miles from Hawkins Bar, beyond some unbelievable hairpin turns, pass a dirt road that forks left to Happy Camp and points north and then climb another 1.2 miles to the top of a spur ridge between the drainages of Trinity River and New River. From there, narrow pavement snakes down the east side of the ridge and then turns northeast through a gap in a spur ridge to a plateau high above New River with a group of houses and some orchards. Reach Panther Creek at 14.5 miles from Highway 299 and continue another 3 miles to Denny Campground straddling the road. The no-fee campground is large and pleasant, with piped water during the summer but no garbage service. The Forest Service's Denny Guard Station is out of sight above the

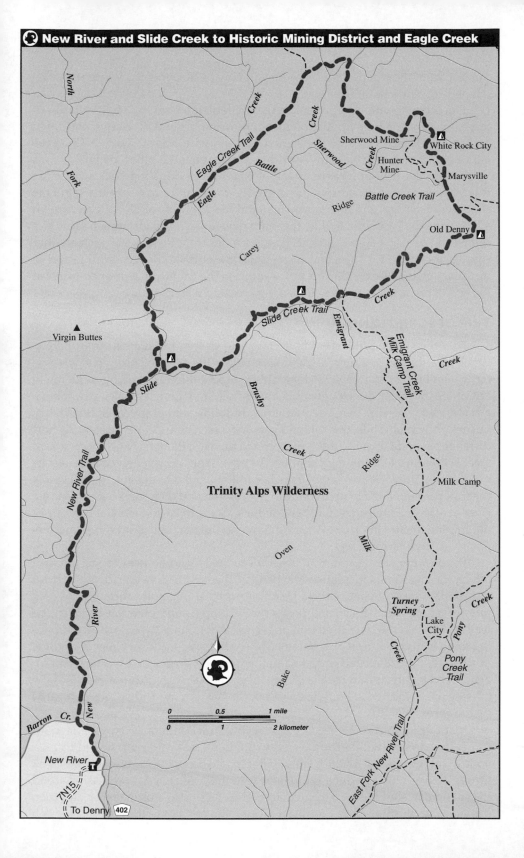

North Fork

Creek

Creek

Sherwood Mine

White Rock City

Eagle Creek Trail

Battle

Sherwood

Creek

Hunter Mine

Marysville

Eagle

Battle Creek Trail

Ridge

Carey

Old Denny

Creek

Virgin Buttes

Slide Creek Trail

Emigrant

Creek

Emigrant Creek Milk Camp Trail

Slide

Brushy

Creek

Ridge

Milk Camp

Trinity Alps Wilderness

New River Trail

Oven

Milk

Turney Spring

Creek

Lake City

Pony

River

Pony Creek Trail

Bake

0   0.5   1 mile
0   1   2 kilometer

East Fork New River Trail

Barron Cr.

New

New River

T

7N15

To Denny 402

upper part of the campground, where you may be able to get a wilderness permit and current trail information.

The actual town of Denny is strung out along the road for a half mile about three-quarters of a mile up the road from the campground. Continue past town and across Quinby Creek to the signed junction with Forest Road 7N15 on the left (if you come to the New River bridge, you've gone 1.3 miles too far).

Follow the well-graveled surface of Road 7N15 doubling back west from Road 402 on a climb away from the river. The road curves north, east around the shoulder of a ridge, and then north again on the west side of New River canyon across from the East Fork. Follow the main road, as lesser roads branch away to a right-hand turn at a signed intersection, 4.7 miles from Road 402. Reach another signed junction at 5.4 miles and turn left, as the surface changes from gravel to dirt (may be impassable during wet weather). The trailhead is in open forest at the end of the road, with a small parking area and a stock tie area.

TRIP DESCRIPTION

Pass the signed wilderness boundary and descend to a crossing of Barron Creek in a thicket of alders. A footlog is below the ford for use when the water is high but generally the ford should be problem-free. Climbing moderately out of the drainage, tall Douglas firs, madrones, and a few tanoaks grow above an understory of vine maples, ceanothus, redbuds, and dogwoods. Blackberry bushes growing in slide areas should provide a welcome treat in season. A short distance beyond Barron Creek, you come to the west bank of New River, where a cable crossing to a mining claim on the east bank, now removed, has left its mark on the trunks of two large firs. After following the west bank for 250 yards, the trail rises moderately up the side of the canyon and then stays away from the river across steep hillsides, flats, and ledges. Good tread follows the contour of old mining ditches in places. A spring flows across the trail about three-quarters of a mile from Barron Creek.

Beyond the spring, the trail rises more steeply to a rocky point, around which the river roars in a horseshoe bend at the base of a steep-sided gulch cut into dark metasedimentary rock. Descend north of this point through the rock piles of an old mining site, and past a large campground on a flat between the trail and the river. A well-used trail on the left that follows the side of an old mining ditch leads only to an old claim on the south bank of Virgin Creek. Continue north across the ditch and drop to a flat, where the Virgin Creek Guard Station once stood before burning to the ground several years ago. Virgin Creek is at the far side of a wide bed of boulders north of the flat, joining Slide Creek 200 yards east to form New River.

Just after a ford of Virgin Creek, the trail junction is marked by a sign attached to a tanoak with directions left to Soldier Creek and right to Old Denny. Follow the trail toward Old Denny, climbing east above the roar of the creek through mixed forest, which thickens where the trail curves northeast. Ascend to the top of a shoulder of a ridge that divides Slide and Virgin creeks and then descend into the Slide Creek drainage. Along the descent to the creek, you catch glimpses of the channel cut through the metasedimentary rock by the rushing waters of Slide Creek. The descent continues until the trail is just a few feet away from and directly above the stream.

Beyond a clearing, immediately switchback away from the creek and climb up to a bench with a campsite. Apparently this spot was the site of some old structure from a bygone era, as the remains of a 20-foot rock wall would indicate. A hundred feet farther up the trail, a small rivulet drifts across the path. About 2 miles from the junction of Virgin and Slide creeks, the trail suddenly gets steeper, makes a couple of switchbacks, and then climbs over a hill and into the gully of a seasonal creek. Traveling three-quarters of a mile farther, you reach the junction between the Eagle Creek and Slide Creek trails, approximately 250 yards above the actual confluence of the two creeks. Here the loop section of the trip begins.

Follow the right-hand trail from the junction and follow a short-legged switchback down to a boulder hop of Eagle Creek (during high water a log footbridge may be available 150 feet upstream). Consider replenishing your water supply here, as the next 3 miles of trail will be dry. There are a few seldom-used campsites on the east side of the creek.

Climb steeply away from Eagle Creek to an ascending traverse high above the level of the creek, at times almost out of earshot of the tumbling stream. Climb through mixed forest to a flat and the remains of a cabin, which, judging from the nature of the debris doesn't appear to be all that old. From the cabin the trail is well graded, gently rolling up and down without gaining or losing much elevation, but remaining high above the creek. Eventually the trail drops down to a large flat next to the creek, with several good, shady campsites and abundant firewood nearby. Plenty of mining paraphernalia lies scattered around the flat, including an intact wood and metal hand truck.

Ascending moderately, you hop over a seasonal creek, cross a steep hillside to an open area, and then wind down to a flowing stream lined with lush vegetation. Proceed away from the stream to a grassy meadow and a somewhat confusing junction, 0.2 mile from the camp area. The confusion dissipates once you proceed on the left-hand trail trending northeast, 40 feet to a sign posted on a pine with information that the other trail leads to Milk Camp and Pony Creek. Continue away from the meadow, perhaps noticing a transition in the vegetation to a predominantly evergreen forest. The trail soon becomes steep and the surroundings dry, remaining so for much of the distance to Old Denny. A clearing along the way provides views up to the crest of the Salmon Mountains. Before reaching Old Denny, trailside mining debris becomes more and more evident. Heading through a dry drainage ravine, you reach a junction at the old townsite in a grove of second-growth oaks and firs, 10.3 miles from the trailhead.

A crude, hand-lettered sign stating simply WATER points to the right (east), where near a meadow you can locate a spring. Since this area once supported a fairly large number of people, you should be able to find any number of decent camping spots spread around the width and breadth of the old town. Please respect the area and leave it as you found it for those who will follow after. Oddly enough, there are some private inholdings upstream from Old Denny, where a few modern-day residents attempt to maintain cabins on a seasonal basis. Please respect these sites as well if you happen to come upon them.

At one time Old Denny had 500 residents and the ground is littered with all types of artifacts, including cast-iron skillets, metal pots, mining equipment, rubber shoe parts, tin cans, bottles, and pottery shards. The miners left a long time ago and their buildings, some as high as three stories, have been replaced with a mature second-growth forest. Tattered old signs pass on some of the town's history: Old Denny was established by the founder, Clive Clements, in 1883, and was originally called New River City. The New River received its name when all the surrounding country had been explored except the rugged terrain around the new river. The quest for gold eventually motivated humans to search for every possible location where precious ore might exist and led to the "discovery" of the last river in the area, hence the name "New River." The last inhabitants left Old Denny in 1920, and decades later only a small number of temporary visitors pass through where once so many lived. Modern-day explorers can spend hours, if not days, poking around the old townsite, uncovering the rich history.

Instead of continuing on the trail up Slide Creek canyon, your route turns north from the junction in Old Denny, following signed directions to Mary Blaine Mountain and Cinnabar Mine. The trail climbs steeply away from the townsite on a well-defined, but little-used, track covered with leaves. Two long-legged switchbacks lead to the top of a divide separating the Slide Creek and Eagle Creek drainages. At this divide, another trail heads east toward Mary Blaine Meadows, while your trail, signed MARYSVILLE, descends into predominantly fir forest and soon reaches the old townsite. Unlike Old Denny, Marysville has little left to show the modern-day traveler.

A short distance from Marysville, you pass an even less often traveled trail on the left that heads west to the ruins of the old Hunter Mine and other mines. The main trail heads up, steeply at times, through mixed forest before breaking into the open just before gaining the top of a ridge. White Rock City is a short distance ahead, a little over a mile from Old Denny. Plenty of potential campsites are scattered around the old townsite at 11.4 miles, firewood is plentiful, and an abundant source of water is 0.2 mile down the trail at Sherwood Creek. For the backpacker, White Rock City occupies a more pleasant setting than Old Denny. Set on the side of a ridge, the townsite has pleasant views to the west and up to the summit of the Salmon Mountains. The wide, level surroundings beneath cedars and pines benefit from cool mountain breezes. Even fewer people reach White Rock City than Old Denny, which may account for artifacts of greater number and quality.

Leaving White Rock City, you head down to Sherwood Creek, climb away, and then traverse a hillside through firs and cedars to a spring. Above the spring on the far side next to a seep is a campsite. As the trail descends, you leave the primarily evergreen forest behind in favor of an oak forest. Poison oak, which hasn't been sighted between the slope above Old Denny and here, begins to reappear in sporadic clumps. As the descent gets steeper, views open up through the trees to the south and east, and the roar of Sherwood Creek is heard in the canyon below. Alert eyes may spy a large, unnatural hump on the steep slope below, which is the closed entrance to the Sherwood Mine. Downslope 50 to 75 feet is the buried opening of the abandoned mine, with an old ore cart, rails, and timbers. Soon after the mine you come upon a sign attached to a tanoak at the junction of the Hunter Mine Trail.

Leaving the Historic Mining District behind, the trail makes a gentle ascent that gets steeper just before rising to the top of a ridge beneath ponderosa pines and incense cedars. Descending from the ridge, you pass under cool fir and pine forest before eventually returning to oak forest, which has dominated at the lower elevations along the route. Rounding a bend, the track narrows and makes a somewhat tedious descending traverse across a rocky hillside until the track widens again under mixed forest. On the approach to Battle Creek, you enter a zone of much denser vegetation, which at times threatens to overgrow the trail. Up to this point, the path has been in relatively good condition and easy to follow, but this particular section runs the risk of becoming lost to the understory if not maintained.

Hop over Battle Creek, a cool and refreshing stream shaded by Douglas firs. Climbing away from the creek, you soon encounter a side stream and then cross a dry, rocky slope dotted with ponderosa pines and cedars, where the track narrows and footing becomes a little tricky. The tread soon widens again and then you ascend to the top of a ridge and a junction with a trail on the right to Rock Lake.

Plenty of artifacts litter the Historic Mining District.

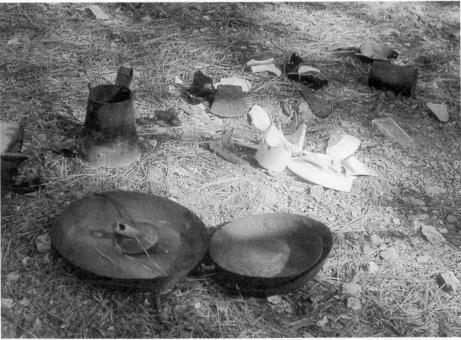

Continue straight ahead at the junction until the trail bends sharply left (south) and heads down from the ridge across a dry and rocky slope. Head back into a forest of Douglas firs, incense cedars, ponderosa pines, and digger pines, as you head down and then up again to the top of another ridge, which separates the Eagle Creek and Battle Creek drainages. Crossing over the ridge, the route then descends into the Eagle Creek canyon under a forest of primarily Douglas firs and incense cedars. Descend, steeply at times, to a clearing, where the trail angles to the right to make a horseshoe bend, switchbacks twice, and then travels west to a clearing at the bottom of the slope. Watch for cairns here, as the trail heads toward Eagle Creek and shortly becomes nearly impossible to follow. Once a dry and open hillside is reached, you can drop down to the creek and pick up distinct tread again where the trail parallels Eagle Creek. Gently graded trail heads downstream under tanoaks, canyon oaks, and Douglas firs.

Soon after passing an old campsite, you reach the crossing of Eagle Creek, which should be an easy boulder hop under most conditions. The creek itself is a delightful stream, with deep green pools suitable for fishing or swimming. The creek rushes downstream on a much steeper course than the trail alongside, which is a dirt, needle-covered path, smoothly graded and quite pleasant to walk on, under Douglas fir forest and alongside lush vegetation. Eventually, the trail becomes basically an up-and-down venture, coming almost to the creek and then climbing away, only to repeat the whole process over and over. Campsites are few and far between along Eagle Creek, which is a shame because the creek is quite delightful. A short climb brings you to the junction of Slide and Eagle creeks at the close of the loop. From there, retrace your steps 6 miles to the trailhead.

BUILD-UP AND WIND-DOWN TIPS

The quaint town of Weaverville offers a few decent options for grabbing a bite to eat before or after your trip. In the historic section of town, the **Garden Café** is a fine place to have breakfast, especially on their shaded patio; they're open for breakfast and lunch every day except Tuesday. Just up the street, the **La Grange Café**, which is open every day except Sunday, serves excellent meals for lunch and dinner. East of the historic section of town, try **Millers Drive-In** for an old fashioned hamburger (although a for sale sign was up during my most recent visit).

30

DEADFALL LAKES, MOUNT EDDY, AND THE SACRAMENTO HEADWATERS

Andy Selters

MILES: 12.2, plus a 2-mile side trip
RECOMMENDED DAYS: 2–3
ELEVATION GAIN/LOSS: 1166´/4490´ (another 1005´/1005´ for side trip)
TYPE OF TRIP: Point-to-point
DIFFICULTY: Moderately strenuous
SOLITUDE: Moderately populated
LOCATION: Shasta-Trinity National Forest
MAPS: USGS 7.5-min. *South China Mountain* and *Mount Eddy*
BEST SEASONS: Summer and early fall

PERMITS

No permits are required for this trip.

CHALLENGES

Completing the entire traverse requires a car shuttle between the two trailheads. Also, the trail along the upper Sacramento River is a bit hard to follow

Photo: Looking west from Deadfall Summit across the Deadfall Lakes basin and to the Scott Mountains in a couple of places, but common sense and careful use of the map will bring you through the short indistinct sections. Maintenance scheduled for 2008 might make these sections clearer.

HOW TO GET THERE • • • • • • • • • • • • •

To reach Parks Creek Summit: Drive north on Interstate 5 for 3.4 miles past the Weed turnoff and take the Edgewood-Gazelle exit. Turn southwest under the freeway to a T-junction, and take the right (northwest) fork. After 0.4 mile turn left (southwest) onto Stewart Springs Road, Forest Road 17. Keep right on this road after 3.9 miles; as it gets steeper, stay on paved Forest Road 17 to the summit, 12.9 miles from the Stewart Springs turnoff.

To get to the eastern trailhead: From downtown Mount Shasta cross I-5 at the main Mount Shasta exit and continue southwest to a T-junction at Old Stage Road (the location of the old hamlet of Sisson). Turn left (northwest) and soon veer right onto W. A. Barr Road, toward Lake Siskiyou. A mile from the Old Stage turnoff, turn right onto North Shore Road, Forest Road 40N27. Drive along the north shore of Lake Siskiyou, keeping left at the only minor fork, and park near where the road ends at a washout, at the North Fork of the Sacramento River. From here the trail takes an old roadbed on the opposite side of the river.

TRIP DESCRIPTION • • • • • • • • • • • • • • •

From Parks Creek Summit you strike southeast on the well-groomed Pacific Crest Trail (PCT), through an open forest with a diversity of conifers like only these Klamath-Trinity Mountains hold. In contouring one long slope, you pass beneath Jeffrey pines, red firs, white firs, Douglas firs, western white pines, and lodgepole pines. However, a mile from the trailhead you come to a logging road established in 2006; the land here is parceled in the checkerboard legacy of 19th-century

TAKE THIS TRIP

Running from subalpine lakes and meadows to transition forest and chaparral, this hike tours the botanically rich north-ernmost Trinity Mountains on a crossing from the Trinity to Sacramento river drainages. It also offers a side trip to the rocky summit of Mt. Eddy, where you can get probably the most overwhelming view anywhere of California's greatest peak, Mt. Shasta. The first half of the hike, to Deadfall Lakes and back, is a popular, mid-summer retreat for fishing and swimming, while the stretch down the head-waters of the Sacramento River sees relatively few hikers.

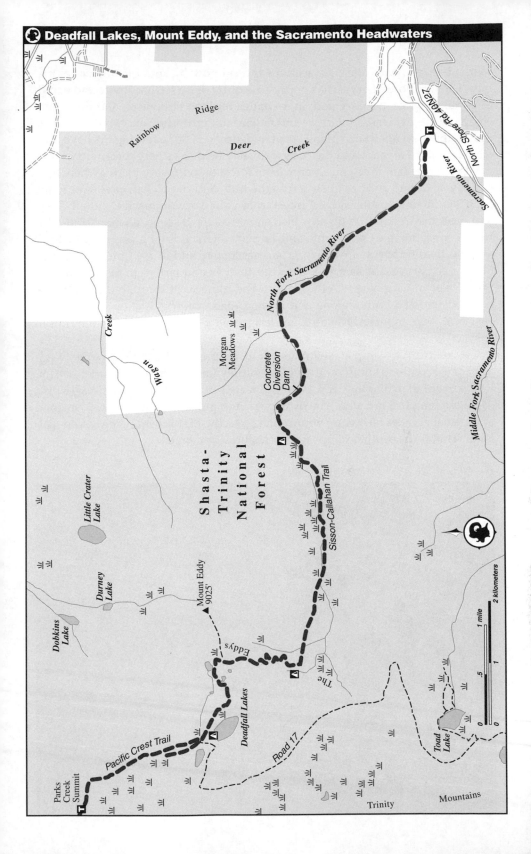

railroad grants, with alternate sections owned now by spin-off timber compa-
nies. The U.S. Forest Service has hoped to acquire these sections (here and in other popular places in this region) in exchange for land elsewhere, and the timber
company has expressed interest—but federal underfunding and political inertia
thus far have stymied such plans. As of midsummer 2007 a few big firs have been
cut near this new road, and the other privately held trees here remain in peril.

In another half mile you emerge from forest onto flowery glades where deli-
cious, year-round springs gush across the trail, and the views open west to the
Scott Mountains. Just ahead, 2.1 miles from your car, you reach Deadfall Creek
and meet the Deadfall Trail, now also signed as the Sisson-Callahan Trail. This
route connecting the Sacramento and Trinity watersheds long was used by Indians and then trappers, prospectors, and cattlemen, and in 1911 the early Forest
Service constructed it as a link between their headquarters in Sisson and the
Scott River mining outpost of Callahan. The route west through the Scotts has
been crisscrossed with logging and mining roads, but the section you'll follow
east from here is intact. It was even designated a National Recreation Trail in
1979.

If you want to camp at, swim in, fish in, or just visit the largest of the Deadfall Lakes, continue south on the PCT a minute farther, cross the outlet stream,
and turn uphill to find the deep, beautiful waters nearby. You might notice a bald
eagle catching fish here too. The fishing, swimming, and camping are also good
at the smaller lakes farther up your route. From the PCT junction, the Sisson-Callahan Trail turns southeast, up another shallow drainage.

Mt. Eddy above one of the Deadfall Lakes

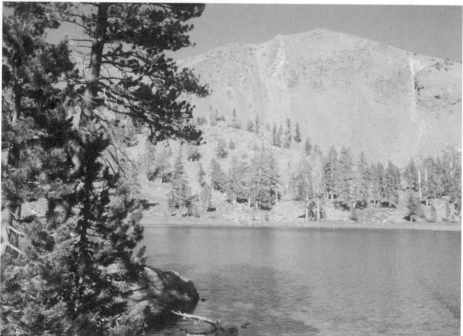

As you climb a subtle ridge you enjoy a view through forest and meadows onto the largest Deadfall Lake, and ahead you see Mt. Eddy. Before long the trail steepens up a shallow ravine and takes you to a bench containing one of the smaller Deadfall Lakes, which you circle along its west shore. Next, hop a stream and rise to a slightly higher bench that cups a medium-sized lake, a subalpine gem reflecting Mt. Eddy's craggy, ochre face. After cruising along the meadowy south shore of this lake, you start the final climb to Deadfall Summit.

A single switchback takes you south out of the last lake's small cirque and up through one of the most diverse stands of conifers you'll ever see; on these slopes grow red fir, white fir, lodgepole pine, western white pine, whitebark pine, and foxtail pine. This area has an unusual number of plant species (including many endemic ones) because, it's thought that, over recent millennia these Klamath-Trinity mountains have maintained a relatively stable climate. During widespread glaciations and droughts, these moist, semi-coastal mountains collected ample precipitation but only small glaciers, and the variety of different altitudes and different-facing slopes have probably offered a variety of shifting subclimates for plants to make their homes in.

The brief, final climb to Deadfall Summit gives you a distant view west beyond the Deadfall basin and across the subalpine ridges of the Scott and Klamath mountains. To the south you can see the high granite peaks that are the core of the Trinity Alps. At the pass, you meet the signed junction with the path to the top of Mt. Eddy.

SIDE TRIP: MOUNT EDDY

This 2.0-mile round-trip climb is a must-do for anyone with just a little stamina to spare. From the Deadfall Summit, the first few switchbacks climb through a stand of foxtail pine, an uncommon relative of the bristlecone pine, which grows only in these mountains and in the southern High Sierra. The switchbacks touch back onto the Trinity-Sacramento divide a couple of times, and then one long switchback cuts back east onto slopes where scattered whitebark pines gradually replace the foxtails. Now a steady bank of tighter switchbacks climbs into the rocky alpine realm of hulsea, phacelia, penstemon, and krummholz whitebark pines.

The rust-colored rock that crunches underfoot is a type of peridotite, a rare stone that derives almost directly from the earth's mantle. In the mishmash of collisions and accretions that formed these mountains, somehow big chunks of material from beneath the earth's crust was pushed up to here.

At Mt. Eddy's summit you'll be at 9025 feet, at eye level with Mt. Shasta. The big peak is just 16 air miles away, so its true scale and grandeur is more than obvious. To the southeast you get a great view of the granitic wonder-world of the Castle Crags. At your feet you also see a few scraps of an old fire lookout, which was last used in 1931.

Continuing on the Sisson-Callahan Trail, you start a steep descent south off Deadfall Summit, braking through duff into a meadowy realm of fir and chinquapin. Before too long switchbacks ease the grade, and on the easternmost of these hairpins you come within 100 yards of a gushing spring, which, along with springs on Mt. Shasta, is one of the sources of the Sacramento River. Depression-era license plates high on the trees mark your trail as an old snow-survey route, and eventually you pass near the remains of the surveyor's old cabin. The cabin burned down in 2003, probably during a visit from a snowmobile party.

Turning southeast here, you continue on a more gradually descending traverse. Here you might notice the original Sisson-Callahan track, the faint trail that runs west back over the divide. The newer eastbound trail becomes a bit obscure also, but numerous tree blazes guide you on a continued downhill traverse to the North Fork of the Sacramento, here just a quiet stream with stones you can hop across. On the other side another old trail heads southwest to climb over to the Middle Fork drainage, and you continue east along the Sacramento, ambling through glades and groves of white fir, lodgepole pine, and surprisingly large incense cedars. As you reach leveler, soggier ground the glades become richer with brodiaea, potentilla, columbine, and yarrow, allowing broader views to ridgelines of rusty-toned peridotite.

At one meadow the grasses have partly overgrown the trail, and you'll want to continue on a straight course across the north side of this meadow to find a dry, rocky creekbed that after a short distance leads into distinct trail. A little farther you come to an old road that crosses the river, and a campsite. The trail follows the old roadbed for a bit, staying near the river's south bank, and then narrows to a single track and veers closer to the water. Your gentle descent continues along the Sacramento for another 0.5 mile, to where a couple of switchbacks start the drop out of the once-glaciated high country into the river's lower canyon. The switchbacks empty onto another old roadbed, which you follow for nearly 0.5 mile before coming to a Sisson-Callahan Trail marker on the north edge of the road. At this post, unfortunately easy to miss without a watchful eye, you drop off the road and start a steady descent along the now-tumbling Sacramento River.

Under sugar pines, Jeffrey pines, and Douglas firs, the trail follows the river canyon's curve to the southeast, passing an old jeep road that climbs south and then descending on a couple small switchbacks. Continue descending past a waterfall and into warmer climes, where beargrass, pipsissiwa, paintbrush, Shasta lily, and azalea catch your eye. As you descend farther, breaks in the forest let you look back for a last glimpse at the eastern summits of Mt. Eddy. Eventually the trail runs onto an old roadbed, which takes you across a tributary creek and curves east down to the washed-out crossing of the main river. Here you can hop rocks or perhaps wet your feet to ford to the eastern trailhead on North Shore Road.

BUILD-UP AND WIND-DOWN TIPS

After your hike, take a swim in **Lake Siskiyou**, the water is great. As you drive back along North Shore Road you might find a good spot via a short walk through the woods, but the more popular beaches, as well as a nice, privately run campground, are off of South Shore Road. With a little exploration along the south shore you will find some out-of-the way spots too.

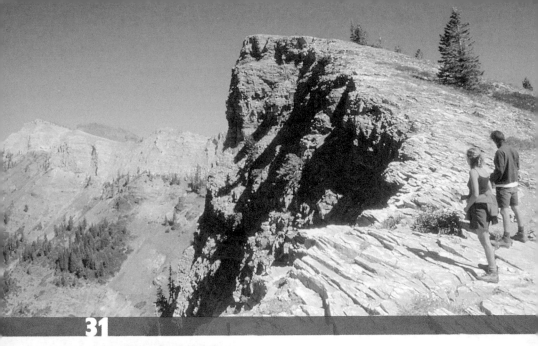

31

MARBLE RIM VIA SKY HIGH LAKES BASIN

Matt Heid

MILES: 17.0
RECOMMENDED DAYS: 2
ELEVATION GAIN/LOSS: 2800´/2800´
TYPE OF TRIP: Out-and-back
DIFFICULTY: Moderate
SOLITUDE: Moderate solitude
LOCATION: Marble Mountain Wilderness, Klamath National Forest
MAPS: USGS 7.5-min. Marble Mountain,
U.S. Forest Service *Marble Mountain Wilderness Map*,
Marble Mountain Wilderness Topographic Map by Wilderness Press
BEST SEASON: Summer

PERMITS ·

No wilderness permit is necessary, but a valid campfire permit is required.

CHALLENGES ·

Marble Mountain Wilderness is located in the far northwest corner of the state and requires a long drive from just about everywhere.

Photo: Looking out from Marble Rim

TAKE THIS TRIP

Designated a primitive area in 1931 and established as one of California's first wilderness areas in 1953, Marble Mountain Wilderness protects nearly a quarter million acres of pristine California. You might think that the deep lakes, striking mountains, lush forest, abundant wildlife, and isolation would attract droves of hikers. But they don't. Come journey past the serene lakes and campsites of Sky High Lakes Basin and stand on the lip of the area's namesake marble cliffs.

HOW TO GET THERE

Take Scott River Rd. 13.4 miles west from Fort Jones on State Highway 3 to Indian Scotty Campground. Turn left (south) onto Forest Service Rd. 44N45, which is posted for Lovers Camp. Bear left at the immediate fork and continue on the sinuous, one-lane paved road as it climbs 6.8 miles to a large parking lot at the road's end.

TRIP DESCRIPTION

From the trailhead at 4150 feet in elevation, start out on the Canyon Creek Trail, passing two established campsites and entering lush forest. Douglas fir, tanoak, and bigleaf maple are common sights overhead; trail markers, wild ginger, and ferns line the path. In 0.1 mile, the trail reaches a confusing intersection of unpaved roads—continue on the trail found diagonally across the road. Passing a wilderness boundary sign hammered to a Douglas fir, you soon reach a posted fork at 0.7 mile in the level trail. The trail to Red Rock Valley heads left, but you continue right on Canyon Creek Trail toward Marble Valley.

While the hike parallels rushing Canyon Creek for several miles, the water remains unseen below you for the duration. After crossing flowing Death Valley Creek, the trail climbs briefly before dropping to cross Big Rock Fork. The logs that litter the bouldery watercourse provide evidence of the ferocity that winter rains and flood bring to the region's otherwise small streams. Shortly thereafter, the trail abruptly turns upslope and begins climbing steeply uphill. Intermittent switchbacks eventually bring you to the junction for Marble Valley at 4.1 miles and 5320 feet. Marble Valley provides faster and more direct access to the Marble Mountains but entirely misses Sky High Lakes Basin. If you are short of time, bear right and continue uphill to the Marble Valley Cabin (closed to the public) and the Pacific Crest Trail (PCT)

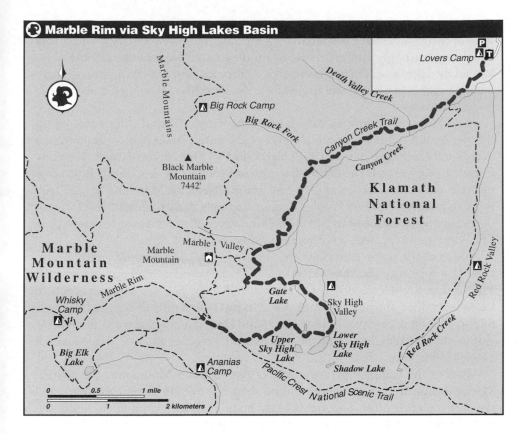

Marble Rim via Sky High Lakes Basin

Lovers Camp

Marble Mountains

Death Valley Creek

Big Rock Camp

Big Rock Fork

Canyon Creek Trail

Canyon Creek

Black Marble
Mountain
7442'

Klamath
National
Forest

Marble   Valley

Marble
Mountain

Marble
Mountain
Wilderness

Marble Rim

Red Rock Valley

Whisky
Camp

Gate
Lake

Sky High
Valley

Big Elk
Lake

Upper
Sky High
Lake

Lower
Sky High
Lake

Red Rock Creek

Ananias
Camp

Shadow Lake

Pacific Crest National Scenic Trail

0   0.5   1 mile

0   1   2 kilometers

junction, and then head south on the PCT until you reach the Marble Rim Trail. This marble-strewn route also makes for an excellent return option to the trailhead from Marble Rim.

Bearing left toward Sky High Lakes, you climb more gradually and soon pass another junction for Marble Valley on the right. Curving east, the trail offers the first views of the Marble Mountains to the west before making a final ascent into Sky High Lakes Basin. After you crest a final rise, diminutive and willow-choked Gate Lake welcomes you to the gently rolling basin.

Carved out by recent glaciation within the past 2 million years, the basin holds several lakes and provides abundant options for camping. Use paths criss-cross the area, but the actual trail leads first to larger Lower Sky High Lake at 6.0 miles in the basin's southeast corner, before turning west toward tiny Frying Pan Lake and then climbing out of the basin. The trees are diverse—white fir, red fir, mountain hemlock, western white pine, and large groves of aspen can all be found. In addition, a rare stand of subalpine fir grows here as well. A common tree throughout the Pacific Northwest, subalpine fir's range extends north to the subarctic. But in Northern California it only occurs here and in scattered locations within nearby Russian Wilderness, and both populations are more than 50 miles distant from the next closest stand in southern Oregon, according to

Ronal M. Lanner in *Conifers of California*. Despite existing at the extreme southern limit of their range, the trees seem to be thriving. Identify them by their narrow spire shape, strongly aromatic crushed needles, and close resemblance to red fir. Within the lakes amphibians thrive: frogs, tadpoles, and the ubiquitous, orange-bellied roughskin newt all entertain along the shorelines. In early October, cattle graze here as well.

Continuing west toward the Marble Mountains, the trail climbs steeply up the slopes and offers superlative views of the entire basin before attaining the divide and reaching a junction with the PCT at 7.1 miles and 6400 feet. The view from the ridge reveals the entire drainage of Wooley Creek within a horseshoe of peaks dominated west-southwest by granite Medicine Mountain at 6837 feet. From its headwaters here, Wooley Creek plummets more than 5000 feet through dense, undisturbed forest to join the Salmon River 20 miles away. Its entire pristine watershed is protected within the wilderness.

Once on the ridge, turn right and follow the PCT descending gently northwest to a four-way junction at 8.6 miles, where you continue straight toward Marble Rim. Right leads down into Marble Valley, the possible shortcut or return route mentioned above. Left drops down in just over a mile to Big Elk Lake, visible southwest in an open grassy area. Now climbing again toward the marble slopes, the trail remains below the divide until it reaches the low, treeless notch along Marble Rim.

Part of the complex geologic mix of the Klamath Mountains, the Marble Mountains most likely originated more than 200 million years ago from coral reefs surrounding an ancient, offshore island or landmass. Over the millenia, the reefs' skeletal remains collected in thick layers that eventually solidified into the sedimentary rock limestone. Smashed into North America, the limestone was transformed to marble and exposed by erosion to form the spectacular cliffs before you. Rainy Valley trails away more than 1000 feet below. Southeast are the jagged peaks of the highest mountains in the wilderness, and the Trinity Alps can often be seen on the distant southern skyline. Return as you came via Sky High Lakes Basin or take the Marble Valley shortcut.

BUILD-UP AND WIND-DOWN TIPS

If you're interested in learning more about the region's history, stop in at the **Siskiyou County Museum** in Yreka before or after your trip. Yreka is about 17 miles north of Fort Jones on State Highway 3. Located at 910 South Main Street in Yreka, the museum has galleries focused on the cultural history and artistry of several Native American tribes; trapping activities in the area in the early 1800s; and 19th-century gold mining activity in the region, as well as an outdoor museum with four recreated historic structures. For more information, call 530-842-3836 or visit them online at www.co.siskiyou.ca.us/museum/index.htm.

32

SHACKLEFORD TO CAMPBELL, CLIFF, SUMMIT, LITTLE ELK, DEEP, AND WRIGHTS LAKES LOOP

Mike White

MILES: 32.0
RECOMMENDED DAYS: 4–6
ELEVATION GAIN/LOSS: 8125´/8125´
TYPE OF TRIP: Loop
DIFFICULTY: Moderately strenuous
SOLITUDE: Solitude
LOCATION: Marble Mountain Wilderness
MAPS: USGS 7.5-min. *Boulder Peak* and *Marble Mountain*;
U.S. Forest Service *A Guide to the Marble Mountain Wilderness & Russian Wilderness*
BEST SEASON: Summer through fall

PERMITS

Wilderness permits are not required, but you will need a campfire permit if you plan to have a campfire (campfire permits are available from any Forest Service ranger station).

Photo: Beautiful Cliff Lake is one of the more popular lakes in the Marbles.

TAKE THIS TRIP

Although Campbell and Deep lakes are some of the most heavily visited destinations in Marble Mountain Wilderness, you may not see another soul on the rest of this 32-mile journey through one of the most remote wilderness areas in California. This trip has all the proper ingredients for a great mountain adventure, including a bevy of scenic lakes, rugged peaks, grand vistas, wildflower-carpeted meadows, shady forests, and cascading streams.

CHALLENGES

Away from the more popular destinations, such as Campbell and Deep lakes, trails in the Marble Mountains are little used and seldom maintained and so may require backpackers to have good route-finding abilities, particularly around Big and Back meadows.

HOW TO GET THERE

From Etna to the south, or Yreka to the north, follow State Highway 3 to Fort Jones and an intersection with Scott River Road near the Scott River Ranger Station. Proceed 7 miles on Scott River Road to a left-hand turn onto Quartz Valley Road and drive another 4 miles to a right-hand turn onto Forest Road 43N21. Follow this dirt road 6.9 miles to the Shackleford Trailhead at the end of the road. Although numerous spur roads branch away, Road 43N21 is well marked and is clearly the most heavily traveled road.

TRIP DESCRIPTION

Head away from the trailhead on a moderate climb along the course of an old roadbed along Shackleford Creek through the shade of a mixed forest of Douglas firs, white firs, Jeffrey pines, and incense cedars to a crossing of dashing Back Meadows Creek. Beyond the creek, gently graded, single-track trail passes into Marble Mountains Wilderness, crosses a rivulet, and then leads to a stock gate near the edge of a grassy meadow. The trail skirts the seep-watered meadow and continues under forest cover, briefly interrupted by a lodgepole-lined clearing. Beyond the clearing, you follow the mildly rising trail across Long High Creek and several tiny seeps and pass another small clearing on the way to a junction with a trail on the right to Log Lake, 2.1 miles from the trailhead.

Veer left at the junction and drop to a crossing of Shackleford Creek. The trail then begins a moderate, switchbacking climb up

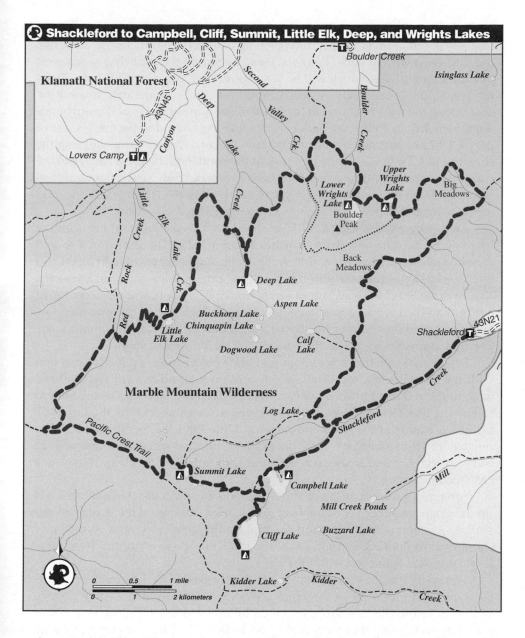

Shackleford to Campbell, Cliff, Summit, Little Elk, Deep, and Wrights Lakes

Klamath National Forest

Boulder Creek

Isinglass Lake

Lovers Camp

Second Valley Crk.

Deep Lake Creek

Lower Wrights Lake

Upper Wrights Lake

Big Meadows

Boulder Peak

Back Meadows

Deep Lake

Aspen Lake

Buckhorn Lake

Chinquapin Lake

Little Elk Lake

Dogwood Lake

Calf Lake

Shackleford   43N21

Marble Mountain Wilderness

Log Lake

Shackleford   Creek

Pacific Crest Trail

Summit Lake

Campbell Lake

Mill Creek Ponds

Mill

Cliff Lake

Buzzard Lake

Kidder Lake   Kidder

Creek

0   0.5   1 mile
0   1   2 kilometers

the canyon of the tributary that drains Campbell Lake. After a mile the grade eases and you reach a Y-junction near the old rock dam at Campbell Lake's northeast shore. The lake is reasonably attractive when full but is much less so later in the season with a lower water level. Spacious, shady campsites may be found down the left-hand trail just across the outlet. Turn right at the Y-junction, pass the north side of the lake to a junction with the trail from Log Lake, and proceed to a T-junction between trails to Summit Lake to the right and Cliff Lake to the left.

Heading toward Cliff Lake, you ascend a low, forested hill and pass a pair of shady ponds, a small, murky, unappealing one and a slightly larger, attractive one covered with lily pads. Between these two, note the trail that heads west toward Summit Lake, which will be your route after you visit Cliff Lake. From the ponds, the occasionally switchbacking trail climbs moderately toward the lake. Along the way, openings in the forest allow fleeting views of the surrounding terrain. Briefly follow the outlet and then swing around to the north shore of deep Cliff Lake, rimmed by the precipitous cliffs of a cirque. Campsites ring the shoreline at 4.7 miles, with the best sites at the south end. Before a change to the current and entirely fitting name, Cliff Lake was once known as Upper Campbell Lake. Similar to its lower neighbor, a dam was built here in the late 1800s to augment the irrigation needs of ranchers in Quartz Valley.

After fully experiencing Cliff Lake, head back to the junction between the two ponds and turn left (west) toward Summit Lake. The trail drops to and crosses a fair-sized meadow and then climbs through pockets of light forest and open, rocky slopes covered with shrubs, zigzagging to and away from a seasonal stream to the left of the trail. About a mile from the junction, you reach the top of a ridge and then follow a moderate descent past flower-filled Summit Meadow and small, shallow Summit Meadow Lake to deeper and larger Summit Lake. The best campsites are across the outlet along the northwest shore.

Follow the main trail across Summit Lake's outlet and soon reach a junction with the Shackleford Creek Trail, which continues ahead toward the trailhead and climbs to the left toward the Pacific Crest Trail (PCT). If you're tempted to follow the Shackleford Creek Trail downstream to a shortcut via the Little Elk Primitive Trail over the ridge and down to Little Elk Lake, be forewarned that much of this trail's tread has disappeared over time and sections of the route are badly overgrown with brush. It is not a trail, but rather a difficult and strenuous cross-country route.

After you turn left at the junction, a moderate, switchbacking climb leads up the slope, passing over a couple of lushly lined streams on the way to an unmarked junction with a very short use trail leading to a vista point on the lip of the cirque overlooking Summit Lake. The moderate climb continues from there to a saddle and a junction with the PCT.

Turn right (northwest) and follow the gently graded PCT through open forest with good views down the remote Wooley Creek drainage. After a grove of thicker forest, the trail drops and then follows a descending traverse across the south-facing slopes of an unnamed peak covered with serviceberry, tobacco brush, huckleberry oak, and manzanita and dotted with Jeffrey pines. Reach a saddle with a momentary view northeast down Rock Creek canyon and then proceed through shady forest to a junction with a half-mile lateral to Cold Spring on the left. From there, gently rising tread leads 0.3 mile to a junction with your route into Red Rock Valley on the right.

Leave the PCT and drop off the ridge on a fairly steep trail that winds through the forest, eventually passing below a pond near the head of the canyon, with a campsite nearby. Break out of the trees and continue to descend through acres

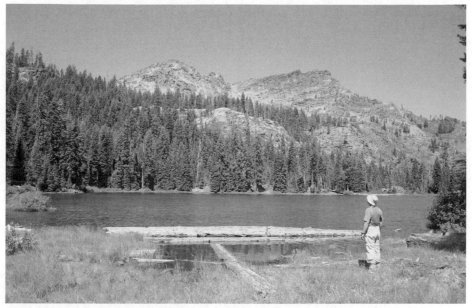

Picturesque Summit Lake

and acres of tall plants and wildflowers, crossing nascent Red Rock Creek and heading downstream along its west bank. Farther down the canyon, the trail continues its descent through more meadows alternating with stands of forest. In one such shady stand, you reach a junction with a trail to Little Elk Lake.

Turn right, boulder hop Red Rock Creek, stroll across a strip of meadow, and then begin a long, forested climb of the ridge dividing the Red Rock Creek and Little Elk Lake Creek drainages. A number of switchbacks get you to the top of the ridge, from where a moderately steep descent leads toward Little Elk Lake. Nearing the canyon floor, you follow cairns across a grassy meadow accented by woolly sunflower and Bigelow sneezeweed to the shallow lake, which is bordered by trees and marshy grasses and is backdropped stunningly by Peak 7605. The chest-deep lake doesn't appeal to swimmers due to the gooey muck covering the basin, but anglers should enjoy the fair fishing, provided they can access the shoreline through the muck and grass. A couple of Spartan campsites scattered around the lake won't make anyone's list of top 10 places to camp, but are more than adequate for a night's stay at 13.6 miles.

Cross the outlet from Little Elk Lake and moderately climb the east canyon wall through lush plants and flowers, hopping over a stream draining Wolverine Lake, with a scenic cascade above the trail. Proceed across a couple of tiny rivulets on the way toward the nose of the ridge dividing the Little Elk Lake Creek and Deep Lake Creek drainages. The trail wraps around the ridge, drops down to an easy boulder hop of Deep Lake Creek, and then starts a moderately steep climb up the canyon. Eventually you break out of the trees and reach a somewhat obscure junction on the top of a moraine covered with drought-tolerant plants, including some scattered mountain mahogany trees.

To reach Deep Lake, bend south at the junction and follow a path across a number of spring-fed seeps that water open slopes carpeted with willows and other water-loving plants. Beyond the seeps, sagebrush and grass covers the dry and open slopes of the upper meadow on the way to a Y-junction, where the right-hand path heads downslope and across the outlet to campsites on the northwest shore, and the path ahead continues toward highly coveted campsites on a peninsula near the southeast shore at 16.9 miles. Cradled into a deep cirque below Red Mountain, aptly named Deep Lake is one of the most scenic lakes in the Marble Mountains, which, along with the excellent fishing and swimming, helps to explain the lake's popularity. Cross-country enthusiasts can spend extra time exploring the rugged "ABCD" (more commonly referred to as ABC lakes) lakes above by climbing the steep slope northeast of Deep Lake and then traversing south into the basin. Although something of a use trail has evolved over the years, only experienced off-trail hikers should attempt the route to Aspen, Buckhorn, Chinquapin, and Dogwood lakes.

After a visit to Deep Lake, return to the junction and follow ducks uphill to more discernible tread, which soon leads to a protracted, rising traverse of the slope above the canyon of Canyon Creek. Along the way are good views across the canyon of the mountains to the north. After passing through a burned area, you reach willow-lined Muse Creek above Muse Meadow. A little way farther is a small sign nailed to a fir tree with an ominous sounding message: STEEP BLUFFS, DISMOUNTING ADVISED. After passing through a small grove of conifers, you follow the trail across steep cliffs and continue the traverse through groves of forest and open terrain to the crossing of Second Valley Creek and a beautiful meadow in the shadow of 8299-foot Boulder Peak. On the far bank is an informal junc-

Back Meadows is both lush and view-packed.

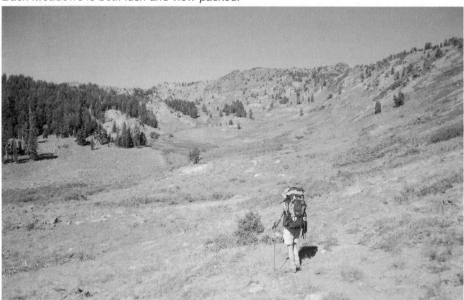

tion with the obscure secondary trail that heads up the canyon of Second Valley Creek to a saddle in the ridge of Red Mountain and then heads northeast along the ridge to reconnect with the main trail above Upper Wrights Lake.

From the crossing the trail veers north to descend across the east side of the creek's canyon before making a short climb over the nose of the ridge dividing Second Valley Creek and Boulder Creek drainages. From there, you descend steeply into a forest of mountain hemlocks, western white pines, and firs to a junction with a trail descending to the Boulder Creek Trailhead. The steep descent continues shortly to a second junction with a trail to that same trailhead.

From the second junction, a much more pleasantly graded section of trail leads across an open flat and then on a rollercoaster route through patchy forest into the canyon of Boulder Creek. Gently graded trail leads through shrubs before a short and steep climb brings you to a crossing of the creek. Well above the east side of the creek bottom, the trail makes a steep ascent through the trees before breaking out into the open to pass through the lush foliage of the meadow below Lower Wrights Lake. The trail climbs to a junction above the lake's northeast shore, where a use trail on the right descends toward it. Situated beneath the towering northeast face of Boulder Peak, Lower Wrights Lake is one of the larger and deeper lakes in the Marble Mountains. The open, windswept, and barren shoreline may seem a bit uninviting to potential campers, but the stunning scenery makes up for the deficiencies of the few campsites on the northeast shore at 22.0 miles. Anglers can ply the waters for rainbow, brown, and eastern brook trout.

From the junction, a stiff, 0.4-mile climb heads east up a steep slope dotted with whitebark pines to the west lip of Upper Wrights Lake's basin, where a cozy campsite is tucked under widely scattered pines. More spacious sites are under the conifers at the far end. Although much smaller than Lower Wrights Lake and lacking its dramatic setting, Upper Wrights Lake, the highest lake in this wilderness area, is set in somewhat more inviting surroundings than its lower counterpart.

Follow the trail around the east shore of Upper Wrights Lake and climb out of the basin to an open saddle at the trip's high point. Here a beautiful, wide-ranging view of the Trinity Alps to the south and Mt. Shasta to the east unfolds. Closer at hand keen eyes may detect the faint tread of the primitive route around Boulder Peak heading southwest. With an extra layover day at Upper Wrights Lake, you could follow this primitive trail for a mile or so to a saddle south of Boulder Peak and then leave the path on a straightforward climb to the summit.

From the saddle, the trail descends generally northeast into a forest belt of foxtail pines, followed by whitebark pines, mountain hemlocks, and finally red firs. Along the way, you hop across a number of spring-fed rivulets before breaking back into the open at the upper limits of flower-covered Big Meadows, where the trail angles sharply southeast to descend 0.75 mile along a lushly lined tributary of Big Meadows Creek. Farther downstream, the stream is bordered with quaking aspens and alders. Reach a T-junction with a little-used trail on the left from Sniktaw Meadow.

Turn right and head southwest on a rising climb across Big Meadows, hopping over numerous streams and negotiating boggy sections of tread before heading back into light forest, which includes an extensive aspen grove. Soon you're back out in the open again, as the trail crosses more meadows and streams. Away from these meadows, the trail climbs shortly over a grassy bench and then drops into the canyon of Back Meadows Creek.

The trail becomes very ill-defined in the lush vegetation of Back Meadows and, further complicating matters, the trail is incorrectly shown arcing high around the head of the canyon on the U.S. Geological Survey map. The fact that cows are allowed to graze in this area, creating additional stock trails in the process, doesn't help matters either when attempting to discern the actual route of the trail. Well-defined tread exits the far side of the meadows around 7000 feet (directly east of the last "s" in "Springs" as shown on the USGS map), but first you have to get there. The first step is to cross the meadows and the creek—doing so on the designated route of the trail would be optimum, but attempting to figure out which of the many faint paths is the correct one can be a frustrating experience. Once across, look for distinct tread climbing up the hillside near a tiny tributary in the vicinity of a low rock hump, which sits just below a larger, low rock hump. In case you need it, a primitive campsite is nearby.

Initially the trail climbs away from Back Meadows extremely steeply via some short-legged switchbacks. Fortunately, the grade eases from sadistic to steep, following longer-legged switchbacks through shady forest. Farther up the slope you break out into the open and follow tighter switchbacks to the top of a ridge with stunning views of the Trinity Alps and down into Shackleford Creek canyon, including Campbell and Cliff lakes.

From the crest, you follow the zigzagging course of the trail down open slopes. The route is easily lost in a patch of lush vegetation about halfway down the slope. If you lose the trail and can't find it again, head for a large cairn well down the hillside on the right-hand side of the clearing near the edge of the forest. Here distinct tread veers into the trees and descends steeply before traversing over to the crossing of a narrow stream. From there, head down a dry, grassy clearing with good views across the canyon and follow cairns across Long High Creek and back into the forest, where you immediately reach a junction with the trail to Calf Lake. If you want to squeeze one more night of camping out of your trip, Calf Lake is a little over a mile and 1000 vertical feet up this trail.

From the Calf Lake junction, your descent continues through light forest. Farther downslope, a series of switchbacks augments the descent on the way to Dog Wallow Meadow and the crossing of a pair of rivulets. More switchbacks lead down to another pair of rivulets just before a junction with a trail west to Log Lake. Veer left at the junction and continue the descent, crossing yet another tiny creek before zigzagging down to a junction with the Shackleford Creek Trail at the close of the loop. From there, retrace your steps 2.3 miles back to the trailhead.

BUILD-UP AND WIND-DOWN TIPS ·

Free overnight camping is allowed near the trailhead. The closest developed campgrounds, **Indian Scotty** and **Bridge Flat**, are accessible from Scott River Road. Although you may be able to procure a few necessities in Fort Jones, you'll have to go all the way to Yreka for most services.

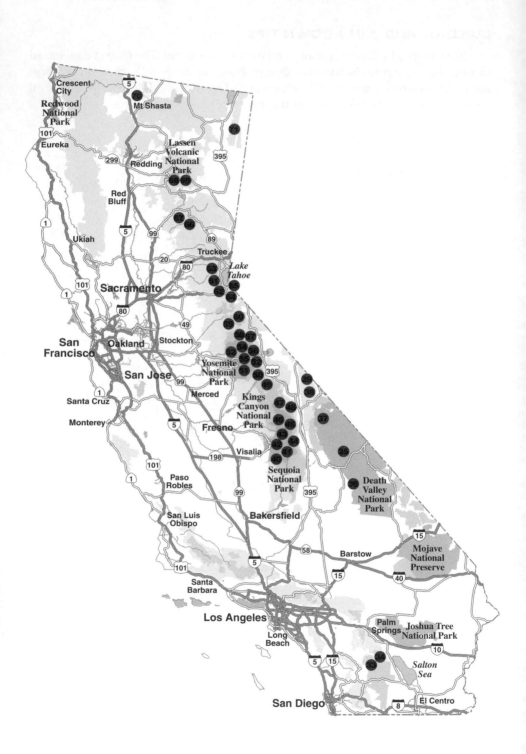

EASTERN CALIFORNIA

DESERT

ANZA-BORREGO DESERT STATE PARK

Anza-Borrego Desert State Park offers a vast landscape of over 1000 square miles spanning the eastern half of San Diego County and portions of Riverside and Imperial counties that rivals many national parks in its diversity and natural resources. Lying adjacent to the famous San Andreas Fault Zone on the eastern edge of the Pacific Plate, the geology of this region is highly influenced by tectonic activity that has raised mountains 2 miles high and dropped nearby basins below sea level to create this rugged yet sublime landscape. In the northern portion of Anza-Borrego, the very active San Jacinto Fault Zone has created vast wilderness panoramas ranging from gaping basins and soaring escarpments to sun-baked dry lakes and occasionally muddy playas to snow-covered winter peaks.

One of the least known and most remote portions of this park is in this northern section bordering the Santa Rosa and San Jacinto Mountains National Monument along the San Diego and Riverside County line. This area lies within both state and federal wilderness areas. The Santa Rosa Mountains Wilderness, at more than 100,000 acres, was part of the original selection creating the California Wilderness Preservation System in 1974. Its boundaries are within the state park. Just north of this area is the Santa Rosa Wilderness, created in 1984. At more than 70,000 acres, it is a very isolated area administered by the Bureau of Land Management. A dramatic entry into the heart of these wilderness areas is through Clark Valley in the northeastern Anza-Borrego. It is a challenging but profound desert experience that offers cross-country backpackers solitude, rock-lined canyons, sweeping views, Indian ruins, shade-covered campsites, and sparse but dependable water supplies.

The best backpacking opportunities in the Anza-Borrego region are found in this same general location due to dependable water supplies, interesting and variable terrain and the general isolation found in wilderness areas. All of the westside canyons along Coyote Creek and off Collins Valley offer good campsites, many with cottonwoods, alders, or palm trees. There are also opportunities for exploration and cross-country travel between canyons.

DEATH VALLEY NATIONAL PARK

Death Valley and the desert ranges surrounding it are protected as Death Valley National Park, located in eastern California and southwestern Nevada, roughly between Owens Valley and the Nevada border. Like most desert valleys in the Basin and Range Province, Death Valley is a long, southwest-trending sink framed on both sides by high-reaching mountains, formed a few million years ago by block-faulting fueled by tectonic forces.

Although it is famous mostly for its high-temperature records, what distinguishes it from other North American deserts is that it is a land of extreme contrast. The lowest point on the valley floor, a few miles from a small salt-saturated pond called Badwater, is 282 feet below sea level—the lowest point in the western hemisphere and most likely the hottest place on Earth. Just 17 air miles to the east rises Telescope Peak, at 11,049 feet the highest summit in the park and often snow-covered in winter. This amazing juxtaposition makes Death Valley the deepest depression in the continental U.S. and twice as deep as the Grand Canyon. This wild range of elevations, combined with a particularly varied and tumultuous geology, has produced an incredible diversity of landscapes. Immense salt flats and exquisite sand dunes dot the wide open valley. On both sides rise rugged, majestic mountains, the home of badlands, extinct volcanoes, fossil beds, mysterious narrows, and deep canyons that wind many miles and thousands of feet up to woodlands of pines and juniper. Although this is one of the driest places in North America, water does come to this bone-dry land in the form of summer storms, winter rains and snow, and underground seeps.

Death Valley has had a long history of human occupation. For centuries, scant populations of Native American tribes migrated from valley floor in winter to higher summits in summer to take advantage of the annual cycle of temperature, vegetation, and wildlife. As early as 1860, and until fairly recently, this region attracted a surprising number of miners, ranchers, fortune seekers, and charlatans in search of unexplored destinations. Of the hundreds of ventures that came to life over the following century, many were as extreme as the land to which they were drawn. In the 1880s a rich industrialist put Death Valley on the map by delivering borax in 20-mule teams. The Keane Wonder Mine erected a heroic mile-long tramway down the precipitous Funeral Mountains and produced nearly 1 million dollars in gold. And in the 1910s, a rich investor built a lavish castle of royal dimensions that would eventually be named after notorious con man Death Valley Scotty.

Few deserts in the world are as colorful, varied, and rich in human and natural history as Death Valley. With such attributes, Death Valley National Park is a tremendous haven for hiking and exploration. It offers unparalleled seclusion, spectacular scenery, and unconventional beauty still seldom appreciated and revered. The sense of freedom when hiking long distances through such quasi-limitless spaces is exhilarating.

But do not underestimate the dangers of backpacking in this desert, especially if you are an adept backpacker familiar with more temperate regions. Death Valley is much rougher, much hotter, and much less forgiving. Trails are almost nonexistent; most of your walking will be cross-country. The terrain is usually rocky and uneven, with slopes averaging 20 percent on the way up to mountains and steeper in the mountains themselves. You will not periodically run across trees to seek shelter, a river or lake to quench your thirst or cool down, or bushes to glean a snack. Vast tracks of this enormous park—about 4½ times Yosemite National Park—hardly ever see humans. If you become stranded, it will likely be days, if not weeks, before someone happens to come by.

Become familiar also with the park regulations; they differ from that of other parks. Camping within 200 yards of any source of water is prohibited. Treat all spring water before drinking. Do not remove or disturb rocks, historic and prehistoric artifacts, plants or animals, including rock art and any mine ruins. Collecting firewood and ground fires are not permitted in the backcountry. Overnight backcountry camping within 2 miles of a major road is prohibited, and some backcountry roads are off-limit to camping as well. Check with the park service for a more complete set of rules.

WHITE AND INYO MOUNTAINS

Rising to the east of Owens Valley, which is itself east of the Sierra Nevada, the White and Inyo mountains are the westernmost of the Great Basin mountain ranges, located along the California-Nevada border. Except to visit either the Schulman and Patriarch groves of bristlecone pines or the summit of White Mountain Peak (one of California's 14ers), very few people venture into these mountains. The region's remote location, lack of constructed trails, and often tedious driving to reach "trailheads" keep most people out. However, those who do visit these mountains will find slot canyons at the lowest elevations, amazing alpine plateaus at the highest elevations, and pinyon-juniper woodlands in-between.

The east and west flanks of the mountains are steep, with the slopes broken by many narrow canyons. In contrast, much of the crest of the White Mountains is rolling hills, covered with large stretches of alpine meadow, sagebrush flats, or in places, talus. There are no lakes within these mountain ranges, but springs exist throughout and many of the drainages sport intermittent or permanent streams.

ADVICE FOR DESERT HIKING AND BACKPACKING

The three main issues one must typically deal with when hiking in the desert are elevated temperatures, lack of native water, and dehydration/stroke. Water sources are generally scarce to nonexistent, and they are often biologically contaminated by wildlife. The absolute golden rule you must *never* break is to always take plenty of water with you, even if you think you are only going a short distance. In the cooler months, count on drinking about as much as you would in temperate regions. When the temperature exceeds 100°F, allow at least one quart per person per hour of walking on level ground, much more on steep climbs. Take mineral/vitamin tablets to offset the loss of these elements through perspiration. Always carry purifying tablets with you, in case you need to drink spring or rain water. If you run low on water, don't save your water but drink it when you are thirsty so you don't get sick. Finally, always stash a few gallons of water in your vehicle for emergency.

Dehydration (and possibly a stroke) is one of your biggest enemies. To reduce the risk of dehydration, drink often and enough, travel in early mornings and late afternoons or later, wear a hat and long-sleeved shirts and pants, and hole up in the shade away from the wind during the day. Learn to recognize the symptoms of dehydration, such as persistent thirst, dark urine, and heat exhaustion, which may evolve into dizziness and vomiting. Pay close attention to these signs: They could be warnings of serious trouble. If you suspect dehydration, rest, cool down, drink, and get back to your vehicle as soon as you are well enough to do so safely.

The desert holds other, smaller dangers, such as rattlesnakes, mine hazards, flash floods, a flat tire, and a disabled vehicle. Even smaller hazards you may read about, from cactus thorns to slippery rocks, twisted ankles, and getting lost, are far less likely to get you in major trouble.

If you are new to the desert, before embarking on a backpacking trip, practice by taking hikes of increasing length and difficulty over a period of a few months. Read a desert survival guide, and memorize its key points. Take these preliminary steps even if you are an adept backpacker; familiarity with temperate regions leaves you wholly unprepared for tackling the desert in summer. Always let someone know where you are going, and arrange for a time by which someone will initiate a search-and-rescue party if you do not call.

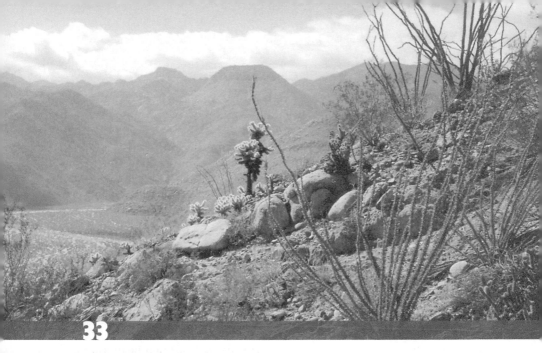

33

BUTLER AND COYOTE CANYON LOOP

Lowell and Diana Lindsay

MILES: 18.0
RECOMMENDED DAYS: 2
ELEVATION GAIN/LOSS: 2160´/2160´
TYPE OF TRIP: Loop
DIFFICULTY: Moderately strenuous
SOLITUDE: Moderate solitude
LOCATION: Anza-Borrego Desert State Park
MAPS: USGS 7.5-min. *Clark Lake, Clark Lake NE, Collins Valley,* and *Borrego Palm Canyon*
BEST SEASON: Winter through spring

PERMITS

No permits are required, but it is wise to check in and out at the Anza-Borrego Desert State Park (ABDSP) visitor center in Borrego Springs (760-767-4205). They will notify a ranger if you don't check back in after a reasonable amount of time has passed.

Photo: View west into Coyote Canyon

TAKE THIS TRIP

If you were to frame the perfect desert backpack, it would have a narrow snaking gorge with steep walls, American Indian sites, running water, spectacular views of both high mountain escarpments and desert lowlands, a register to record your crossing over Alcoholic Pass, and segments of total solitude and silence. All of these await you on this trip—a high-quality escape that's close to civilization. After a day's workout winding down shaded desert canyons, Coyote Creek will be a refreshing place to cool off. Enjoy the chorus of frogs at the water's edge.

CHALLENGES

The most challenging portion of this trip is at the beginning, working your way up the mouth of the rocky gorge of Butler Canyon and identifying the route up to the playa on the ridge. Carry sufficient water during the day as the only available water on this trip is Coyote Creek on the far side of the Butler/Box Canyon ridge. The Coyote Canyon segment of this trip is along a jeep route and later a high-clearance vehicle route—watch out for passing vehicles.

HOW TO GET THERE

From State Highway 86 (Salton City), travel west 21.3 miles on County S-22 to the paved turnoff just east of mile marker 26. Turn north (right) and proceed northeasterly toward Clark Dry Lake. From Borrego Springs, travel east 7.2 miles on Highway S-22 to this turnoff on the north (left) side.

A high-clearance vehicle is recommended for the road to Rockhouse Canyon. Drive northeast (leaving pavement after 0.7 mile and passing a gravel pit on the left) to the signed Rockhouse Canyon turnoff after 1.6 miles from Highway S-22. Turn northwest (left) at this junction and drive another 7.7 miles around Clark Dry Lake and past the northeast wedge of Coyote Mountain. Beware of sand traps north of here and continue to the junction of Butler and Rockhouse canyons and park. (Do not attempt to cross Clark Dry Lake if it is wet or muddy—you will get stuck.)

TRIP DESCRIPTION

From the junction of Rockhouse and Butler Canyons at 1200 feet in elevation, begin by following vehicle tracks a mile northwest (left) up to the entrance of Butler Canyon (the lower end of Dry Wash). Proceed up-canyon working around granitic boulders as the walls close in on the twisting, climbing passageway. Note the slick surfaces carved out by flash floods

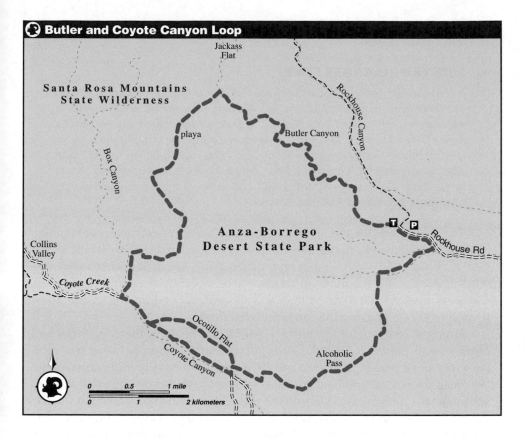

Butler and Coyote Canyon Loop

that have periodically spewed out from Dry Wash and Jackass Flat. Gradually the canyon opens up and flattens out at a huge saddle-shaped boulder in the wash at 4.4 miles and 2020 feet. (A long-abandoned two-wheel cart marked this point as late as 2007.) In less than another half mile, search the west (left) slope of the canyon at 4.8 miles and 2080 feet just before (south of) a steep gully entering

DESERT LAND NAVIGATION

Cross-country trips demand special pre-trip preparation and careful study of the hike's route. Be sure to trek deliberately when following faint trails, diverging routes, or rock cairns (ducks). Evidence of ancient Indian and mining trails is intermittent and scattered in the desert. While ducks may be helpful, they should be used with discretion considering that they occasionally end abruptly with no clue as to where to go next. Consult your map constantly, compass frequently, and take notes often. Even if the notes are not critical to the current trip, they could be lifesavers for the next. They may also be entertaining to your survivors.

from the west (left) for a trail, actually an ancient Indian trail, proceeding south-westerly up the slope.

SIDE TRIP: JACKASS FLAT

If you intentionally or inadvertently pass this Butler Canyon checkpoint (2080) and continue north another half mile, you will enter Jackass Flat, which sprawls to the east and north against Buck Ridge. The eastern edge of the flat is the site of a former Cahuilla Indian village. Look for scattered pottery shards and morteros, or grinding holes. A major summer solstice site is also located on the flat. All Indian artifacts are protected. Look and wonder, but please don't disturb anything. Return to the Butler Canyon checkpoint (2080) and climb up the slope. This side trip adds about 2.5 miles to your total distance.

The objective at the top of the slope is a broad near-level area, containing a shallow depression or "playa" (at 2620 feet in elevation), in the west half of Section 12 on the *Collins Valley* topographic map. Such elevated, undrained playas, while uncommon in mountainous areas, can be found in several places on these Coyote Canyon and Dry Wash ridges and are evidence of dramatic seismic activity and recent uplift along the San Jacinto fault zone.

From the east side of the playa, continue south along the vague trail and cross a small saddle at 6.4 miles and 2730 feet in elevation between two pica-chos (or "small peaks" 2760 west and 2810 east). You have joyfully crossed into the vast Coyote Creek watershed and now want to descend southerly and then southwesterly, staying generally on the ridgeline into the Box Canyon drainage. Avoid dropping from the ridgeline into small but deep canyons on either side until you near the bottom of Box Canyon. As the ridgeline turns clearly west at 2000 feet in elevation, arc a bit to the northwest (right) and descend into shallow tributary canyon to exit west (left) onto the floor of Box Canyon at 8.4 miles and an elevation of 1610 feet. Turn south (left) and descend Box Canyon to enter Coyote Canyon at 9.7 miles and an elevation of 1190 feet between Lower Willows and Third Crossing at 9.9 miles of Coyote Creek.

Camp nearby or hike west (right) into Collins Valley to find a more isolated campsite along gurgling Coyote Creek. From Third Crossing it is a leisurely 2.8-

HIKING DISTANCES IN THE DESERT ARE FARTHER THAN THEY SEEM

Cross-country travel estimates in the desert are not equivalent to travel on established trails like the Pacific Crest Trail or even on city sidewalks. Allow extra time. An estimated pace of 1 to 2 miles per hour should be used for planning purposes, especially when bouldery and brushy terrain is expected (which is almost always). If you underestimate the time it will take to reach your destination, you may find yourself caught in the dark or short of water. Always carry a light and extra batteries and water.

mile hike downstream following the jeep route to the Alcoholic Pass turnoff 0.5 mile southeast of (beyond) Desert Gardens. The gardens are marked by a table and bench and commemorate the work of the Anza-Borrego Committee (now Foundation) to acquire private landholdings within the park for public benefit. (Alternately you could hike a couple additional flat miles on the Ocotillo Flat horse trail, which loops northeast from Second Crossing along the colorful Coyote Badlands and then southeast to First Crossing to rejoin the road.)

The Alcoholic Pass Trail at 12.7 miles and 920 feet is an Indian route between Coyote Canyon and Rockhouse Canyon. Follow the trail up the rocky ridge and discover a trail register en route to the saddle, which is at 13.9 miles and 1550 feet. Three miles farther, down a prominent wash, is the Rockhouse Canyon Road. Turn northwest (left) and continue about a mile to the Rockhouse/Butler Canyon junction to complete the loop.

BUILD-UP AND WIND-DOWN TIPS

For last-minute hiking gear, go to **True Value Hardware** just east of Christmas Circle or to **Borrego Outfitters** in the mall near **Kendall's Restaurant**, which is open early for breakfast. For last-minute food supplies, there's the **grocery store** hidden across the street from the mall behind the shops on the north side of the street. For a great inexpensive dinner after your trip, try a taco at **Hilberto's** just west of Christmas Circle in Borrego Springs. Borrego midnight is 9 PM. The only place open for a late meal or drink is **Carlee's**, across the street from Hilberto's.

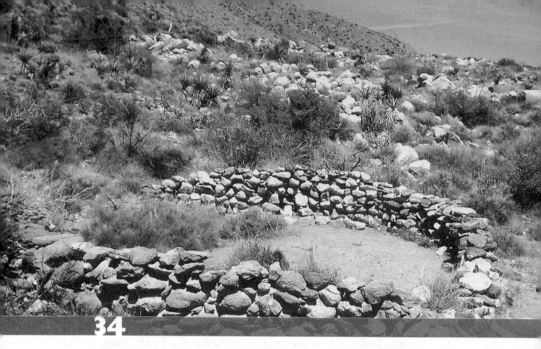

34

ROCKHOUSE VALLEY LOOP

Lowell and Diana Lindsay

MILES: 24.7 (almost all cross-country)
RECOMMENDED DAYS: 2–3
ELEVATION GAIN/LOSS: 3650´/3650´
TYPE OF TRIP: Loop
DIFFICULTY: Strenuous
SOLITUDE: Solitude
LOCATION: Anza-Borrego Desert State Park;
Santa Rosa and San Jacinto Mountains National Monument
MAPS: USGS 7.5-min. *Clark Lake NE* and *Collins Valley*
BEST SEASON: Winter through spring

PERMITS ·

No permit is required, but it is essential to check in and out at the Anza-Borrego Desert State Park (ABDSP) visitor center in Borrego Springs (760-767-4205). They will notify a ranger if you don't check back in after a reasonable amount of time has passed.

Photo: View from Old Santa Rosa southeast into Rockhouse Valley

CHALLENGES

Excellent cross-country navigation skills are required as sign (evidence) of the ancient Indian and mining trails is, at best, vague and intermittent. The only reliable water is an isolated spring in Nicholias Canyon, *but be sure to carry sufficient water for an unplanned day's travel* back to the road if you don't locate this spring. "Seeps" shown on topographic maps are iffy. Dry waterfalls (which are class 3 and require some chimneying but are not exposed) and thick brush in Nicholias Canyon require care and transit time allowed in hours per mile. This is the desert, after all; it's different out here.

HOW TO GET THERE

Go east from Borrego Springs or west from Salton City on County Highway S-22 to mile marker 26 (near the Pegleg Lost Mine monument.) Turn northeast onto the briefly paved road just east of mile 26 into Clark Dry Lake and Valley and Rockhouse Canyon. A high-clearance vehicle is recommended for the road to Rockhouse Canyon.

Drive northeast to the signed Rockhouse Canyon turnoff after 1.6 miles from Highway S-22. Turn northwest (left) at this junction, and drive another 7.7 miles around Clark Dry Lake (don't cross Clark Dry Lake if it is wet or muddy—you will get stuck) and past the northeast wedge of Coyote Mountain. Beware of sand traps north of here and continue to the junction of Butler and Rockhouse Canyons and park (9.3 miles from Highway S-22). Unless you are a very experienced off-road driver and choose to drive 3.1 rugged miles up the trail in a four-wheel-drive vehicle, commence hiking up-canyon northerly (right) from here.

TAKE THIS TRIP

For total wilderness solitude within a short distance of civilization, this trip can't be beat. Visiting the Old Santa Rosa Indian ruins perched on the edge of Rockhouse Valley is a trip back into a timeless past. One can almost feel the intrusion of grubbing miners who left their rusting tools so close to village sites. Camping in the shaded cottonwood grove beneath Toro Peak with a running spring nearby should tempt you to delay your departure for another day or more.

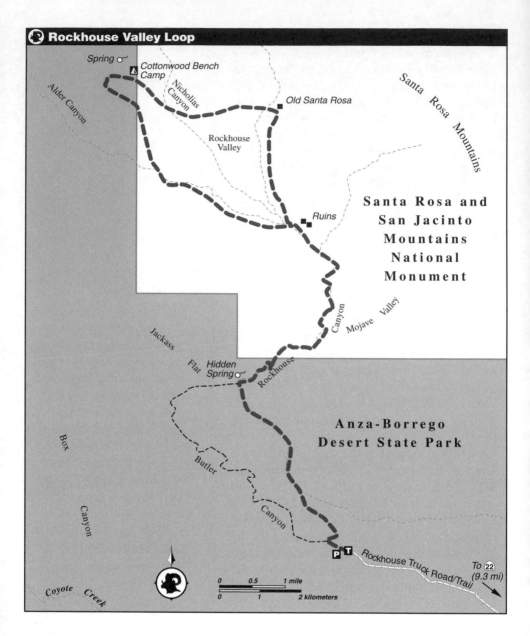

Rockhouse Valley Loop

Spring

Cottonwood Bench Camp

Nicholias Canyon

Alder Canyon

Old Santa Rosa

Santa Rosa Mountains

Rockhouse Valley

Santa Rosa and San Jacinto Mountains National Monument

Ruins

Canyon

Mojave Valley

Jackass

Flat

Hidden Spring

Rockhouse

Box

Butler

Anza-Borrego Desert State Park

Canyon

Canyon

Canyon

P T

Rockhouse Truck Road/Trail

To (22) (9.3 mi)

Coyote Creek

0   0.5   1 mile
0   1   2 kilometers

TRIP DESCRIPTION

Hike from the junction at 1200 feet in elevation to signed Hidden Spring at 3.6 miles and 2040 feet on the west bank (left) of the canyon. Its paltry water production is owned by too many bees and salts for your liking, but any water is a highlight in this arid area. Jackass Flat (described in the Butler and Coyote Canyon Loop, Trip 33) is atop this bank and is accessible by a steep but short trail slightly south (left) from the spring.

Continue up-canyon from Hidden Spring to a granitic barrier across the wash at 4.1 miles and 2200 feet. From a point about 15 yards before the barrier, carefully ascend a route up and around on the north (left) side. After another pleasant, sandy mile the canyon opens up where Mojave Valley enters from the east (right). Bear north (left) up Rockhouse Canyon.

From Hidden Spring, it is 3.5 miles to the grand entrance into Rockhouse Valley at 7.1 miles and 2800 feet, backdropped by the soaring massif of Toro Peak, at 8716 feet the high point of the Santa Rosa Mountains. Proceed northwesterly up Alder Canyon wash, close against Buck Ridge. After another half mile the first group of rock houses are northeast (right) on a rocky bench atop a long narrow ridge that divides Alder Canyon wash from a smaller, more north-trending wash. Three major rock houses with walls two to three feet in height soon emerge like phantoms to the discerning eye. From here, 7.6 miles and 2970 feet in elevation, you have two options to reach Cottonwood Bench (grove) in Nicholias Canyon (labeled "Old Nicholas Canyon" on the 1942 USGS topo map).

The "high road" route (more brushy and rocky) is to ascend northwest (right) through the valley toward a low ridge between Nicholias Canyon and herein-named "White Cliff Wash." A ducked trail is visible intermittently leading via the southwest (left) slope of the ridge into Nicholias Canyon and the grove campsite. (The return route involves this trail after leaving the campsite as described below.)

For your outbound leg, follow "the low road" route (more sandy and open) west-northwest (left) via Alder Canyon wash 2.5 miles to its junction with Nicholias Canyon, at 10.1 miles and 3680 feet. The trick is identifying the turnoff to Nicholias because Alder, the larger canyon, continues straight on northwest. Nicholias is the small, steep canyon to the northeast (right) just before a large dry waterfall in Alder Canyon at 3700 feet in elevation. Immediately after you turn right into Nicholias Canyon, the canyon angles to the left and the first of three dry waterfalls that you must scale is visible; each of them is about 10 feet tall and has good hand- and footholds. It would be good to carry a short line with you to haul up your backpack if you are unsteady climbing the dry waterfalls while wearing a backpack. One dry waterfall requires climbing up a small chimney. After the waterfalls the canyon opens up and becomes very brushy. Farther up look for abandoned mining equipment near the site of an old mine at 4500 feet.

DESERT PLANTS CAN HURT YOU

In the desert you are guaranteed to get pricked and scratched, especially hiking in brushy or cactus-covered areas. Hike in long-sleeved shirts and long pants to protect against thorny and prickly plants. Especially irritating and nasty are the microscopic barbs (glochids) on beavertail cactus. Carry first aid supplies, including a comb, tweezers, pliers (a Leatherman is great), and masking tape (which works better than Scotch tape) to remove glochids.

From the mine ruins, climb the ridge northwest to the second site of rock house ruins. East of these ruins at 12.1 miles and 4850 feet is a flat area known as Cottonwood Bench (grove), a great campsite or base camp for several days of exploration in this rich area. A mile-long trail leads northwest from the grove and then northeast (right) down into the thick vegetation in a gully to the spring that, according to meager reports, is potable and runs year-round.

To complete the loop back down via the Old Santa Rosa Indian ruins and then through Rockhouse Valley to the roadhead, follow the ducked trail from the grove to the southeast over a small rise. Contour some 2.5 miles easterly at about 4200 feet via intermittent trail traces and ducks in the upper reaches of "White Cliff Wash" to find the third set of rock houses—the Old Santa Rosa village group at 14.6 miles. As with most rock houses, and indeed most archaeological treasures, they are strangely felt before they are seen.

From the village site, you can see south across the valley to the low point, marked by a light-colored sandy area, at the confluence of Rockhouse Valley washes into the canyon. Select the trace trails of your choice to descend 3 miles across the valley to complete the loop, at 17.6 miles and 2800 feet, and descend 7.1 miles through the canyon to the roadhead at the Butler/Rockhouse Canyon junction.

BUILD-UP AND WIND-DOWN TIPS

If you have at least five days available, combine this loop with the Butler and Coyote Canyon Loop (Trip 33). Both trips begin at the same point, and you can restock at your car. If you are looking for a late meal after your trip, go to **Carlee's** in Borrego Springs, just west of Christmas Circle. Borrego Springs shuts down early, but Carlee's stays open until midnight. For an early breakfast, try a stack of blueberry pancakes at **Kendall's** in the mall. For supplies you have forgotten, try **Borrego Outfitters** in the mall or **True Value Hardware** just east of the circle. The **grocery store** is hidden behind stores across the street from the mall on the north side of Highway S-22/Palm Canyon Drive.

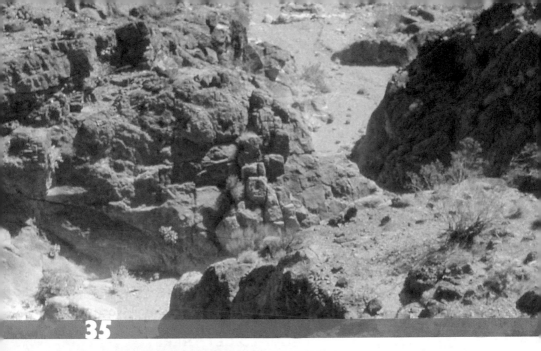

35

MARBLE CANYON TO COTTONWOOD CANYON LOOP

Michel Digonnet

MILES: 26.5
RECOMMENDED DAYS: 3
ELEVATION GAIN/LOSS: 3750´/3750´
TYPE OF TRIP: Loop
DIFFICULTY: Moderately strenuous
SOLITUDE: Solitude
LOCATION: Death Valley National Park
MAPS: USGS 7.5-min. *East of Sand Flat*, *Cottonwood Canyon*,
and *Harris Hill*
BEST SEASONS: Spring and fall

PERMITS

A permit is not required, but check with a park ranger (760-786-2331) in case regulations change.

CHALLENGES

If you are new to desert backpacking, first read up on the particular dangers this area presents—heat exhaustion and strokes, dehydration, mines, rattlesnakes, flash floods, hantavirus—and how to best avoid them. Then practice

Photo: Side canyon in lower Marble Canyon

by taking a few dozen dayhikes of increasing length and difficulty. Always let someone know your itinerary, and stick to it. And be sure to keep several gallons of water in your car because they might save your life that one day you return parched from too many water-less miles in three-digit temperatures. Check with the park for a complete set of regulations because they differ from those of other parks.

The only reliable water is at the springs in Cottonwood Canyon. So lugging a heavy pack through trailless desert country is one challenge. The others are bushwhacking through the springs and route-finding from Dead Horse Canyon to Cottonwood Canyon.

HOW TO GET THERE

In Stovepipe Wells, look for the Cotton-wood Canyon Road on the left side of the campground entrance. Follow it 8.6 miles to an open area on the edge of the wide wash of Cottonwood Canyon. This road is sandy at first, then a washboard for several miles, and it has a little soft gravel near the end, but a passenger car can usually make it this far. The road continues roughly west up the wash 2.2 miles to the junction with Marble Canyon. Along the way, it winds through the lower narrows of Cottonwood Canyon, a deep pas-sage framed by awesome walls. Just past the narrows' abrupt end, the road veers left and follows the south wall (do *not* drive up the wide canyon straight ahead, which is usually blocked off by a sign and a log). The junction with Marble Canyon is 0.8 mile farther. It is easy to miss: Look for the old MARBLE CANYON sign on the north side of the wash. Park with-out blocking the way but within a few feet of the road.

This final 2.2-mile stretch is rougher and requires good clearance. If you are driving a standard-clearance vehicle, start hiking from the open area, which will add 4.4 miles to the total hiking distance.

TAKE THIS TRIP

This is a Death Valley clas-sic, and one of the park's best backpacking routes. From the western edge of Death Valley, this loop first goes up through spec-tacular Marble Canyon, where long, tight narrows adorned with beautiful petroglyphs will guide you deep into the mountain. You will then look for a cross-country route across a rarely traveled ridge to upper Cottonwood Canyon, the wildest and only challenging part of this hike. In Cottonwood Canyon, you will hike down through three amaz-ing springs, lush islands of cottonwoods, willows, and grapevine miraculously irrigated by a perennial creek. The inner canyon below the springs wind through a meandering gorge and offers several exciting side canyons for further exploration.

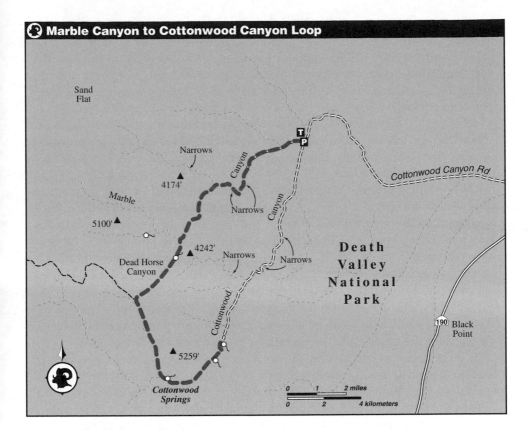

Marble Canyon to Cottonwood Canyon Loop

Sand Flat

Narrows

Canyon

4174'

Marble

5100'

Narrows

Canyon

Dead Horse
Canyon

4242'   Narrows   Narrows

**Death
Valley
National
Park**

Cottonwood

5259'

Cottonwood Canyon Rd

190 Black
Point

Cottonwood
Springs

0   1   2 miles
0   2   4 kilometers

TRIP DESCRIPTION

At the junction, the Marble Canyon Road is the one that goes up the open wash on the right. The other one is the Cottonwood Canyon Road, the way you will be coming back. The first 2.4 miles along the Marble Canyon Road are up over coarse alluvia and not very exciting, except for the views of the rugged high slopes of the Cottonwood Mountains. Then you enter Marble Canyon's first narrows, and your surroundings change abruptly. For the next mile or so, you walk through a colorful corridor framed by vertical walls underneath massive tilted strata that shoot up to the distant rim. At places, the walls are less than 10 feet apart. This scenic, more shaded corridor ends at an enormous boulder wedged between the walls. You might need a 20-foot rope to hoist your pack to the top. The second narrows, a short distance farther, rank among the most impressive in the park. They begin as a tight channel in gray dolomite, gradually deepen, open up for a short distance, then tighten again. The polished walls lean high above the gravel wash, folding into a serpentine passage where light changes continuously throughout the day.

The section of more open canyon above it skirts impressive high walls of colorfully stratified limestone and dolomite. This area is sprinkled with little surprises—constrictions, side canyons, and a few good exposures of fossil shells, especially on the polished, slanted walls of dark dolomite on the south side. The first side canyon on the north side above the second narrows has unusual walls packed with large nodules, scattered fossils of large gastropods, and eventually some amazing narrows. The third narrows, shorter and less spectacular, go through high black-and-white banded walls and end at another huge boulder. This area contains finely polished displays of marble, white grading into gray, which might be this canyon's namesake. From here it is a short distance to Dead Horse Canyon, where you will leave Marble Canyon. If for some reason you desperately need water while in this vicinity, the closest reliable water is at Goldbelt Spring, 5.8 miles up-canyon.

While hiking through Marble Canyon, keep an eye open for petroglyphs, figures pecked in the rock by the aboriginal cultures that lived here centuries ago. Such sites are common in the Southwest, but they are generally smaller in Death Valley, a reflection of the harsher climate. Marble Canyon, however, is blessed with one of the highest densities of petroglyphs in the park. The local rock art varies greatly in subject matter, size, and level of detail. Some beautiful figures adorn walls and boulders, abstract drawings and pregnant bighorn sheep, lizards, birds, and anthropomorphic images. Many of these sites have been badly damaged by vandalism. Remember that petroglyphs are part of a sacred cultural heritage. Do not touch or deface them; they are protected by federal law.

To cut across to Cottonwood Canyon, head up into Dead Horse Canyon. You first go through a narrow stretch, then a constriction, and finally reach a little spring in a long right bend in the canyon. This is the start of the crux. About 0.9 mile from Marble Canyon, you reach the thickest part of the spring, at the southernmost point in the bend. On the spring's south side, a ravine climbs to the south-southwest. Follow it to the ridge top (0.6 mile, very steep at the end, elevation of about 4220 feet) then drop down the far side into a drainage (300 yards). This small canyon has several forks in this vicinity. Hike up the main one, which has a spring and heads roughly southwest. About 1.2 miles beyond the spring, shortly after a long meander, take the side canyon that points to the southwest, and stay with it in this general direction until it tops an open crest overlooking a broad south-trending valley, which is the upper drainage of Cottonwood Canyon. Climb down the steep slope to the valley floor, and you are done with

DANGERS OF THE DESERT

To bring the dangers of the desert into proper perspective, here are some of my personal statistics. In thousands of miles of hiking in the California desert, I have seen less than a half dozen rattlesnakes, and all the ones who were awake gave me a fair warning. I have seen no flash floods, mountain lions, scorpions, or rock falls, but I have had many flat tires and have been dehydrated numerous times, even though I never ran out of water.

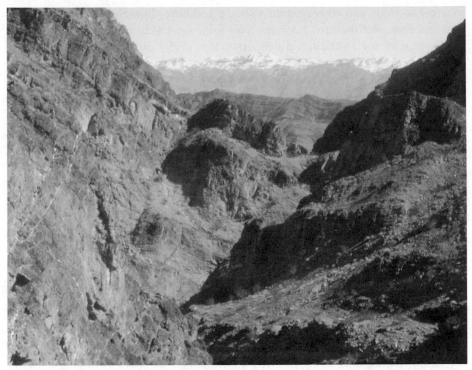

Narrows in side canyon of Marble Canyon

the crux. The quadrangle map definitely helps minimize backtracking. If you get lost, retrace your steps and hike back to your car.

The next stretch, down the valley, is open and uneventful, but it is downhill over easy terrain, and the scenery is about to change dramatically. After 3.3 miles, you reach the head of Cottonwood Creek, an amazing desert stream that gives rise to three luxuriant oases. The uppermost oasis, known as Cottonwood Springs, starts at the bottom of the valley, where it veers abruptly east and squeezes into a real canyon trapped between 1000-foot desert hills. A profusion of healthy trees block the entrance to the canyon, and for the next mile you have to find a passage through the dense vegetation. For easier walking and to avoid damaging this unique riparian system, bypass portions of it on the faint trail 30–50 feet above the wash on the north side. The going is not always easy, but the rewards match the efforts. Here in the heart of an overwhelmingly dry land, you stroll along a vigorous stream, under the canopy of old cottonwoods and tall willows covered with hanging grapevine. In the summer, you find welcome shade, coyote and bighorn tracks along sandy bottoms, and a surprising variety of birds. In the fall, look for the golden gourds of coyote melons, or a lone tarantula tiptoeing across the sand. Later in the season, the yellowing trees and carpets of dead leaves give a rare autumn flavor to this refreshing scenery.

At the east end of Cottonwood Springs, the creek goes underground and the vegetation ends abruptly. The transition from spring to desert is stunning:

In a few seconds you emerge from a shady and humid jungle into bright water-less expanses. For the next 1.1 miles you follow a sandy wash, until you reach the middle spring. Although much drier, it is still a delightful place, invaded by dark, muddy swamps where plants totally unexpected in the desert thrive, like watercress and a large mushroom called desert puffball. Below this smaller spring, there is another 0.5-mile length of open wash to the lower spring. This one has several good runs of flowing water, on average a couple of inches deep and 1 or 2 feet wide. In late October I once estimated its flow at a hefty 30 gallons per minute. In the shade of tall trees, grasses, cattails, cane, and willow shoots jostle for sipping rights along the creek. Here as at the middle spring, you might get wet crossing the brush-choked stream. Following the animal tracks on either side of the groves helps reduce bushwhacking.

The lower spring ends at the upper end of the Cottonwood Canyon Road. The rest of the canyon is dry, so fill up in preparation for the home run. Remember that camping is allowed anywhere in Cottonwood Canyon except within 200 yards of the springs. Water at the springs is usually abundant year-round, but treat it before drinking.

The rest of Cottonwood Canyon down to the Marble Canyon junction (8.4 miles) is fairly wide, straight, and less eventful—except for the narrows and the side canyons. The narrows start 1.5 miles below the lower spring. For no less than 2 miles, the wash meanders tightly beneath rugged stone walls. The scenery changes gradually along the way as the gorge first cuts through dark-gray dolomite, then tilted strata of interbedded dolomite and limestone, and finally limestone. In the west wall about 1.4 miles down the narrows, there is a nice breccia of angular limestone blocks cemented with calcite, stream-polished into a fine panel of black and white mosaic.

Cottonwood Canyon has about a dozen side canyons. They are often narrower and windier than the main canyon, and all very different. A short hike into one of them may well turn out to be a highlight of your hike through this canyon. Try the side canyon on the west side just above the narrows. It is quite pretty, it has two beautiful tight narrows, and finding a route around its high falls and chockstones poses a stimulating challenge.

Don't miss the unusual 70-foot deep overhang in the east wall about 1 mile below the narrows. From there it is 3.9 miles down to the junction where you parked. It is open the whole way but the surrounding hills are quite scenic, and because the grades are uncommonly gentle the walking goes at a good clip—a good thing if you are low on water.

BUILD-UP AND WIND-DOWN TIPS

For a good meal in an old-west setting, go to the one and only restaurant in **Stovepipe Wells**. If you are new to Death Valley, check out the **Death Valley Dunes** just east of the small town and at least the lower reaches of nearby **Mosaic** and **Grotto canyons**. See also the recommendations on page 236.

36

SURPRISE CANYON

Michel Digonnet

MILES: 24.0

RECOMMENDED DAYS: 4

ELEVATION GAIN/LOSS: 9600´/8350´

TYPE OF TRIP: Point-to-point or out-and-back

DIFFICULTY: Moderately strenuous

SOLITUDE: Solitude

LOCATION: Surprise Canyon Wilderness (Bureau of Land Management) and Death Valley National Park

MAPS: USGS 7.5-min. *Ballarat*, *Panamint*, and *Telescope Peak*

BEST SEASONS: Spring and fall

PERMITS

A permit is not required, but check with a park ranger (760-786-2331) in case regulations change.

CHALLENGES

If you are new to desert backpacking, first read up on the particular dangers this area presents—heat exhaustion and strokes, dehydration, mines, rattlesnakes, flash floods, hantavirus—and how to best avoid them. Then practice by taking a few dozen dayhikes of increasing length and difficulty. Always let

Photo: Spring in Johnson Canyon

TAKE THIS TRIP

If there is one place in Death Valley National Park that makes sense to explore with a backpack, it has to be Surprise Canyon. In a desert world-famous for its extreme dryness and record-high temperatures, this anomalous canyon is blessed with several streams, and for a change you do not have to carry massive amounts of water. It is also exceptionally beautiful.

From the end of the road in the lower canyon, you hike through a series of idyllic springs coursed by spirited creeks to Panamint City, one of the most remote and historically significant mining centers in the California desert. Lost in seldom-visited high-desert country, within walking distance of perennial streams, this legendary site is a wonderful camping location from which to explore the area on leisurely hikes for two days. Miles of roads zigzag up into the surrounding mountains to scenic side canyons and dozens of fascinating historic sites—cabins, mills, and tunnels—left over from Panamint City's historic silver-mining boom of the 1870s. You will see lots of birds, run into burros every day, soak in cool springs, and walk through fragrant pine forests.

You complete your trek by continuing up canyon to spectacular Panamint Pass, then dropping along the famous "fresh vegetable route" into Johnson Canyon. This well-watered canyon takes you through verdant oases and the ruins of a historic Shoshone ranch all the way to the edge of Death Valley.

someone know your itinerary, and stick to it. And be sure to keep several gallons of water in your car because they might save your life that one day you return parched from too many waterless miles in three-digit temperatures. Check with the park for a complete set of regulations because they differ from those of other parks.

In spite of the reliable springs conveniently distributed along the way, you must still carry plenty of water, just in case, so one of the challenges is carrying a heavy pack. Bring a filter or purification tablets, and treat all water before drinking, as most sources are contaminated by wildlife. Another challenge is bushwhacking at some of Johnson Canyon's springs. In Surprise Canyon, since the road closure in 2001 the springs have been locally reclaiming the road, and some bushwhacking is also required. Except for summer, bring a warm sleeping bag, as nights are often surprisingly cold.

Avoid taking this trip in winter, since you need to walk in a creek, and there will likely be snow around Panamint City. From mid-June through September, days are hot but manageable because of the high elevations, which range from 2630 to 8070 feet.

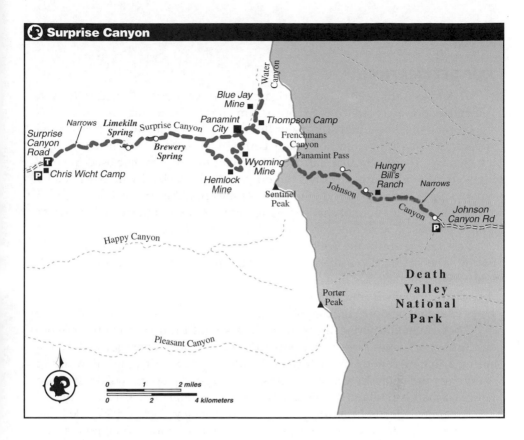

Surprise Canyon

HOW TO GET THERE •

To get to Surprise Canyon, drive to the junction of State Highway 190 and Panamint Valley Road in Panamint Valley. This is 2.5 miles east of Panamint Springs Resort, and 28.1 miles west of Stovepipe Wells. Both places are your last chance for gas and food. Stay on the Panamint Valley Road 13.8 miles until it ends on the Trona-Wildrose Road and make a right. Continue 9.4 miles to the Ballarat turnoff, on the left just north of a wide left bend. Drive this road 3.6 miles to Ballarat. From Ballarat's general store, head north on the graded Indian Ranch Road 1.9 miles to a small sign that points right to Surprise Canyon. The Surprise Canyon Road climbs 2.3 miles to the canyon and ends 1.7 miles inside the canyon at the site of Chris Wicht Camp, the starting point of your journey. The canyon road is a little steep. It is sometimes passable with a passenger car, but to be safe plan on driving a high-clearance vehicle. Two old-timers still lived at the historic oasis of Chris Wicht Camp until their cabin burnt down in 2006.

The end point of your trip is Wilson Spring in Johnson Canyon, on the Death Valley side of the mountains. It is accessed by a primitive road that starts on the West Side Road 20.9 miles from its north end, or 15 miles from its south end. The Johnson Canyon Road climbs the fan 6.4 miles, then drops steeply into the broad canyon wash, and continues up-canyon for 3.7 miles to end at Wilson Spring.

This route requires high clearance on the fan, and four-wheel drive as well in the canyon.

TRIP DESCRIPTION

This hike starts with a bang. Irrigated by a lively stream lined with lush vegetation, the lower stretch of Surprise Canyon is a long idyllic oasis that holds some of the most beautiful scenery in this range. You walk by the tree-shaded stream, crossing it over and over and getting wet—a rare treat in Death Valley country. The spectacular narrows just a half mile up are enclosed in striking walls of white marble nearly 1 billion years old. The banks are bordered by willow, grass, rush, and slender orchids. At the crux, the stream spawns seven waterfalls, slippery but not challenging to climb, an exciting place where water sluices down sculpted chutes and foams into dark potholes.

Past the narrows, the water fun continues for another mile to Limekiln Spring. The stream flows alternatively on the road and underneath large willows. You will likely see butterflies, dragonflies, and little frogs parked by the water. At Limekiln Spring, the stream comes gushing from under a huge mat of grapevine spilling down the canyon wall.

Above Limekiln Spring, the road meanders along the open canyon. At Brewery Spring, 1.3 miles farther, it scoots through a shady tunnel formed by the spring's arching canopy. A swift creek floods the road, irrigating sidewalks of watercress and nettle. In warmer months, this is a good place to cool off. It is also your last chance to fill up: the remaining 2.4 miles to Panamint City are dry.

Panamint City is beautifully situated in a valley enclosed by 3000-foot mountains. The steep slopes are peppered with pinyon pines and junipers, and profusely decorated with wildflowers from spring through early fall. The first signs of the ghost town will be dozens of stone ruins lining the wash, then the tall smokestack of its famous smelter. Just beyond it is "downtown"—a two-room plywood cabin nicknamed the Panamint City Hilton because of its glass windows and working tap, a large workshop, and a quarried-stone quadrangle.

Good campsites are plentiful. When choosing one, keep in mind the proximity of water. Water is available at the main cabin, the workshop, and the largest cabin on the north side (if the taps still work), at Slaughterhouse Spring, in Water Canyon, and at the spring in Sourdough Canyon.

Start your next day with a stroll through Panamint City. Other than its isolation, what makes this place so special is its many well-preserved structures spanning well over a century. This area was feverishly mined for silver from 1872 until 1876. The involvement of two Nevada senators and the large number of deposits triggered one of the region's biggest rushes. By 1874, the rough camp of Panamint City had a population of 2000, by far the largest for 100 miles around. The company controlling the mines completed its monumental mill in June 1875 and was soon shipping silver bullion by 20-mule team. To protect this tempting treasure from robbers, the silver was cast into 400-pound ingots, much too heavy to be lifted, and there never was a single robbery! By 1876, the richest mines had mostly played out. A few dozen workers remained until 1882. Some of the old claims were revived in the 1890s, 1920s, late 1940s, and as recently as the 1970s through the mid-1980s. But all in all, Panamint City returned only about $600,000, most of it before 1876, for an investment exceeding $1,000,000—for all its glamour, it was a spectacular loss.

The smelter's towering smokestack is the town's crowning jewel. Built of a half million bricks, it is a magnificent tower tapering to an ornate crown, and a priceless landmark in American West history. The oldest ruins are the dozens of rooms, walls, dugouts, and canvas-tent platforms along the wash, once the houses and businesses of Main Street. Had you been strolling through here in 1875, you could have shopped for fresh food, garments, and medication, consulted a doctor, boarded a stagecoach to L.A., or sipped wine at a French restaurant.

The "downtown" buildings were put up during the 1970s–1980s revival, and so was the milling complex up behind the smelter—the best example of a modern mill in the park. It was powered by the large diesel generator inside the workshop, while the ingenious waterwheel at the easternmost cabin supplied the town's electricity. The mill might have exploited ore from the amazing straight tunnel behind it—at 750 yards possibly the park's longest.

The next destination is Water Canyon. Walk up the road, past the waterwheel and tank at Slaughterhouse Spring, until it angles left into Water Canyon. Year-round, a creek flows along this canyon's willow-shaded wash, feeding swamps of watercress, rush, and monkeyflowers. The scenery is dwarfed by the canyon's spectacular eastern wall, a 3000-foot high, mile-long tableau of giant granite fins. Thompson Camp, just inside the canyon, was named after the couple who lived and mined here in the 1930s. Its decrepit cabin looks out to Sentinel Peak from under large cottonwoods festooned with vine. Do not miss the camp's water tank, hidden among willows where the road crosses the creek 130 yards above the camp. In the warm season, it's a pleasure to sit on its rim and relax to the sound of the overflow cascading below. You can continue up the road, first along the willow-shaded creek, then up the west slope to the five tunnels of the Blue Jay Mine (1 mile). Even if mines leave you cold, come here for the views.

Another interesting site is Stewart's Wonder Mine, claimed in 1873 by one of the original discoverers, and the area's third largest producer. From the smelter, walk down Surprise Canyon 0.3 mile, and make a right on Sourdough Canyon Road. In 0.2 mile it reaches an eclectic camp of trailers, sheds, and trucks from the

FINDING YOUR CAR

When hiking back a long distance across open desert to the road where your vehicle is parked, if you cannot see your vehicle or remember its exact location, apply the principle of purposeful error: Aim for a point well to the right (or left) of where you think your vehicle is parked, and when you reach the road head left (or right) on the road. This approach statistically minimizes the time it takes to find your car.

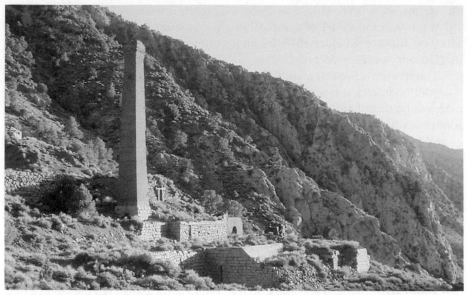

Smelter tower at Panamint City

1950s to the 1960s. The side road to the right leads to a picturesque wood-and-stone cabin, landscaped with pines and flowerbeds. Visitors sometimes stay here overnight. There is usually water at the spring up-canyon. The well-preserved mill across the road is an interesting piece of machinery from the 1960s. The colorful blue-green quartz scattered around is silver ore. The trail to Stewart's Wonder Mine starts a few steps below the mill, on the west side. Supported by well-engineered walls and paved with flat rocks, it is almost perfectly level for 0.65 mile and offers plunging views into Surprise Canyon. After 0.5 mile the trail angles into Wonder Gulch. Soon after, take the right fork, then after it ends scramble up the rocky slope to the historic mine. The impressive upper tunnel is a monstrous crack held open by tree trunks harvested more than 13 decades ago. Enjoy the ore, which is quite colorful, and the views.

On the third day, your destination is a partly shaded and fragrant loop of mining roads in the mountains south of Panamint City that will take you to the area's two richest mines. Start on the Wyoming Mine Road, which heads up the slope just south of the workshop. At the fork 0.35 mile out, turn right. The road winds steeply through pine and offers good views of Panamint City. The first tunnel, in a sharp left turn, belonged to the Wyoming Mine, as did all remains along the next 0.7 mile. The plywood workshop next to it dates from the 1970s. It still houses the electric blower that circulated fresh air into the tunnel, and the dusty air duct still follows the 1000-foot tunnel. The Wyoming Mine Tramway, hidden in the trees 50 feet to the west, is a gem. Erected in the winter of 1874–1875 and refurbished in 1925, its stocky towers of roughly hewn timber are simply designed but surprisingly sturdy.

An interesting mix of modern and historic remains are scattered around the end of the road. The 350-foot tunnel was known as Tramway. A rail track links it to a trestle bridge, where the ore was dumped into the tramway terminal below it and lowered 1100 feet to the 20-stamp mill. There is a deep shaft partway in, so keep out. Most of the Wyoming ore came from two tunnels. The Kennedy Tunnel is about 250 feet higher up the slope, near the top of the ridge to the south. To reach the Limestone Tunnel, take the level constructed trail past the road and level with it. It ends in 0.2 mile at a wide tailing. Then scramble 80 feet up the slope to a second level trail, and follow it south a short distance to its end. Scramble another 80 feet up to a third level trail. The Limestone Tunnel was located in this vicinity. It is now obscured by later mining, but this area is rich in old workings and colorful tailings.

To continue the loop to the Hemlock Mine, follow the third trail 0.6 mile to a sharp right bend at the Marvel Canyon wash crossing. Except for a few places, this trail is well built and hard to lose. Across the wash, the trail splits. Take the left fork, which winds up a steep forested slope. It is faint, so you may end up trying a few dead ends. At the top, be very careful: the trail comes dangerously close to the abrupt edge of the Hemlock Mine's trench.

The Hemlock Mine was the district's largest producer—and it shows. The trench is a long gash framed by vertical walls. The sheer height of the two tailings cascading down the long slope below it is particularly impressive. Made of fine material with about the angle of repose of sand, they are both exhilarating to climb down! The tunnel at the top of the lower tailing was the main producer.

To complete the loop, head down the ravine below the lower tailing about 100 yards to the upper end of the Hemlock Mine Road. After a quarter mile it angles sharply left, then wiggles down Marvel Canyon 1.3 miles to the Surprise Canyon Road. From this junction it is about 1 mile up-canyon to downtown.

On the fourth day, head east up the road. Below Water Canyon, take the right fork in the wash, which is Frenchmans Canyon. This heavily forested drainage climbs steeply to Panamint Pass, a pronounced notch at the crest of range. The going is a little rough, but the reward matches the efforts: The views of Johnson Canyon and southern Death Valley are spectacular.

In the mid-1870s, to satisfy Panamint City's need for fresh produce an enterprising man named William Johnson started a ranch he called Swiss Ranch in Johnson Canyon. He built terraces and irrigation ditches, and planted gardens of beans, squash, and corn, as well as a fruit and nut orchard. He made a profit on the vegetables, but the boom was over before the trees matured. By the spring of 1877, Johnson had moved on. Some years later, a Shoshone named Hungry Bill took over Swiss Ranch. He and his family cleared a few additional acres, planted more trees, and tended vegetable gardens. They lived here until Hungry Bill passed away, probably in 1919.

Below Panamint Pass's eastern rim, look for an aging trail that drops into the canyon. This is the "fresh vegetable route," the trail Johnson used to haul his harvest to Panamint City. It switchbacks down to the canyon floor, offering fine views of the range's pine-covered summits. At the bottom, simply walk down the wash. At first it is steep and strewn with boulders, and progress is tedious. But the walking soon becomes easier, along partly shaded game trails

wandering among granitic boulders. The scenery is beautifully rugged, dominated by a healthy conifer forest livened by birds and rodents, brightened by
blooming cacti in late spring.

Johnson Canyon's four closely-spaced springs make delightful rest areas.
The highest one is a thick grove of willows. At the next one, near timber line,
masses of vines hang down the sheer canyon walls and impenetrable thickets
choke the narrow wash. Bypass it on the narrow trail on the north side. The 10-
acre field 0.2 mile farther on the south side was Swiss Ranch. Almost completely
enclosed by walls, it is still lined with the historic orchard trees. In late spring,
it turns to a striking meadow of bright vermillion globe mallow. Hungry Bill's
Ranch starts a little below. Its large cleared fields enclosed by monumental stone
walls give this area an unexpected rural flavor. Several feet high, up to 6 feet
thick and hundreds of feet long, these walls are lasting works of art. The lowest
set of large walls, on the north side, is thought to have been Hungry Bill's camp.
The Shoshone lived here in wickiups well into the 1900s.

The most exceptional part of Johnson Canyon starts right below the ranch:
For the next 1.5 miles, you cross one of Death Valley's most luxuriant springs.
The canyon narrows and almost completely fills up with vegetation. A strong
stream flows through it, often hidden, occasionally plunging over a waterfall.
To minimize frustration, avoid this jungle on the higher trails along the gorge's
rims. Although steep, rocky, and unpredictable, they are your best bet. Stay on
the south side, which has the most continuous trails, except at the sharp jog in
the canyon, where the creek must be crossed twice. It is slow going, but it is
a great hike, overlooking the lively ribbon of shrubs, grapevine, and trees that
snakes down the gorge, within earshot of the creek.

Below the spring, a well-defined trail will take you about 0.3 mile to the upper end of the road at Wilson Spring, a cluster of willows and tall cottonwoods
irrigated by a little creek.

BUILD-UP AND WIND-DOWN TIPS ·

At either end of your trip, camp in **Ballarat** and explore the remains of this
scenic ghost town. It boomed around 1890 and before World War I, as a supply
center for miners working in the Panamint Mountains. Check out the general
store, the old cabins, the cemetery, and little-known Post Office Spring 0.8 mile
south on the southern extension of Indian Ranch Road. The closest place for a
good meal is **Panamint Springs**, a family-owned resort with a nice country atmosphere and very friendly staff. If your travels take you west on Highway 190, try
to make the short detour through **Darwin**. It is one of California's largest ghost
towns, and its many old cabins, extensive mining camp, and funky residents will
take you back in time well over a century.

37

UBEHEBE COUNTRY LOOP

Michel Digonnet

> **MILES:** 23.0
> **RECOMMENDED DAYS:** 3
> **ELEVATION GAIN/LOSS:** 4900´/4900´
> **TYPE OF TRIP:** Loop
> **DIFFICULTY:** Moderately strenuous
> **SOLITUDE:** Solitude
> **LOCATION:** Death Valley National Park
> **MAPS:** USGS 7.5-min. *Ubehebe Peak*, *West of Ubehebe Peak*,
> and *Teakettle Junction*
> **BEST SEASONS:** Spring and fall

PERMITS

No permit is required, but check with a park ranger (760-786-2331) in case regulations change.

CHALLENGES

If you are new to desert backpacking, first read up on the particular dangers this area presents—heat exhaustion and strokes, dehydration, mines, rattlesnakes, flash floods, hantavirus—and how to best avoid them. Then practice by taking a few dozen dayhikes of increasing length and difficulty. Always let

Photo: Saline Valley and the Inyo Mountains from the Copper Queen Trail

237

TAKE THIS TRIP

This is the quintessential desert hike. From the edge of the eerie Racetrack, you will ascend the dizzying heights of Ubehebe Peak, then drop into remote Saline Valley along a tilted ridge commanding breathtaking views, and finally return along a labyrinthine canyon blessed with a mile-long narrow corridor as straight as an arrow. Along the way, you will pass by several interesting historic mines and camps, including a locally famous lead mine and a forgotten copper property with striking blue ore. You will wiggle your way up tight narrows, cross fields of sparkling granitic boulders, marvel at 300-million-year-old fossils, scramble up dry falls, put your orienteering skills to the test across ankle-twisting fans, and play hide-and-seek with elusive mining trails that have not seen much traffic in over a century. Few places in the desert offer such a stunning diversity of landscapes and natural attractions in less than 25 miles.

someone know your itinerary, and stick to it. And be sure to keep several gallons of water in your car because they might save your life that one day you return parched from too many waterless miles in three-digit temperatures. Check with the park for a complete set of regulations because they differ from those of other parks.

This entire route is devoid of springs, so you will need to carry about three gallons, which is very heavy. The Copper Queen Trail is extremely faint at places and staying on it can be challenging. The cross-country hike to Corridor Canyon requires decent map-reading and orienteering skills. Finally, this route involves climbing a 10-foot class-5 fall. If you are a novice or afraid of climbing, come here with a good climber who can help you. Bring a short rope to lift your pack.

HOW TO GET THERE · · · · · · · · · · · · · ·

The starting point is in Racetrack Valley, the long, north-south trending high-desert valley filled with a dry playa world-famous for its moving rocks. Drive to the Ubehebe Crater overlook. At the start of the loop, take the primitive road on the right, which is the Racetrack Valley Road. Stay on it 19.7 miles, past healthy stands of Joshua trees, to Teakettle Junction. It is marked by a tall sign festooned with kettles left by visitors, a decades-old tradition. Continue straight toward the Racetrack 2.2 miles to a spur on the right. This rutted high-clearance side road ends in 0.7 mile at the Ubehebe Mine, the way you will hike out of Corridor Canyon. If you want to cache water for your trip, do so near the mine. Then drive another 2.2 miles to the Grandstand turnout, on the west side near the north end of the Racetrack playa. Much of this road is a bad washboard, and it has deep gravel at places. However, unless there has been a recent washout due to rain, people with experience driving desert roads can usually make it with a standard-clearance vehicle.

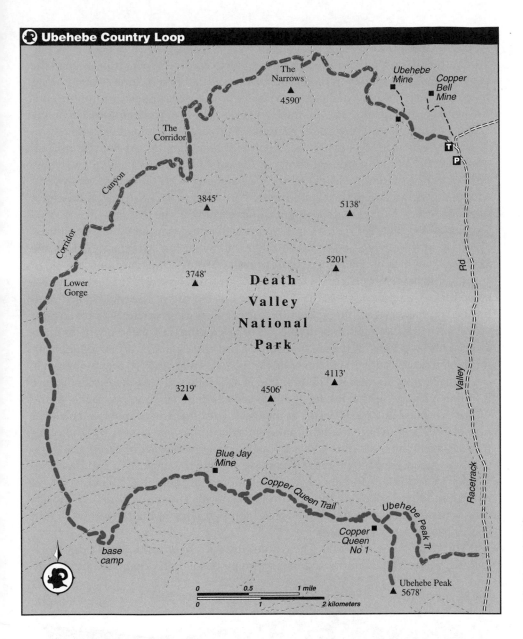

Ubehebe Country Loop

The Narrows
▲ 4590'

Ubehebe Mine

Copper Bell Mine

The Corridor

Canyon

3845' ▲

5138' ▲

Corridor

Lower Gorge

3748' ▲

Death Valley National Park

5201' ▲

3219' ▲

4506' ▲

4113' ▲

Blue Jay Mine

Copper Queen Trail

Ubehebe Peak Tr.

Copper Queen No 1

base camp

Racetrack

Valley Rd

Ubehebe Peak
▲ 5678'

0   0.5   1 mile
0   1   2 kilometers

TRIP DESCRIPTION

The first part of this trip is a trail climb of Ubehebe Peak, the highest summit towering over the west side of the Racetrack playa. At the Grandstand turnout, the trail is identified by rock alignments. It first heads west up a fan, then veers and continues generally northwest about 1 mile before switchbacking to a low saddle at the divide of the Last Chance Range. This good little trail crosses beautiful fields of quartz monzonite, a Mesozoic granitic formation containing large sparkling crystals of orthoclase. It commands increasingly fine views of

Racetrack Valley. In the warmer months it is best tackled in the late afternoon, when the upper trail is in deep shade.

At the divide the trail forks. The more conspicuous leftmost trail ascends the peak. If time allows, do try it (take water with you!). At first it climbs steeply along the ridge. Then it skirts a nameless secondary peak and becomes very faint to non-existent near the saddle between the two peaks. The best route, marked by a few cairns, is a little west of the ridgeline, much of it very steep and over loose rocks.

The views from this route are absolutely breathtaking. At the summit, on one side you will look straight down at the pristine Racetrack playa and its island of dark rounded rocks called the Grandstand, with the high Cottonwood Mountains sprawling in the background. Turn around and you are on the brink of Saline Valley, with its salt lake and dunes shining in the distance, nearly 4000 feet down and dwarfed by the 2-mile-high wall of the majestic Inyo Mountains.

Back at the divide, look for the other, fainter of the two trails. This is the Copper Queen Trail. From here it descends 2.1 miles, mostly along the ridge framing the nameless canyon to the north, to the canyon wash. It goes down five steep rock-strewn slopes separated by more level terraces. The trail is fairly well defined on the terraces, but on the three upper slopes its switchbacks are so faint you'll have to believe it is there to see it. Try to spot the trail ahead of you as often as possible, and look for the small historic cairns that mark it. If you wander off, follow the ridge and you will never be far from it. There are two areas where it is particularly easy to miss it. The first one is 0.15 mile south of the divide, where it makes a sharp right. Look for it at the second bench below the divide, at the whitish serrated outcrop 50 yards to the west. The other tricky spot is at an elevation of 3880 feet, where the trail makes a critical but very faint turn. The other trail visible to the south, just across a wash 300 feet below, is the wrong trail. The Copper Queen Trail actually makes a sharp right to the northwest and descends steeply to a saddle. After about 1.4 miles, at an elevation of 3710 feet, you will reach a saddle overlooking the canyon to the north. The trail forks. Take the left fork, which zigzags down 0.7 mile across an open slope to the canyon wash (the last 100 yards are washed out).

The scenery is spectacular. The whole way you are on an exposed ridge overlooking Saline Valley, immersed in a supreme desolation dominated by deeply

The Racetrack playa and the Grandstand from near Ubehebe Peak

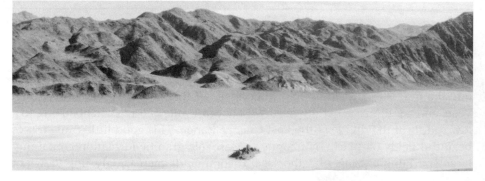

chiseled slopes and monzonite outcrops. If you are on the right track, at the halfway point you will cross a scenic field of rounded boulders crowned by an oddly tilted pinnacle. A little farther there is a little copper mine with a primitive wooden headframe, hidden against a low knoll.

Up-canyon from the trail there is an interesting historic mine called Blue Jay and imposing narrows, both well worth checking out and located in a good general area to camp. Discovered in 1902, this area was mined off and on by a single miner for at least three decades. In 1915 alone, it produced 4000 pounds of copper and nearly 1200 ounces of silver. To get to it, walk 400 yards up the wash and take the right fork. The mine's many workings extend for 600 feet, on both sides of the wash, in the vicinity of the impressive whitish limestone cliff that looms 400 feet over the area. Several of them have striking blue ore, mostly malachite and chalcocite. At the next fork, look for an old grade switchbacking up to the south. The road-cut at its upper end is covered with beautiful porphyritic samples sparkling with pink calcite, quartz, epidote, garnet, and chalcopyrite. Beyond the mine, the canyon narrows abruptly as it cuts through a hard plug of monzonite. These narrows are short but dark and chaotic, interrupted by boulders and short falls that make for fun scrambling. They end at a nearly vertical fall, more than 40 feet high and unscalable for most people.

To cut across to Corridor Canyon, retrace your steps down the wash to the trail, then past it about 0.6 mile to the canyon mouth. Along the way, do not miss the historic camp of the Blue Jay Mine, on the south bank shortly after the second right bend. It has a small wind shelter and a prominent stone house, two tiny roofless rooms erected against a large boulder. Once out of the canyon, head west down the rough fan about 2.3 miles, at which point you should have cleared the west end of the ridge to the north. Then veer northwest and follow the base of the mountain about 1 mile, past the mouths of two secondary canyons, to the very wide wash of Corridor Canyon. Then follow this wash up about 0.6 mile northeast to the mouth of the canyon. The walking is hard, over uneven fans dissected by many small washes, but it is a beautiful area, tucked between the bright crisp edge of Saline Valley and the variegated foothills of the Last Chance Range.

The lower canyon is a broad gorge that winds between colorful desert hills, wrinkled and scantily vegetated. There is no particular difficulty here, but as with any up-canyon travel, you need to pick the right direction each time the canyon forks. Fortunately, the right way is almost always obvious; just stay with the main wash, and consult the map often.

After around 3 miles the canyon gradually narrows. If you have hiked desert mountains before, you will know something momentous is likely about to happen. You first run into a wide, smoothly polished slanted chute. Then, in a tight bend, you come face-to-face with an impressive deeply notched strata rising vertically several hundred feet. A couple of sharp bends later you enter the highlight of this canyon—the Corridor. For nearly 1 mile, the wash squeezes through a straight channel trapped between vertical walls often less than 30 feet apart. In all the California deserts, there are no other narrows like it. Except for two small jogs, they are almost perfectly straight. At places the walls are so smooth that they seem to have been cleaved with a giant blade. Look for ripples exposed on vertical surfaces 15 feet above the wash—they bear witness to the Pennsylvanian sea in which these rocks were deposited. At its upper end, the Corridor is forced to make a sharp left by a vertical stratum. Further progress is impeded by a series of high and potentially dangerous falls, but if you are a good climber you will find an equally spectacular passage above.

Fortunately, there is an easier route out. Just below the first jog, 0.65 mile up from the Corridor's lower end, a side canyon branches off to the east. It starts right away as a deep and dark slot, no more than 4 feet wide, curving gently beneath highly polished walls crisscrossed with white veins. Shallow potholes line the exposed bedrock. Halfway through these exciting narrows there is a 10-foot polished fall that you must climb. The holds are good (low 5's), but a rope will come in handy to hoist your pack.

Above the narrows the scenery gradually opens up as you approach the crest of the range. After 1.2 miles, look carefully for an opening in the soaring eastern wall. This side canyon leads soon to short narrows in light-gray limestone sculpted by erosion. Then it meanders up 1.5 miles to the end of the Ubehebe Mine Road. It is a nice little canyon, narrow at places, bounded by well-stratified high cliffs, easy to walk. Just pay close attention to the direction you take at the many side canyons along the way. Also keep an eye open for fossils, which are locally fairly abundant. The most obvious and striking ones are Mississippian crinoids and corals from a time when Death Valley was a tropical reef.

The picturesque wood cabin near the road was part of the Ubehebe Mine, the longest active historic mining venture in this district. It operated mostly from 1906 to 1908, in the 1910s and 1920s, then off and on until 1968, eventually leaving its mark as one of Death Valley's top lead producers. The hill north of it is crawling with old workings and the remains of a tramway. Look around for other remains—an old car carcass, stone walls and foundations, and a lone rusted stove.

The final stretch (2.9 miles) is first on the Ubehebe Mine Road to the Racetrack Valley Road, then on the latter to your starting point. Although exposed to the sun, this part is easy, slightly downhill most of the way, in full view of the Racetrack and its scenic ring of mountains.

BUILD-UP AND WIND-DOWN TIPS ·

To experience the ultimate in secluded bare-bones desert camping, try **Home-stake Dry Camp** at the end of the Racetrack Valley Road (camping elsewhere south of Teakettle Junction is prohibited). Check out the interesting remains of the historically important **Lippincott Mine** (lead) starting a half mile south. To return, take the dusty Big Pine Road across northern Death Valley to visit the impressively high **Eureka Dunes**. This scenic, desolate road continues across Eureka Valley, then crosses the forested crest of the Inyo Mountains as a paved road, and drops to Big Pine on U.S. Highway 395. At the picturesque town of Independence 26 miles south, treat yourself to a tasty traditional French meal at the **Still Life Cafe**, a casual restaurant owned and operated by a friendly couple from France.

38

BLACK CANYON

Elizabeth Wenk

MILES: 10.6 (with an additional 3.9 miles for trip to the Schulman Grove of Bristlecone Pines)

RECOMMENDED DAYS: 2

ELEVATION GAIN/LOSS: 2300´/2300´ (with an additional 1700´ for trip to the Schulman Grove of Bristlecone Pines)

TYPE OF TRIP: Out-and-back

DIFFICULTY: Moderately strenuous

SOLITUDE: Solitude

LOCATION: White Mountains, Inyo National Forest

MAPS: USGS 7.5-min. *Westgard Pass, Blanco Peak* (for trip to the bristlecone pines), and *Poleta Canyon* (for the drive to the trailhead)

BEST SEASONS: Spring or fall

PERMITS

No permits are required for this trip.

CHALLENGES

You must walk 0.3 mile upstream of the suggested campsite to reach water; the sections of the canyon with flowing water are generally steep and narrow or choked with wild roses, making camping impractical.

Photo: When heading down Black Canyon, you enjoy sporadic views of the Sierra Nevada.

TAKE THIS TRIP

The first miles of this walk are reminiscent of a desert canyon, a miniature of Death Valley's Titus Canyon, yet it is just a 20-minute drive from the town of Bishop and accessible by two-wheel-drive vehicle. The walk up a little-used dirt road leads you through a steep narrow canyon of dark metamorphic rock, past sections of exquisitely folded layers, through a band of limestone eroded into pinnacles, and up into rolling flats of western junipers and pinyon pines. Two perennial springs provide water.

HOW TO GET THERE

From the intersection of Line St. and Main St. in Bishop, drive 2.5 miles south on U.S. Highway 395 to Warm Springs Rd. Turn east on Warm Springs Rd. and drive 4.6 miles to an intersection shortly after you cross Owens River. Continue straight ahead, following the road, now called Black Canyon Rd., as it bends to the south. After 2.7 miles you reach another intersection where you bear right and begin the climb into Black Canyon. All passenger cars should be able to ascend at least 2.2 miles, while a high-clearance car can make it an additional 0.8 mile. (Note that Black Canyon can legally be ascended by four-wheel-drive vehicles or off-road vehicles, but few motor vehicles enter this secluded area.)

TRIP DESCRIPTION

Located in the southwestern White Mountains, this hike follows a rugged road up Black Canyon. But don't worry, you are unlikely to encounter a vehicle as this is a little-used, difficult to navigate, dead-end road. This description begins at the confluence of Black Canyon and Marble Canyon, but those in a low-clearance car are advised to park about 0.8 mile down-canyon.

You ascend a narrow canyon with steep, dark walls of metamorphic rock. The flat slabs are bedding planes along which the shale fractures. One old mine shaft along the southeast side of the road will likely catch your attention. After about 1.5 miles, you note a trickle of water running down the road, and around the next corner is the first spring. (The USGS topographic maps incorrectly indicate that there is a permanent stream down the entire length of Black Canyon; except in the vicinity of the spring at the 1.5-mile mark, the lower reaches of the canyon are generally dry.) The tangles of wild roses indicate that this is a permanent water source. If you wish to have a

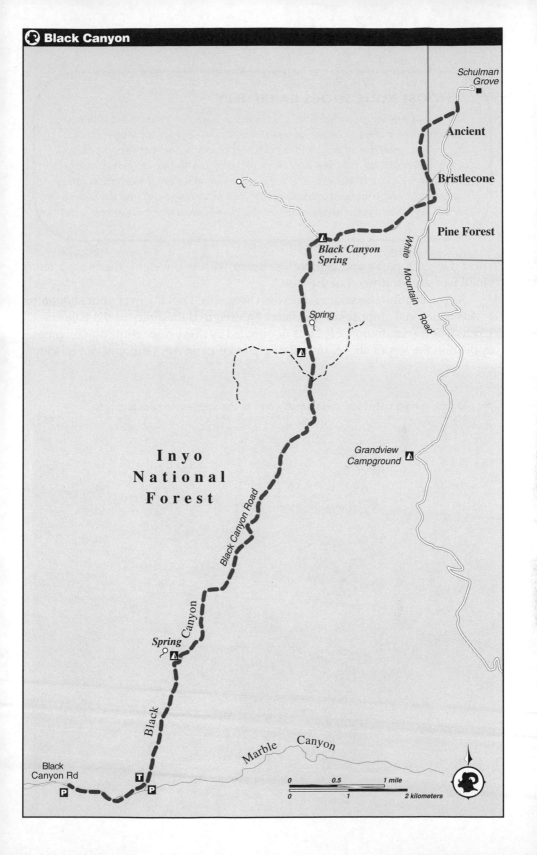

Schulman
Grove

Ancient

Bristlecone

Pine Forest

White Mountain Road

Black Canyon
Spring

Spring

Grandview
Campground

I n y o
N a t i o n a l
F o r e s t

Black Canyon Road

Spring

Canyon

Black

Marble   Canyon

Black
Canyon Rd

0   0.5   1 mile

0   1   2 kilometers

CHOOSE YOUR SHOES CAREFULLY

Don't bow to peer pressure when choosing shoes. Veteran backpackers usually have a strong opinion of what constitutes appropriate footwear for a given hike, yet different people have different opinions on what is appropriate. So they should, as different people would rank the following considerations in different orders: ankle and arch support and shoe weight, breathability, and waterproofness. You need to try different types of footwear and over the course of several hikes decide what shoes suit you best in each hiking situation.

short day with packs and explore upstream with less weight, there are a few small tent sites northwest of the road.

As you continue ascending, the wash broadens. Looking over your shoulder yields occasional glimpses of the Sierra Nevada in the vicinity of the Palisades. Underfoot is a community of plants dominated by sagebrush, while pinyon pines appear on the slopes above. (In fall of a good pinyon nut year, you can quickly

An old rock mining cabin you pass shortly before the suggested camping area

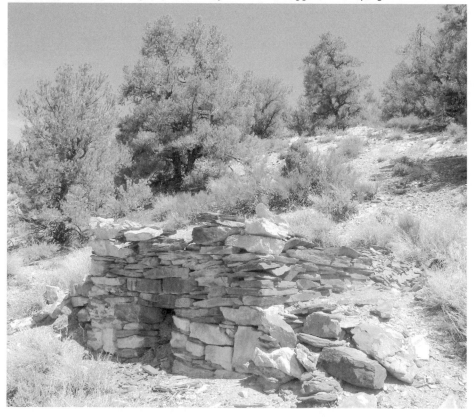

collect a tasty topping for your dinner. Just crack open the outer shell and pull out the tasty, off-white colored pine nut.)

About 2.5 miles above the first spring the canyon narrows again and you find yourself walking between towering marble pinnacles. Beyond this constriction you suddenly find yourself in rolling pinyon-juniper woodland, the characteristic mid-elevation vegetation community in the White and Inyo mountains.

Shortly, you pass a small mine shaft (and the side drainage that leads up to Grandview Campground), and about 1.0 mile above the marble formations reach a fork in the path. Take the left-hand fork, and after a few steps reach another junction. This time, head right, following the less traveled of the two forks, and indeed a trail that is not shown on current USGS topographic maps. The grade is now negligible, and you walk through open woodland. High above you to the east is a visible line, the White Mountain Road leading to the bristlecone pine forests.

Before long, note a collapsing cabin to your right, built of burnt orange rock. A few more minutes of walking brings you to an open flat dotted with picturesque juniper trees, a recommended campsite, located 0.3 mile beyond the previous trail junction. It is dry, but clear spring water is just 10 minutes (0.3 mile) ahead. Walk just another minute past the first wet seeps to encounter a road junction and running water. In early summer, this area sports a colorful collection of flowers.

If you can take the time the next morning, I encourage you to follow the water to its source, Black Canyon Spring, 1.0 mile upstream of the junction with running water. For much of the distance, the stream runs down one of the tire tracks, part of the reason environmental groups are hoping this route will one day be closed to vehicles. Trending right each time the road forks leads you to a small cabin near Black Canyon Spring. As rose thickets cover the stream banks, the only camping option is the sloping area beside the cabin.

If you wish to take an even more ambitious dayhike or do the hike as a point-to-point trip, continuing upstream an additional 2.9 miles and 1700 feet takes you to the Schulman Grove of Bristlecone Pines. Note that vehicles are *not* permitted on this last stretch of trail.

BUILD-UP AND WIND-DOWN TIPS

If you return from your trip with time to spare, the two photo galleries in town are well worth perusing: **Vern Clevenger's gallery** at 905 North Main Street in Bishop, toward the north end of town near Starbucks, and **Galen Rowell's gallery** at 106 South Main Street in Bishop, on the southeast corner of the intersection of Main and Line streets. Plus, the bar menu at **Whiskey Creek** (524 North Main Street, just south of the Bank of America) is half price before 6 PM on weekdays.

39

COTTONWOOD BASIN LOOP

Elizabeth Wenk

MILES: 9.4 (add 5.5 to explore Tres Plumas Meadow and Tres Plumas
    Creek as a dayhike)
RECOMMENDED DAYS: 2 (3 with side trip)
ELEVATION GAIN/LOSS: 1600´/1600´ feet for basic loop (with an addi-
    tional 1000´/1000´ for optional dayhike)
TYPE OF TRIP: Loop
DIFFICULTY: Moderate for basic loop; Strenuous for loop with side trip
SOLITUDE: Moderate solitude
LOCATION: White Mountains, Inyo National Forest
MAPS: USGS 7.5-min. *Mount Barcroft*
BEST SEASON: Summer

PERMITS ·

No permits are required for this trip.

CHALLENGES ·

Expect the drive from Big Pine to take at least 1½ hours. Do not be tempted
to drive fast along the dirt roads—the sharp rocks on the White Mountain Road
are infamous for their tire-eating capabilities.

*Photo: The view north as you descend the four-wheel-drive road to the South Fork of
Cottonwood Creek*

HOW TO GET THERE ·············

From 0.6 mile north of Big Pine turn east onto Highway 168, toward Westgard Pass. After 14 miles turn left (north) onto the White Mountain Road. Continue on a paved road for 9.7 miles, to the Schulman Bristlecone Pine Grove. Continue straight ahead beyond the grove, now on a well-graded dirt road for 10.8 miles. Turn right at the Crooked Creek junction. Passing a junction to the White Mountain Research Station, continue straight ahead for 3.1 miles. Now bear left and climb up to a pass overlooking Cottonwood Basin. There is a parking area to the right. Passenger cars should find the road passable up to this point. High-clearance four-wheel-drive vehicles can continue along the road, cutting 1.7 miles off the hike. (This last section of road is not passable to Subarus or many low-clearance SUVs.)

TRIP DESCRIPTION ···············

Cottonwood Basin is the best-known backpacking destination in the White Mountains, but due to its remote location you can still expect a high degree of solitude. The trip description begins at the large parking area on the pass south of the Cottonwood Basin, the location from which most people begin this hike. You begin by descending a steep four-wheel-drive road, passing through scattered bristlecone pines and limber pines. After a little over a mile, you pass through a small grove of cottonwoods and emerge into a flatter meadow through which Poison Creek flows.

You continue along the four-wheel-drive road across two stream crossing (both easy step-across crossings) and then trend left to follow an old dirt road up the South Fork of Cottonwood Creek, 1.7 miles from the parking area. The road quickly diminishes into a well-traveled use trail. Alongside this first section, you are at the point where dolomite and granite meet. The dolomite, to your left,

TAKE THIS TRIP

Cottonwood Basin is a magical place deep in the White Mountains. Remarkably flat, easy walking along a good use trail, abundant flowers, and a wonderland of granite towers are among its attractions. The distance into attractive camping areas is relatively short, leaving you lots of time to explore the meadows containing Cottonwood Creek and its tributaries or to explore passageways between the granite formations.

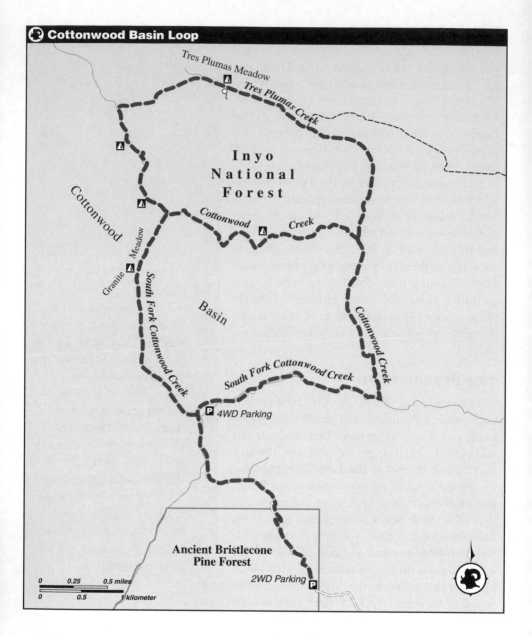

Cottonwood Basin Loop

Tres Plumas Meadow

Tres Plumas Creek

Inyo National Forest

Cottonwood

Cottonwood   Creek

Meadow

Granite

South Fork Cottonwood Creek

Basin

Cottonwood Creek

South Fork Cottonwood Creek

🅿 4WD Parking

Ancient Bristlecone Pine Forest

2WD Parking 🅿

| 0 | 0.25 | 0.5 miles |
| 0 | 0.5 | 1 kilometer |

is the main substrate on which bristlecone pines grow, and this is the only place along this hike that you will encounter it (or these trees). After a bit over 0.5 mile the main meadow trends left, while the use trail follows the narrower right-hand fork. Passing between walls of granite, you climb over a shallow saddle and drop into Granite Meadow. The spring-fed creek should always have flowing water, and during midsummer its banks are densely lined with colorful flowers. A few drier sections of the meadow provide camping possibilities where you won't damage vegetation.

Although only a few miles from the start, Granite Meadow is an undeniably picturesque location to spend a night, and you can easily spend an afternoon exploring the many nearby meadows and granite formations. You can alternatively continue up Cottonwood Creek, as described in the beginning of the side trip below. (Note that fishing in Cottonwood Creek is prohibited to protect the rare Paiute Cutthroat Trout.)

At the north end of Granite Meadow (1.7 miles since leaving the dirt road) you join the northern fork of Cottonwood Creek. Cross the creek and turn right, descending through meadows and occasional sections of forest. The use trail is marked sporadically with fence posts and is well maintained; the brushy willows are cut back at each of the many creek crossings, so passage is easy. As you descend note how much more forested the north-facing slopes (to your right) are, since they receive less sun and are therefore cooler and moister. There continue to be enticing granite towers throughout this section and camping possibilities in most of the small meadows through which the trail passes.

SIDE TRIP: **TRES PLUMAS MEADOW AND CREEK**

For the most adventurous hikers, this 5.5-mile loop provides a chance to climb up onto a high sagebrush-covered plateau. Do not attempt to descend Tres Plumas Creek with a full pack unless you have experience and are comfortable scrambling on rocks—you encounter the trickiest section when you are just a short distance from Cottonwood Creek and will not wish to retreat the way you came.

From the north end of Granite Meadow head up Cottonwood Creek. For the first 0.9 mile this route continues on a use trail along the creek, passing in and out of beautiful groves of quaking aspen. A few small benches alongside the creek serve as tent sites. After 0.8 mile you pass a side drainage to your left. Just thereafter is a small, but steep knob. As you pass the knob, turn right (east) and note a relatively open slope above you. Head due east, not northeast as is initially tempting, and you will contend with little brush. After climbing a little more than 400 feet you will find yourself at the crest of a nearly bare slope, with views into Tres Plumas Meadow, a broad, flat meadow perched above Cottonwood Basin. A use trail exists along the east side of the meadow, in the low sagebrush, but walking is easy anywhere. Most years, springs will be flowing near large granite pinnacles, a beautiful campsite.

Toward the southern end of the meadow you will intersect a road that climbs up to Tres Plumas Flat. Where the road leaves the creek you begin a steep descent back to Cottonwood Creek. An old fence, a grove of aspens covered with initials carved in the mid-1900s, and pieces of a horse skeleton indicate that you aren't the first person to pass this way. However, this route is little used and there is only a faint and often difficult-to-follow use trail down the drainage. Instead of trying to follow it, it is easiest simply to remain along the west bank of the creek. This engaging descent winds past ever-taller granite pinnacles, and you are never able to see far downstream.

A bit below 9600 feet the canyon pinches yet farther and the last third of a mile to Cottonwood Creek is trickier. One possible route is to climb 50 feet to the west to avoid a steep slab and then descend class 2 talus back to the drainage.

Thereafter, you will contend with several rose thickets, but no difficult scrambling. Alternatively, you can climb high to the east to bypass the cliffs before descending directly to the confluence with Cottonwood Creek. When you reach Cottonwood Creek, go approximately 200 feet downstream of the true drainage junction to a place where the willow thicket vanishes, allowing you easy access to the trail on the southwest side of the creek.

After 1.7 miles you reach the junction where Tres Plumas Creek merges with Cottonwood Creek. Here Cottonwood Creek (and the trail) bend to the south. The drainage is now more open. The granite walls begin to diminish in size and the meadows through which you pass are large and open. For the first time, juniper trees occasionally dot dry knobs and slopes. In the meadows, where the trail sometimes vanishes, it is best to stay on the east (left) side of the creek near the border between grass and sagebrush. Continuing down you reach the junction with the South Fork of Cottonwood Creek after 1.2 miles. Contrary to what is shown on the USGS 7.5-minute map, the four-wheel-drive road does not descend this far. Instead, the use trail trends west up the stream drainage. After 0.6 mile you see the terminus of the four-wheel-drive road to the north, but the trail you have been following continues along the south bank of the creek, passing

Its rugged granite pinnacles are one of Cottonwood Basin's many charms.

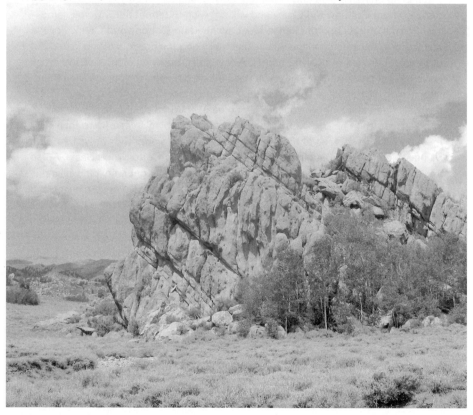

THE REAL REASON NOT TO CAMP NEAR WATER

Dew dripping from your tent and drenching your sleeping bag is an excellent way to ruin a good night's sleep. To avoid this (and to follow the regulations in most wilderness areas), do not camp along the banks of streams or lakes or in a meadow. Instead, climb a few feet up a little knob or step back into the forest. You will be warmer and will have dry gear in the morning.

through some stands of aspen and small meadows. If you wish to avoid getting your feet wet, it is best to stay on the south side of the drainage until you leave Cottonwood Basin behind (0.6 mile after first reaching the four-wheel-drive road) and begin retracing your steps up the four-wheel-drive road to the pass, a 1000-foot climb.

BUILD-UP AND WIND-DOWN TIPS

If you have spare time at the end of your trip, be sure to visit either the **Schulman** or **Patriarch groves** of bristlecone pines. There are short nature walks at both locations with signs and pamphlets providing information on the biology of the world's oldest trees and their importance in learning about past climate patterns. **Grandview Campground**, located at 8600 feet along White Mountain Road, is a beautiful place to spend the night before or after your hike—but there is no water so be sure to have a jug in your car.

SOUTHERN SIERRA NEVADA

The Sierra Nevada reaches a climax toward the southern end of its 400-mile range, in an area referred to as the High Sierra. A sizable portion of the High Sierra lies within the boundaries of Kings Canyon and Sequoia national parks, John Muir Wilderness, Golden Trout Wilderness, and Ansel Adams Wilderness. Within these jurisdictions are some of the range's most significant geographical features—14,494-foot Mt. Whitney, the highest peak in the lower 48, and the largest groves of *Sequoiadendron giganteum,* more commonly known as giant sequoias, the world's largest trees. This region also provides passage to a trio of famous routes: a section of the 2600-mile Mexico-to-Canada Pacific Crest Trail, part of the 218-mile Whitney-to-Yosemite Valley John Muir Trail, and the entirety of the trans-Sierra, 69-mile High Sierra Trail. Along with these legendary features, the High Sierra is blessed with acres and acres of terrain for which the area is famous: glistening granite peaks, crystalline lakes, dashing streams, wildflower-carpeted meadows, and glaciated valleys.

Thankfully, this region is mostly devoid of major roads. Between Tioga Pass Road through Yosemite and Highway 178 well to the south—a distance of roughly 170 air miles—no highways cross the Sierra, leaving a huge, roadless tract of land for the enjoyment of backcountry visitors. The Southern Sierra features vast wilderness lands, including 863,714-acre Sequoia-Kings Canyon—90 percent of which is managed as wilderness; 580,323-acre John Muir Wilderness—California's largest wilderness area—which wraps around the northern and eastern boundaries of the parks; and the 303,511-acre Golden Trout Wilderness, located along the southern boundary of Sequoia. Smaller pockets of wilderness adjoin the parks on the west side, including Monarch, Kaiser, Dinkey, and Jennie Lakes wildernesses. Farther north, between the John Muir Wilderness and Yosemite National Park, the Ansel Adams Wilderness (formerly Minarets Wilderness) protects another 231,005 acres of rugged backcountry.

254

All told, the two national parks and three wilderness areas in this section, spanning an area from Horseshoe Meadows in the south to the Ritter Range in the north, contain more than 1500 miles of maintained trail, offering plenty of opportunities to escape the crowds. Eleven distinct trips are described in this section, beginning at trailheads on both the west and east side of the range. Seven of the trails are primarily within the majestic backcountry of Sequoia and Kings Canyon national parks, with four more exploring the High Sierra of the John Muir and Ansel Adams wilderness areas.

SEQUOIA AND KINGS CANYON NATIONAL PARKS

Although slightly less famous than Yosemite to the north, Sequoia and Kings Canyon national parks contain much of the Sierra Nevada's most impressive features. On the extreme eastern side of Sequoia is Mt. Whitney, at 14,494 feet the highest summit in the lower 48. The 10,760 feet between Mt. Whitney and the town of Lone Pine in Owens Valley at the eastern base of the Sierra is the greatest relief between mountaintop and valley in the lower 48 as well. The Kings River gorge, just west of the confluence of the Middle and South forks, is one of the deepest canyons in North America, measured at just over 8000 feet from the top of Spanish Mountain to the river. The biggest living organism on the planet, the General Sherman Tree, also resides within Sequoia, at over 52,500 cubic feet the largest giant sequoia in existence. Along with these extraordinary features, some of the most magnificent backcountry in the Sierra Nevada is found in and around these two parks. Several summers could be spent backpacking in this area and there would still be more placid lakes, crystalline streams, flower-covered meadows, and granite peaks to see and experience.

From western trailheads, Trails 40–43 venture into the heart of the parks' backcountry, including Trail 41, which follows the High Sierra Trail on an epic adventure from the big trees in Giant Forest to the big mountain of Mt. Whitney. Trails 44–46 start at eastern trailheads, crossing the Sierra Crest and journeying through the rugged terrain on the eastern fringe of the parks. Trails 47–49 also begin on the east side of the range, visiting the scenic high mountain terrain of the John Muir and Ansel Adams wilderness areas north of Kings Canyon National Park. Trail 50 is accessed from the west side of the range and travels into the heart of the Ansel Adams Wilderness just south of Yosemite National Park.

ANSEL ADAMS WILDERNESS

Ansel Adams Wilderness adjoins the east and southeast boundaries of Yosemite National Park, and it can be split into two landscapes. The eastern lands almost coincide with a belt of metamorphic rocks, so this area has a very different feel: deep, near-crest canyons painted in various earth hues of metamorphic rocks that dominate over the gray granitic rocks. Here you'll find arguably the finest mountain scenery in the Sierra Nevada, the sawtooth Ritter Range and sparkling, reflecting lakes along its east base (Trip 49). In the west part of this wilderness the landscape is more granitic than metamorphic, and the relief is less, and therefore offers relatively easy hiking to its many lakes (Trip 50).

40

MINERAL KING AND LITTLE FIVE LAKES LOOP

Mike White

MILES: 40.5
RECOMMENDED DAYS: 5–7
ELEVATION GAIN/LOSS: 10,710′/10,710′
TYPE OF TRIP: Loop
DIFFICULTY: Strenuous
SOLITUDE: Moderately populated
LOCATION: Sequoia-Kings Canyon national parks
MAPS: USGS 7.5-min. *Mineral King*, *Chagoopa Falls*, and *Triple Divide Peak*
BEST SEASON: Late summer through early fall

PERMITS

A wilderness permit is required for entry into the backcountry of Sequoia and Kings Canyon national parks. Trailhead quotas are in effect from about the end of May to the end of September, and approximately 75 percent of the daily trailhead quota is available by advanced reservation between March 1 and September 15. Get a permit application from the park website (www.nps.gov/seki) and submit the completed form by mail (Sequoia and Kings Canyon National Parks, Wilderness Permit Reservations, 47050 Generals Highway #60, Three Rivers, CA, 93271) or fax (559-565-4239). A $15, nonrefundable fee is assessed per

Photo: Several granite domes are visible from a section of the High Sierra Trail.

reservation and can be made by credit card, check, or money order.

Applicants will receive a reservation confirmation by mail, which must then be turned into the nearest issue station to your departure trailhead in order to obtain the actual wilderness permit. Confirmation or pick up of your permit must occur before 9 AM on the departure day, otherwise the permit is cancelled and becomes available to other parties on a walk-in basis. Free walk-in permits may be obtained after 1 PM on the day before departure, and unclaimed reserved permits become available after 9 AM on the day of departure. Fees are charged for entrance into the park as well ($10 for a 7-day pass, $30 for an Annual Park Pass to Sequoia and Kings Canyon, and $80 for an America the Beautiful Pass that provides year-long access to all national parks and recreation areas).

CHALLENGES ·

Gas is not available beyond Three Rivers, so make sure you have enough fuel to get to Mineral King and back. The marmots of Mineral King are notorious for chewing on engine hoses and stowing away in engine compartments. Make sure you check your vehicle for leaks and stowaways before departure. Campfires are banned in several places along this route, so plan on using a stove. Bears are active throughout Sequoia National Park, and while bear canisters are not required, they are highly recommended. In lieu of canisters, make use of the bear boxes at locations noted in the description. Bear-bagging food has proved to be largely ineffectual, compounding the bear problem.

HOW TO GET THERE · · · · · · · · · · · · · ·

Near the east end of Three Rivers, leave State Highway 198 to follow the Mineral King Road east for 23.5 miles to the Mosquito-Eagle Trailhead parking area. The narrow and winding road has unpaved sections and will

TAKE THIS TRIP

While this trip, with great elevation gains and losses and the crossing of two major Sierra passes, is not for the fainthearted, the incredible scenery along the way is more than ample reward for all your hard work. Panoramic views, alpine basins, cirque lakes, flower-covered meadows, tumbling creeks, serene forests, and numerous lakes are just some of the visual treats. With an extra layover day or two, you can fully explore such delightful spots as Little and Big Five Lakes basins. You can also reverse the direction of this loop, or, by traveling over Sawtooth Pass, reduce this to a 27-mile, three- to four-day loop trip.

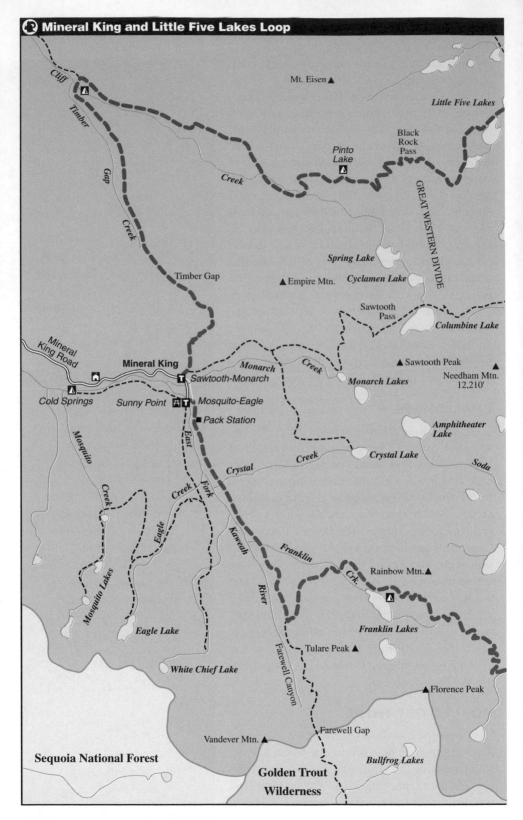

Cliff

Timber

Gap

Creek

Mt. Eisen ▲

Little Five Lakes

Black Rock Pass

Pinto Lake

Creek

GREAT WESTERN DIVIDE

Spring Lake

Timber Gap

▲ Empire Mtn.

Cyclamen Lake

Sawtooth Pass

Columbine Lake

Mineral King Road

Mineral King

Monarch

Creek

▲ Sawtooth Peak

Needham Mtn. 12,210'

Sawtooth-Monarch

Monarch Lakes

Cold Springs

Sunny Point

Mosquito-Eagle

Amphitheater Lake

Pack Station

Mosquito

East

Crystal

Creek

Crystal Lake

Soda

Creek

Fork

Creek

Eagle

Crystal

Kaweah

Franklin

Crk.

Rainbow Mtn. ▲

Mosquito Lakes

River

Franklin Lakes

Eagle Lake

Tulare Peak ▲

White Chief Lake

Farewell Canyon

▲ Florence Peak

Sequoia National Forest

Vandever Mtn. ▲

Farewell Gap

Bullfrog Lakes

Golden Trout

Wilderness

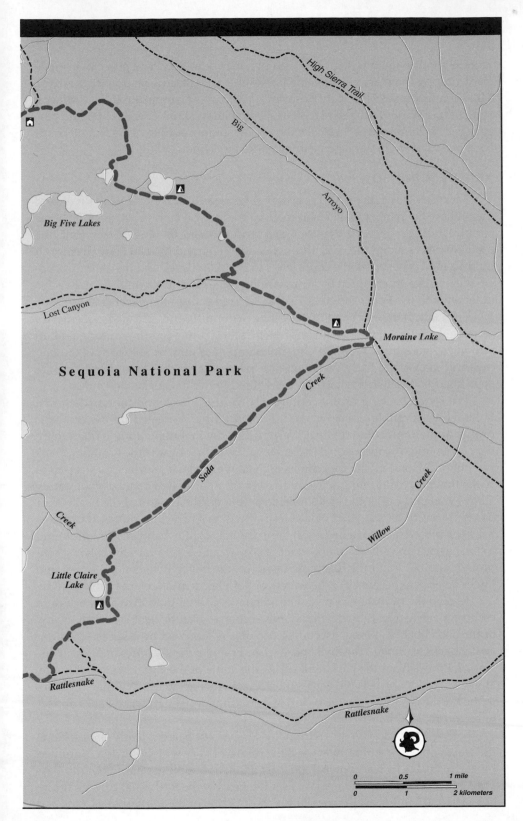

Big Five Lakes

High Sierra Trail

Big

Arroyo

Lost Canyon

Moraine Lake

Sequoia National Park

Creek

Soda

Creek

Willow

Creek

Little Claire
Lake

Rattlesnake

Rattlesnake

| 0 | | 0.5 | | 1 mile |
| 0 | 1 | | 2 kilometers |

259

require about one-and-a-half hours to negotiate—more if you encounter much traffic. Along the way, you pass the Lookout Point entrance station (fee), Atwell Mill Campground, Silver City Resort, Cold Springs Campground, and Mineral King ranger station. Any extra food or scented items should be placed in the storage shed (24-hour access) opposite the ranger station, as both bears and marmots have been known to damage vehicles parked in Mineral King.

TRIP DESCRIPTION

Backtrack down the road, cross the bridge over East Fork Kaweah River, and then follow the pack station access road up the canyon (southeast) past the horse corral. After a mile, ford Crystal Creek and proceed on single-track trail (the road continues along the river through Aspen Flat and over to Soda Spring). A mild-to-moderate, 0.75-mile climb leads to Franklin Creek and the start of steeper switchbacks, interrupted by an ascending traverse near the midpoint. Reach a junction with the Franklin Lakes Trail at 3.25 miles from the parking area.

Turn left (northeast) and make a long, ascending traverse across the northwest flank of Tulare Peak, with impressive views down to Mineral King and up red-and-orange-hued Franklin Canyon. Sharp eyes may be able to spot the tailings and shaft of the Lady Franklin Mine, perched atop the slope above a pair of switchbacks. Reach a crossing of willow-lined Franklin Creek at 4.4 miles.

The switchbacking ascent continues toward the rock-and-mortar dam that holds Lower Franklin Lake, where a fine backdrop is created by the dramatic profile of the multicolored Great Western Divide, including aptly named Rainbow Mountain. A short use trail accesses campsites alongside the tumbling creek just below the outlet. The trail climbs high above the lake's surface, past a pair of paths that descend to petite, overused, foxtail-pine-shaded campsites on sandy ledges stamped out of the steep hillside on the northeast side of the basin (bear boxes). A pit toilet screened by a clump of willows near the southernmost area has been placed here to help protect the extremely shallow and sterile soils found in the basin. You can escape some of the crowds at Lower Franklin Lake by continuing another half mile to exposed sites on the bench between the upper and lower lakes. Anglers can ply the waters of both lakes in search of brook trout.

Ascend the trail above Lower Franklin Lake to well-graded switchbacks and climb above the trees, across open slopes of coarse, granitic pebbles. From the top of the switchbacks, a long, ascending traverse is followed by a series of shorter switchbacks leading to the final approach to Franklin Pass (approximately 11,760 feet), 7.4 miles from the parking area. At the spine of the Great Western Divide, alpine splendor spreads out across the horizon, including Mt. Whitney, 18 miles to the northeast, above the deep cleft of Kern Canyon. The Kaweah Peaks appear to the north, less than 10 miles away.

Follow winding path down from the pass, across barren, sandy slopes; along the way, you will eventually witness the return of very widely scattered, stunted pines. Switchbacks lead downslope, past a junction with the faint Shotgun Pass Trail, and around a small meadow near the head of the Rattlesnake Creek drainage. About 0.5 mile past the meadow is the junction of the Rattlesnake Creek and

Soda Creek trails, at 10 miles from the trailhead. Follow the left-hand path (east) and proceed through lodgepole pine forest on a mildly rising ascent 0.5 mile to grass- and pine-rimmed Forester Lake, where fine campsites and the chance to fish for brook trout may tempt overnighters.

A moderate climb away from the lake leads past a small meadow to the top of a rise, followed by a moderate descent to the east side of Little Claire Lake. On the south shore, a large, sandy slope dotted with foxtail pines provides a fine camping area, complete with an excellent view of 12,210-foot Needham Mountain across the surface of the lake. Additional campsites may be located along the north shore, near the outlet, close to the lip of Soda Creek's steep canyon. Good-size brook trout in Little Claire Lake will lure any anglers in your party.

From Little Claire Lake, the trail drops 900 vertical feet in a mile of switchbacks down a steep, forested slope to a ford of Soda Creek. The next 3.25 miles is along a featureless descent alongside the creek through a lodgepole pine forest, broken only by intermittent avalanche swaths that have swept the wall of the canyon. Near the Lost Canyon junction, red firs, western white pines, and Jeffrey pines join the lodgepoles.

Fortunately, the Park Service has rerouted the section of trail up Lost Canyon from the junction. Formerly, the merciless route was exposed to the hot and scorching sun before eventually entering cool forest along Lost Canyon Creek. Turn left to follow sometimes steep switchbacks northwest along a zigzagging course through light forest, across the creek, and up to a meadow with a campsite nearby (bear box). This is followed by a more moderate climb to the Big Five Lakes junction.

Turn right (northeast) and follow long-legged switchbacks up a hillside carpeted with chinquapin and dotted with lodgepole pine. A tepid tarn situated on a bench partway up the slope offers a refreshing swim, along with secluded campsites above the heather-lined shore. The moderate ascent amid boulders

THE ULTIMATE CAMP SHOES

Even with light and comfortable backpacking footwear, your feet are apt to be tired after several hours on the trail. An extra pair of lightweight sandals or flip-flops will provide a welcome respite at camp. Such footwear, when suitable for use in water, also keeps hiking boots from getting soaked at stream crossings. I reluctantly purchased a pair of the somewhat effeminate-looking Crocs on the advice of several backpackers, who assured me they were the best camp shoes on the planet.

After setting up camp, my friend and I changed into our Crocs for a leisurely afternoon stroll. Soon our hyperactivity led to a scramble route to an upper lake requiring a 15-foot, Class 3 rock climb. Still clad in our Crocs, we went up and down this obstacle without ill effect, dubbing our trusty Crocs "the go anywhere, do anything" shoes. Despite such a ringing endorsement, don't chuck your hiking boots altogether.

and slabs resumes beyond the pond, to the apex of a ridge that overlooks the Big Five Lakes basin. A steep and rocky descent drops from the ridge to the first of the lakes, 2 miles from the junction in Lost Canyon. Good campsites are located near the outlet and along the north shore. Continue along the north side of the lake to an informal junction, and take the right-hand fork up a short, steep, zig-zag to a T-junction with the trail to Little Five Lakes (the left-hand path travels to the highest and prettiest of the Big Five Lakes).

Bound for Little Five Lakes, head north and follow the trail's rolling course for the next mile, with occasional views of the Kaweahs. Drop down to the crossing of a small stream and then climb through lodgepole pine forest. After a while, Lake 10476 springs into view, and you soon reach the peninsula on the northeast side of the lake, where there are several overused campsites (bear box). A use trail on the right provides access to the more remote, northernmost lakes.

Proceed ahead (southwest) on the left-hand trail and climb through open terrain toward the highest of the Little Five Lakes. A couple of view-packed campsites sit well above the lake and away from the trail. From the lake, the trail veers west and makes a sometimes steep climb to Black Rock Pass (approximately 11,700 feet) at a gap in the Great Western Divide. As you catch your breath, enjoy the sweeping views of both Five Lakes basins dropping into Big Arroyo and backdropped by the Kaweah Peaks. In the eastern distance, Mt. Whitney can be seen atop the Sierra Crest.

A steep, switchbacking descent leads away from the pass across open, rocky slopes that provide stunning views into the cirque basins of Spring, Cyclamen, and Columbine lakes at the head of rugged Cliff Creek canyon. More sedate

View of Upper Cliff Creek Basin from the Black Rock Pass Trail

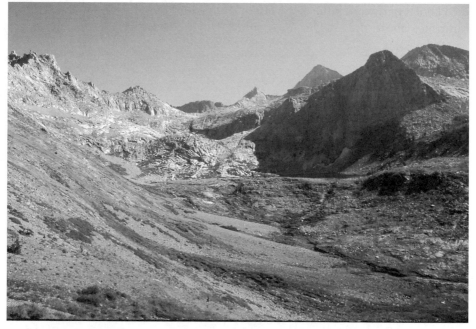

scenery waits ahead, as you descend toward the meadows bordering Cliff Creek on the way to diminutive Pinto Lake, tucked off the trail in a thicket of willows. The lake offers surprisingly warm swimming. A use trail on the left just beyond the lake leads to campsites (bear box).

Away from the vicinity of Pinto Lake, the trail drops on rocky switchbacks through dense shrubs before the grade eases near a view of ribbon-like Cliff Creek Falls. The descent continues down a boulder-filled wash, where the creek follows a subterranean course. You then leave the open terrain in favor of scattered fir forest. Hop across a number of lushly lined rivulets before arriving at a boulder hop of Cliff Creek (difficult in early season), a junction with the trail to Redwood Meadow, and campsites with a bear box.

Veer ahead (left, south), cross the creek, and follow the trail toward Timber Gap, a nearly 2400-foot, 2.75-mile climb. Forested switchbacks lead up a ridge to a long, flower-filled, sloping meadow well watered by numerous seeps. This charming, verdant vale seems to mute the otherwise stiff climb toward the gap. Just below Timber Gap, reenter forest, which inhibits any kind of rewarding view.

Fortunately, a view eventually comes, as the trail beyond Timber Gap soon breaks out of the trees onto brush-covered slopes, the result of a fire back in the 1990s. Here, the entire sweep of the Mineral King area lays at your feet, as the moderately steep trail propels you toward the Sawtooth-Monarch Trailhead. Just before the trailhead, you reach the junction with the trail east to Monarch Lakes and Sawtooth Pass; proceed on the right-hand trail from there a short distance to the trailhead.

BUILD-UP AND WIND-DOWN TIPS ·

Rustic **Silver City Resort** (559-734-4109, www.silvercityresort.com) offers breakfast, lunch, and dinner, Thursday through Monday, but their main attraction is the fresh-baked pies that are available every day of the week. Choose from apple streusel, chocolate walnut, blueberry, boysenberry, fruits of the forest, blackberry, mixed berry, and pecan. All pies are available à la mode. Visit the resort's website at www.silvercityresort.com.

Back in Three Rivers, there are plenty of restaurants, as well as several lodging options. The best dining can be found at the **Gateway Lodge** (559-561-4133, 45978 Sierra Dr.), the last commercial establishment before the Ash Mountain entrance on the extreme eastern edge of town. It offers both exquisite fare and stunning views of the scenic Kaweah River. A wide range of entrees allows patrons the opportunity to drop several bills on such delights as filet mignon, broiled salmon, or braised lamb shanks, or to choose something more economical, like a cheeseburger or the Gateway veggie pizza. For more details, check out the lodge's website at www.gateway-sequoia.com.

Since just getting to Mineral King requires a long drive from just about anywhere, camping at either the **Atwell Mill** or **Cold Springs campgrounds** provides a chance to get a good night's rest and acclimatize before starting your backpack trip.

41

CRESCENT MEADOW TO WHITNEY PORTAL VIA THE HIGH SIERRA TRAIL

Mike White

MILES: 68.5
RECOMMENDED DAYS: 8–14
ELEVATION GAIN/LOSS: 13,350´/11,850´
TYPE OF TRIP: Point-to-point
DIFFICULTY: Strenuous
SOLITUDE: Moderately populated to Moderate solitude
LOCATION: Sequoia-Kings Canyon national parks
MAPS: USGS 7.5-min. *Lodgepole, Triple Divide Peak, Mt. Kaweah,*
Chagoopa Falls, Mt. Whitney, and *Mt. Langley*
BEST SEASON: Late summer through early fall

PERMITS

A wilderness permit is required for entry into the backcountry of Sequoia and Kings Canyon national parks. Trailhead quotas are in effect from about the end of May to the end of September, and approximately 75 percent of the daily trailhead quota is available by advanced reservation between March 1 and September 15. Get a permit application from the park website (www.nps.gov/seki)

Photo: A successful summiteer returns on the Mt. Whitney Trail.

and submit the completed form by mail (Sequoia and Kings Canyon National Parks, Wilderness Permit Reservations, 47050 Generals Highway #60, Three Rivers, CA, 93271) or fax (559-565-4239). A $15, nonrefundable fee is assessed per reservation and can be made by credit card, check, or money order.

Applicants will receive a reservation confirmation by mail, which must then be turned into the nearest issue station to your departure trailhead in order to obtain the actual wilderness permit. Confirmation or pick up of your permit must occur before 9 AM on the departure day, otherwise the permit is cancelled and becomes available to other parties on a walk-in basis. Free walk-in permits may be obtained after 1 PM on the day before departure, and unclaimed reserved permits become available after 9 AM on the day of departure. Fees are charged for entrance into the park as well ($10 for a 7-day pass, $30 for an Annual Park Pass to Sequoia and Kings Canyon, and $80 for an America the Beautiful Pass that provides year-long access to all national parks and recreation areas).

CHALLENGES

Gas is not available within Sequoia or Kings Canyon—make sure you have enough gas to get into and out of the parks. Campfires are banned in several places along this route, so plan on using a stove. Bears are active throughout Sequoia National Park and surrounding national forest lands, requiring you to observe proper food-storage guidelines at all times. Bear canisters are required on the Mt. Whitney Trail, so you'll probably have to carry one on the rest of the trip anyway. Speaking of Mt. Whitney, as of 2007, all human waste must be packed out of the Mt. Whitney area. Pack-out kits are available at the visitor center in Lone Pine and the Crabtree ranger station and may be disposed of at the human-waste receptacle at Whitney Portal.

TAKE THIS TRIP

While it's lesser known than the 218-mile John Muir Trail, which runs the length of the Sierra from Mt. Whitney to Yosemite Valley, the 68.5-mile High Sierra Trail, traversing the Sierra from Giant Forest to Mt. Whitney, deserves equal consideration. While hordes of peakbaggers set their sights on Mt. Whitney from the east, and a good number of backpackers visit Bearpaw Meadow and Hamilton Lakes from the west, few others experience the majesty of the land in between. Wonderful treasures such as the alpine heights of Nine Lakes Basin, the meadows of Big Arroyo, the serenity of Moraine Lake, the glacier-carved depths of Kern Canyon, and remote lakes below the Sierra Crest await.

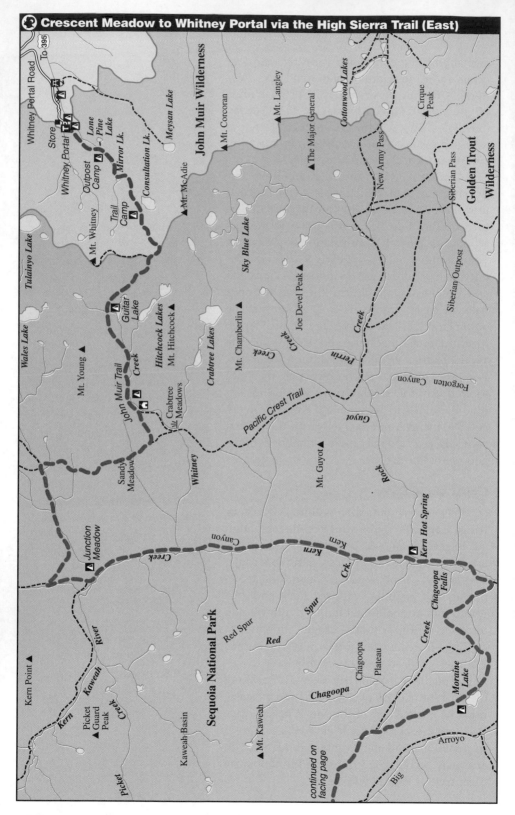

To 395

Whitney Portal Road

John Muir Wilderness

Meysan Lake

Mt. Corcoran

Mt. Langley

Cottonwood Lakes

Cirque Peak

New Army Pass

Siberian Pass

Golden Trout Wilderness

Store

Whitney Portal

Lone Pine Lake

Outpost Camp

Consultation Lk.

Mirror Lk.

Trail Camp

Mt. McAdie

The Major General

Siberian Outpost

Mt. Whitney

Tulainyo Lake

Guitar Lake

Sky Blue Lake

Joe Devel Peak

Perrin Creek

Forgotten Canyon

Wales Lake

Mt. Young

Hitchcock Lakes

Mt. Hitchcock

Crabtree Lakes

Mt. Chamberlin

Creek

Creek

Creek

John Muir Trail

Creek

Crabtree Meadows

Whitney

Guyot

Pacific Crest Trail

Sandy Meadow

Mt. Guyot

Rock

Junction Meadow

Kern Hot Spring

Kern

Canyon

Kern

Chagoopa Falls

Creek

Crk.

Red Spur

Spur

Chagoopa Plateau

Moraine Lake

Kern Point

Kaweah River

Red

Chagoopa

Sequoia National Park

Picket Guard Peak

Creek

Mt. Kaweah

Kaweah Basin

Kern

Picket

Arroyo

continued on facing page

Big

Crescent Meadow to Whitney Portal via the High Sierra Trail (West)

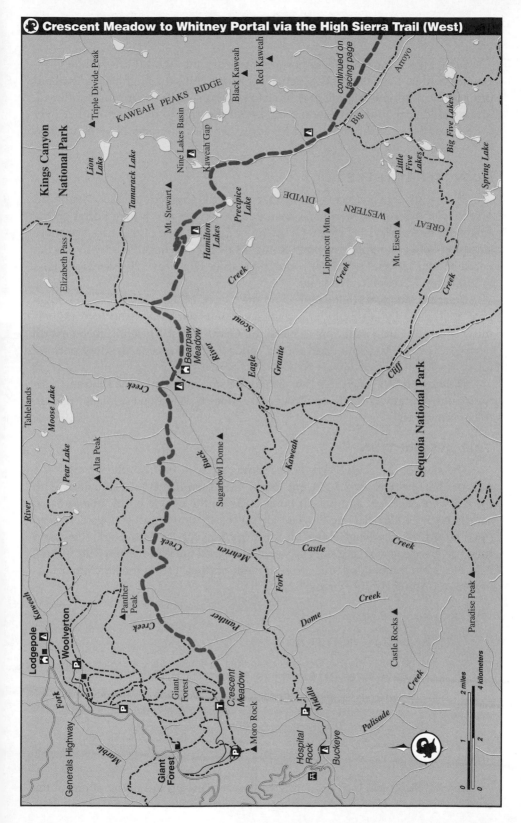

continued on facing page

Kings Canyon National Park

Triple Divide Peak ▲

KAWEAH PEAKS RIDGE

Black Kaweah ▲

Red Kaweah ▲

Arroyo

Big

Lion Lake

Nine Lakes Basin

Kaweah Gap

Big Five Lakes

Tamarack Lake

Little Five Lakes

Spring Lake

Mt. Stewart ▲

Precipice Lake

WESTERN DIVIDE

Hamilton Lakes

Lippincott Mtn. ▲

Mt. Eisen ▲

GREAT

Elizabeth Pass

Creek

Scout

Creek

Creek

Tablelands

Bearpaw Meadow

River

Eagle

Granite

Cliff

Moose Lake

Creek

Sequoia National Park

Pear Lake

Alta Peak ▲

Buck

Creek

Sugarbowl Dome ▲

Kaweah

River

Creek

Creek

Mehrten

Castle

Creek

Panther Peak ▲

Fork

Panther

Dome

Creek

Paradise Peak ▲

Lodgepole

Woolverton

Creek

Castle Rocks ▲

Kaweah

Fork

Giant Forest

Crescent Meadow

Middle

Creek

Marble

Moro Rock ▲

Buckeye

Polisade

Generals Highway

Giant Forest

Hospital Rock

2 miles   4 kilometers

0   1   2

Competition for wilderness permits for entry into the Whitney Zone is exceedingly high. Unlucky backpackers who wish to hike the High Sierra Trail but can't obtain a Whitney permit may have to select an alternate terminus trailhead. The most logical alternative would be to exit the area to the south, either over Cottonwood Pass to the Horseshoe Meadow Trailhead, or over New Army Pass to the Cottonwood Lakes Trailhead.

HOW TO GET THERE

Making arrangements to get dropped off at the Crescent Meadow Trailhead on the west side of the Sierra and then get picked up at Whitney Portal on the east side several days later may be the most difficult part of this trip. For those shuttling between trailheads, State Route 58 over Tehachapi Pass (between Bakersfield and Mojave) is a faster route than either Highway 120 over Tioga Pass or Highway 178 over Walker Pass.

Crescent Meadow Trailhead: Follow the Generals Highway from the Lodgepole area (where you should have picked up your wilderness and parking permits) south toward Giant Forest. Near the Giant Forest Museum, turn east on narrow Crescent Meadow Road for 2.5 miles to the Crescent Meadow parking lot.

Whitney Portal: Take U.S. Hwy. 395 to the small town of Lone Pine and turn west onto Whitney Portal Road. Proceed 13 miles to Whitney Portal and park in the overnight lot.

TRIP DESCRIPTION

The start of the High Sierra Trail follows a paved path southeast, crosses a pair of short bridges over Crescent Creek, and then heads past junctions with the Crescent Meadow and Bobcat Point trails on the way to a fork in a forested saddle near the Burial Tree. Proceed ahead (east), as the trail swings across an open hillside perched high above Middle Fork Kaweah River, to Eagle View, and then traverses south-facing slopes to a junction with the Woolverton Cutoff Trail, 2.5 miles from the parking area. A short walk northeast from the junction brings you to refreshing Panther Creek.

IMAGINING A HIGH TRAIL

The High Sierra Trail was the brainchild of former park superintendent Colonel John White, who envisioned a trail connecting the two main features of Sequoia National Park, the big trees (giant sequoias) and the big peak (Mt. Whitney). Constructed by members of the Civilian Conservation Corp in the 1930s, the High Sierra Trail has been dazzling visitors ever since.

Beyond the creek, the undulating trail moves in and out of the seams of the creek's tributaries for the next couple miles before climbing over Sevenmile Hill.

At 5.5 miles, you hop over Mehrten Creek, where a short use trail climbs steeply up the hillside to the first legal campsites along the HST (bear box).

Continue east past the Sevenmile Trail junction and make a short traverse beneath light forest cover to an easy ford of a tiny tributary of Mehrten Creek. A pronounced descent then leads to the twin-channeled crossing of the first of many Buck Creek tributaries. At 8.25 miles, near another twin-branched tributary, is the next developed campsite (bear box). Beyond the streams, the trail bends around the mostly open slope of Buck Canyon and then drops to a bridge over the main channel of Bucks Creek. From the bridge, a switchbacking climb attacks the east wall of Bucks Canyon on the way to the top of a low ridge and a junction with the 200-foot lateral south to Bearpaw Meadow Campground. The overused campground has numbered sites sheltered by dense timber. There are also bear boxes, a spigot with treated water, and a pit toilet. Campfires are prohibited.

While heavily shaded Bearpaw Meadow Campground looks somewhat gloomy, Bearpaw Meadow High Sierra Camp, 0.2 mile east on the HST, is the exact opposite. Perched high atop the canyon wall, the open setting, near the lip of Middle Fork Kaweah River canyon, offers stunning views of the glacier-scoured surroundings to the east, including Eagle Scout Peak and Mt. Stewart on the Great Western Divide, the Yosemite-esque cleft of Hamilton Creek, and Black Kaweah above Kaweah Gap. Similar to the famed High Sierra Camps in Yosemite's backcountry, guests at Bearpaw Meadow sleep in tent cabins and enjoy hot meals for breakfast and dinner (by reservation only). The nearby ranger station offers emergency services.

Follow a descending traverse east, away from the activity at Bearpaw Meadow, to cross the precipitous north face of River Valley, where you will enjoy excellent views of the canyon along the way. At the canyon bottom, a concrete culvert spans usually rowdy Lone Pine Creek. A short climb above the creek leads to a small bench and a junction with the trail to Elizabeth Pass. Decent campsites can be found near the junction.

Head southeast for a stiff, switchbacking climb across dry slopes covered with manzanita, sagebrush, and scattered black oaks. The trail curves into the canyon of Hamilton Creek; the stunning, view-packed topography in this granite sanctuary is absolutely amazing. North of the trail, the towering wall of Angel Wings rivals any of Yosemite Valley's better-known walls. The white domes of Hamilton Towers top the ridge on the opposite sides of the canyon. You soon ford tumbling Hamilton Creek and climb over shards of rock above Lower Hamilton Lake to the outlet of Upper Hamilton Lake at 8235 feet. At the north end of the lake, there are good but overused campsites offering fine views of a waterfall at the east end (two-night limit, and no fires). Anglers may enjoy the challenge of trying to land a brook, rainbow, or golden trout.

Now you face the 2500-foot ascent to Kaweah Gap. The trail is something of an engineering marvel, blasted right out of solid rock in places. From the outlet of Upper Hamilton Lake, the trail zigzags up the north wall of an enormous cirque and then veers south past a tarn on the way to Precipice Lake, at the base of the impressive north face of Eagle Scout Peak. A 0.75-mile climb past a smattering of miniature tarns finally leads to Kaweah Gap, where there is a grand view of the Kaweah Peaks, Nine Lakes Basin, and Big Arroyo.

Glacier-scoured Nine Lakes Basin is a special place, worthy of at least one layover day for those who have the extra time and energy. The U-shaped basin at the convergence of the Great Western Divide and Kaweah Peaks Ridge, culminating at Triple Divide Peak, presents unparalleled alpine scenery. To visit the basin, descend a few switchbacks from Kaweah Gap and then leave the HST to head north cross-country to the first lake, at about 10,455 feet. From there, off-trail travel to the upper two lakes is straightforward. The route to a set of lakes to the east crosses more difficult terrain and requires advanced route-finding skills.

From Kaweah Gap, the trail steadily descends down the west side of Big Arroyo. Halfway down the canyon, you cross Big Arroyo Creek and follow the east side of the canyon through alternating pockets of meadow and granite, crossing numerous side streams along the way. The open terrain permits fine views of the canyon and the multihued Kaweah Peaks to the north. Near a tributary draining an unnamed tarn are some campsites (with a bear box), about a quarter mile before the Little Five Lakes Trail junction, 3 miles from Kaweah Gap. Little Five Lakes is another area worthy of a side trip.

From the junction, head southeast to embark on a long, sustained, ascending traverse of Big Arroyo. The timber along this section is sparse, which allows a flourish of shrubs such as sagebrush, chinquapin, and manzanita, accented by splashes of color from a host of drought-tolerant wildflowers. After crossing several tributaries, pass a small tarn and then begin a mild descent away from the lip of the canyon. Head through alternating sections of meadow and lodgepole and foxtail pine forest, and shortly arrive at a large meadow with a junction with the trail to Moraine Lake.

Although the designated route of the HST continues across Chagoopa Plateau, the alternate route to Moraine Lake offers better scenery and the opportunity to camp at the lake. Veer right (south-southeast) at the junction and leave the meadow behind on a descent through dense stands of foxtail and lodgepole pines. Returning to the edge of Big Arroyo provides fine views of the canyon and the impressive peaks of the Great Western Divide. The descent gets steeper on the way to the wooded shore of Moraine Lake, where excellent campsites offer an overnight haven; campsites along the south shore offer the best views of the Kaweah Peaks.

Hop across the outlet of Moraine Lake, traverse the moraine at the east end, and drop down to lovely, flower-filled and grass-covered Sky Parlor Meadows, with additional views of the Kaweah Peaks and Great Western Divide. Rejoin the HST near the eastern edge of the meadow, just beyond a ford of Funston Creek.

A moderate, then steep descents leads into the deep, U-shaped trench of Kern Canyon. Along the way, white fir and Jeffrey pine replace the trees from above and, farther down, an occasional juniper or black oak stands above the manzanita and snowbush understory. Tight, rocky switchbacks parallel the tumbling course of Funston Creek, which you cross a couple times before bottoming out on the floor of the canyon. Reach a junction with the Kern Canyon Trail, 5 miles from Moraine Lake and 4000 feet below Kaweah Gap.

Turn left (north) and follow the Kern Canyon Trail upstream through a marshy area, a pair of meadows, and a stretch of forest composed of Jeffrey pines and incense cedars. Hop across Chagoopa Creek, catching a glimpse through the trees of the falls high on the west side of the canyon. Gently graded trail continues upstream to the stout bridge across the Kern River. Now on the east side of the gorge, you soon reach the ford of Rock Creek. Shortly beyond the ford, around a point, is Kern Hot Spring, a popular backcountry destination, despite the fact that days of hiking are required to reach it from the nearest trailhead. Hot water fills a crude cement bathtub downstream from the spring, providing a warm oasis that has soothed the tired muscles of many a hiker for several decades. The designated campground (bear box) northeast of the spring is cramped and overused; solitude seekers should look for campsites farther afield.

Head north from Kern Hot Spring, ford the upper branch of Rock Creek, and then proceed upstream on a gravelly path past some campsites. For the next 7 miles, the trail follows the east side of the U-shaped Kern River trench, beneath the towering walls of the canyon. Glacial action has left many hanging valleys on either side of the canyon, resulting in scenic cascades spilling down the walls toward a union with the Kern River and requiring numerous fords as you continue north. Some of these fords may be difficult in early season, particularly on the stream draining Guyot Flat, Whitney Creek, and Wallace Creek. The ascent of the canyon is gentle for the most part, resulting in straightforward travel through generally open terrain until you approach the ford of Wallace Creek, where you enter a Jeffrey pine forest accented by a smattering of lodgepole and western

The research hut on the summit of Mt. Whitney was built in 1909.

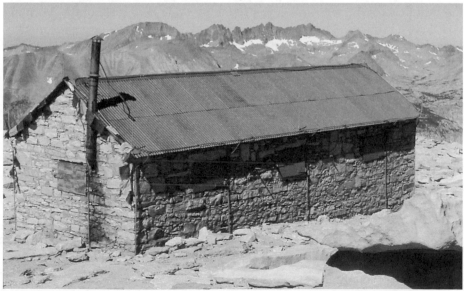

white pines. Continue through the trees to shady campsites near Junction Meadow (bear box). A short distance up the trail is a junction with the Colby Pass Trail, heading west toward the Kern-Kaweah canyon.

Continue up Kern Canyon (north) from the junction, climbing moderately through stretches of mixed forest alternating with manzanita- and currant-covered clearings, which offer fine views of Kern-Kaweah canyon and the Kern River trench. After 1.2 miles, the HST climbs out of Kern Canyon on an ascending traverse toward Wallace Creek. A mile farther, the path veers northeast, up Wallace Creek canyon, and climbs another mile to the ford of Wright Creek. Continuing the climb, you reach a junction with the shared route of the famed John Muir and Pacific Crest trails.

Turn right (south) on the JMT/PCT, which immediately leads to a ford of Wallace Creek. Campsites near the ford (bear box) offer the possibility of a layover day for exploration of upper Wallace Creek and Wallace, Wales, and Tulainyo lakes. Gently graded trail proceeds through groves of lodgepole and foxtail pines before climbing over a saddle to the west of Mt. Young. Continue past Sandy Meadow to a junction, where the JMT bends northeast and the PCT continues its southbound journey toward the Mexican border.

Turn left to follow the JMT toward Crabtree ranger station (pick up a human-waste pack-out kit for Mt. Whitney) and nearby campsites along Whitney Creek (bear box). The route of the JMT differs from what is shown on the USGS 7.5-min. *Mount Whitney* map, remaining well up the north bank of Whitney Creek until it reaches a picturesque meadow just below Timberline Lake (no camping). The trail climbs moderately through open, rocky terrain to Guitar Lake, a popular camping area for those interested in a next-day Mt. Whitney summit bid. The Hitchcock Lakes to the south generally provide more secluded camping.

From Guitar Lake, you climb through moist alpine meadows to a series of long-legged switchbacks up the west face of the Sierra Crest to a junction with the trail to Mt. Whitney. Unless you're the first one here early in the morning, you'll see a number of backpacks stowed away in rock clefts near the junction. You should feel reasonably comfortable adding your backpack to the pile and carrying a small daypack with valuables and necessities to the summit.

Here, the 2-mile slog to the summit begins. A steady climb leads along the west side of the ridge, with the trail periodically entering notches in the crest that provide acrophobic vistas straight down the near vertical east face. Proceeding up the rocky trail, sharp eyes may detect the summit's research hut, built by the Smithsonian Institution in 1909. As you approach the final slope, the grade increases, as multiple paths follow serpentine routes toward the top. Cairns may aid some in finding the route, but the way is unmistakable—head for the highest point! Soon, the roof of the hut pops into view, and you quickly gain the broad summit, which is filled with jumbled slabs and boulders. Don't forget to sign the summit register located near the hut. To proclaim the sweeping view from the summit as fantastic seems wholly inadequate.

Although the John Muir Trail technically ends at the 14,496-foot summit of Mt. Whitney, the terminus to your trip still lies several trail miles away. After returning to the junction and retrieving your pack, turn right (southeast) to make the short ascent to Trail Crest (at 13,620 feet), at the boundary between Sequoia National Park and John Muir Wilderness. Now begins the mind-numbing descent down the "100 switchbacks" toward Trail Camp. About halfway down is a shaded area notorious for being covered with ice—steel cables provide handholds if necessary.

The knee-pounding switchbacks finally end near the outskirts of Trail Camp, where a preponderance of colorful tents and brightly clad summit hopefuls from around the globe often creates a circus-like atmosphere. Don't expect a serene wilderness experience if you plan to camp in this vicinity. Some campers venture off to the south, toward sites around Consultation Lake, which tends to diminish the crowds only slightly. Due to the overwhelming number of visitors, coupled with the shallow soils and the inability of composting toilets to digest significant amounts of waste at this altitude, regulations now require campers to pack out all human waste. Despite the crush of human activity, the scenery at Trail Camp is stunning, with an amphitheater of towering peaks dwarfing the immediate surroundings.

Away from the hubbub of Trail Camp, the trail drops steeply on rock steps and pebbly tread through a sea of boulders, fords Lone Pine Creek, and then traverses Trailside Meadow, a verdant grassland punctuated with colorful wildflowers, including columbine, paintbrush, and shooting stars. Beyond this oasis, the trail continues descending through rocky terrain on the way to switchbacks that lead down to mellower terrain near Mirror Lake (no camping), a smallish body of water occupying a cirque below the south face of Thor Peak. Boulder hop across the outlet and then descend more switchbacks to a ford of Lone Pine Creek, just before Outpost Camp, the only legal place after Trail Camp to pitch a tent.

Skirt a willow-covered meadow just beyond Outpost Camp, make a pair of creek crossings, and then follow more switchbacks to a junction with a lateral to Lone Pine Lake. Veer left (north-northwest) to stay on the main trail, cross the creek once more, and begin the last set of long and dusty switchbacks. Other than when you make a couple more crossings of Lone Pine Creek, the trail lacks shade until you enter the cool forest surrounding Whitney Portal at trail's end.

BUILD-UP AND WIND-DOWN TIPS ·

After eight to 14 days on the trail, you'll enjoy the chance to taste real food again at the **Whitney Portal Store**. Although the selection is limited, a hamburger and a milkshake should be satisfying. The tiny town of **Lone Pine** offers a handful of restaurants serving fare ranging from burgers and pizza to steaks and seafood. A nearly equal number of budget motels offer hot showers and real beds.

42

LODGEPOLE CAMPGROUND TO DEADMAN CANYON LOOP

Mike White

MILES: 52.0
RECOMMENDED DAYS: 6–12
ELEVATION GAIN/LOSS: 14,000´/14,000´
TYPE OF TRIP: Loop
DIFFICULTY: Strenuous
SOLITUDE: Moderate solitude
LOCATION: Sequoia-Kings Canyon national parks
MAPS: USGS 7.5-min. *Lodgepole, Mt. Silliman, Sphinx Lakes,*
and *Triple Divide Peak*
BEST SEASON: Late summer through early fall

PERMITS

A wilderness permit is required for entry into the backcountry of Sequoia and Kings Canyon national parks. Trailhead quotas are in effect from about the end of May to the end of September, and approximately 75 percent of the daily trailhead quota is available by advanced reservation between March 1 and September 15. Get a permit application from the park website (www.nps.gov/seki) and submit the completed form by mail (Sequoia and Kings Canyon National Parks, Wilderness Permit Reservations, 47050 Generals Highway #60, Three Riv-

Photo: Ranger Lake backdropped by Twin Peaks

ers, CA, 93271) or fax (559-565-4239). A $15, nonrefundable fee is assessed per reservation and can be made by credit card, check, or money order.

Applicants will receive a reservation confirmation by mail, which must then be turned into the nearest issue station to your departure trailhead in order to obtain the actual wilderness permit. Confirmation or pick up of your permit must occur before 9 AM on the departure day, otherwise the permit is cancelled and becomes available to other parties on a walk-in basis. Free walk-in permits may be obtained after 1 PM on the day before departure, and unclaimed reserved permits become available after 9 AM on the day of departure. Fees are charged for entrance into the park as well ($10 for a 7-day pass, $30 for an Annual Park Pass to Sequoia and Kings Canyon, and $80 for an America the Beautiful Pass that provides year-long access to all national parks and recreation areas).

CHALLENGES

Gas is not available within Sequoia or Kings Canyon—make sure you have enough fuel to get into and out of the parks. Campfires are banned in several places along this route, so plan to use a stove. Bears are active throughout Sequoia National Park and surrounding national forest lands, requiring you to observe proper food-storage guidelines at all times. While bear canisters are not required, they are highly recommended. In lieu of canisters, use the bear boxes at locations noted in the trip description. Bear-bagging food has proved to be largely ineffectual.

HOW TO GET THERE

Access Generals Highway within Sequoia National Park from either State Highway 198 east from Visalia or State Highway 180 east from Fresno, and follow it to the Lodgepole turnoff. Pick up your wilderness and parking permit at the visitor center and proceed past

TAKE THIS TRIP

This 50-plus-mile loop takes you to one of the most scenic canyons in the California, glacier-carved Deadman Canyon. Here, classic High Sierra scenery is abundant, with glistening granite walls rimmed by towering summits and extensive flower-covered meadows below. And best of all, the crowds are light. The trail passes through a wide range of environments in addition to the dramatic canyon, including mid-elevation forests, subalpine, and alpine zones.

Extra days can be spent adventuring into equally scenic areas off the main route. Before the shuttle-bus season ends (usually after Labor Day), it's possible to hike out the last 9 miles along the more scenic High Sierra Trail to the Crescent Meadow Trailhead, rather than following the described route back to Lodgepole. From the trailhead at Crescent Meadow, catch the bus to the Giant Forest Museum and transfer to the bus to Lodgepole. Buses usually run between 9 AM and 6 PM.

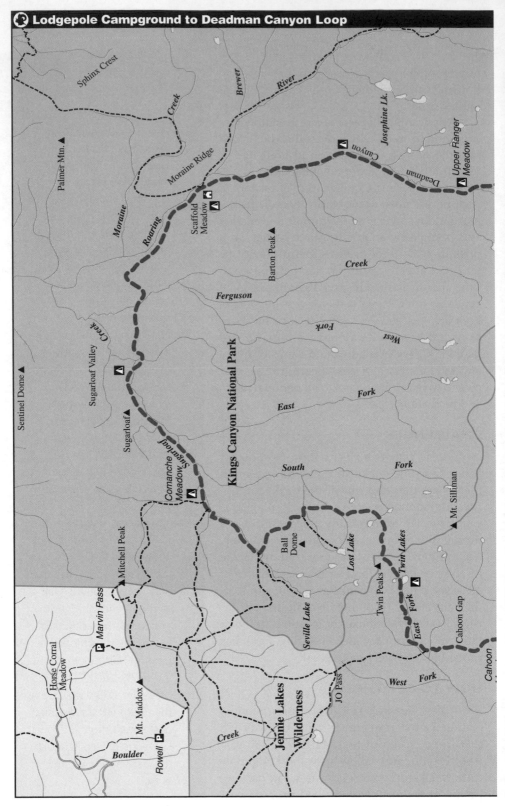

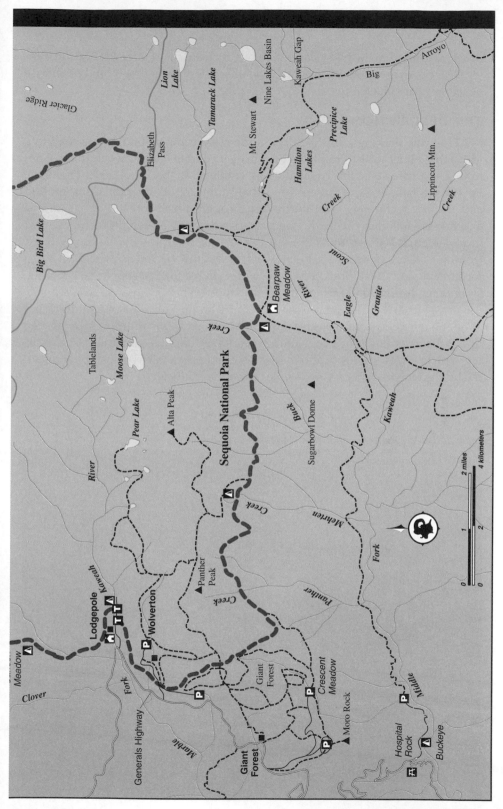

the campground to the hiker parking lot across from the Walter Fry Nature Center. Bear boxes are available for any food or scented items that would otherwise be left in your vehicle.

TRIP DESCRIPTION

From the parking area, head back down the campground access road to a fork and go left (north), crossing a bridge over Marble Fork Kaweah River. Continue a short way past the Topokah Falls Trailhead to the Twin Lakes Trailhead. Follow the Twin Lakes Trail north-northwest through Lodgepole Campground and then start climbing west-northwest through mixed forest over a moraine and into the Silliman Creek drainage. Cross a tiny, spring-fed brook and almost immediately reach a T-junction with the Wuksachi Trail to Wuksachi Village. Continue ahead, cross a rock-filled wash, and climb via rocky switchbacks to a ford of Silliman Creek (the creek is the water source for Lodgepole, so camping, swimming, fishing, and picnicking are not allowed here).

Away from the creek, the ascent continues around the nose of a south-facing spur and then heads northeast to Cahoon Meadow. A few campsites are nestled under the trees along the fringe of the meadow. Continue climbing past a clearing with fine views across Cahoon Meadow and past a fair-sized, sloping meadow on the way to Cahoon Gap, 4 miles from the trailhead.

Lush and lovely Ranger Meadow in Deadman Canyon

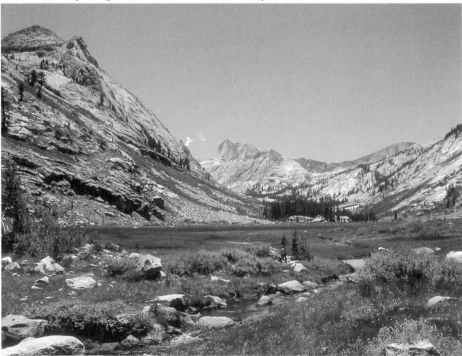

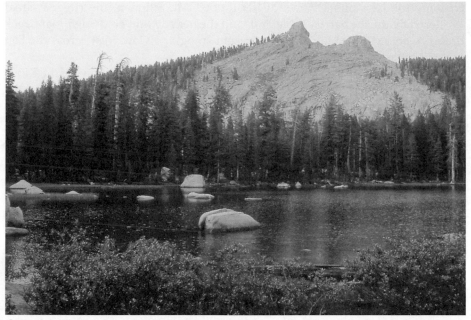

One of the Twin Lakes with Twin Peaks above

A mild to moderate descent from the gap parallels East Fork Clover Creek and then crosses a tributary stream via an easy boulder hop to campsites (bear box) on the far side. Proceed through fir forest for 0.3 mile to a junction with the trail to JO Pass, with campsites nearby.

Bear right (northeast) at the junction and continue climbing, following East Fork Clover Creek to a ford. The grade increases as you veer away from the creek and climb up the steep hillside, where lodgepole and western white pine join the forest, and a host of wildflowers provide an array of color in season. Beyond a series of switchbacks, the grade finally eases on the approach to Twin Lakes. The two lakes are more like fraternal than identical twins. The southernmost lake is quite a bit larger than the other, and they bear no physical resemblance to each other in shape. The rugged towers of Twin Peaks are visible from spots along the shore of the larger lake. A pair of bear boxes is located on the strip of forest between the two lakes, near a number of overused but shady campsites. Slightly less-used sites are spread around the shoreline of both lakes, and a pit toilet is located west of the smaller twin. Swimming in the shallow lakes can be pleasant, particularly on customarily hot afternoons.

From Twin Lakes, you begin a switchbacking, 700-foot climb northeast toward Silliman Pass. The trail crosses back and forth over the diminutive inlet, providing welcome opportunities to slake your thirst during the stiff ascent. Between sporadic clumps of lodgepole pines, you have improving views of the lakes below and Twin Peaks above. The grade eases near the crest, as you stroll over to Silliman Pass (at approximately 10,185 feet), which marks the boundary between Sequoia and Kings Canyon national parks. Through widely scattered conifers, the pass offers views of flat-topped Mt. Silliman, the rugged Great Western Divide, the barren Tableland, and the heavily timbered Sugarloaf Creek drainage below. If not for the ever-present smog, the view west across the San Joaquin Valley would be equally impressive.

Steep switchbacks descend away from the pass, with good views of the Kings River country along the way, including Tehipite Dome and the peaks along the Monarch Divide. Soon, the blue surfaces of Beville and Ranger lakes spring into view to the east, as the steep, serpentine descent continues, ultimately leveling off at the basin's floor, where you pass a pair of junctions with short trails north to Ranger Lake and south to Beville Lake. Beville Lake offers only marginal campsites, while Ranger Lake has five designated campsites, two bear boxes, and a summer ranger cabin. Anglers can ply the waters of the lodgepole-rimmed lake in search of rainbow trout.

From the Ranger Lake junction, proceed northeast over granite slabs, around boulders, and beneath widely scattered pines on a general descent, interrupted briefly by a short climb over the crest of a ridge. Just past a verdant pocket meadow well watered by a flower-lined stream, you pass a junction with the Lost Lake Trail. Continue north over the lushly lined outlet, and proceed through mixed forest around the southeast flank of Ball Dome. Crest a ridge and drop through a

A stunning view from below Elizabeth Pass

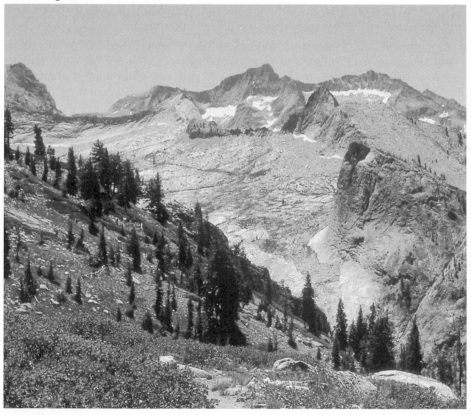

grassy vale to the bottom of Belle Canyon and the broad fork of Sugarloaf Creek; there is a junction here with a trail to Seville Lake and Rowell Meadow.

Turn right (northeast) and follow a gently graded descent to a crossing of an unnamed tributary. Contrary to its appearance on the USGS Mt. Silliman map, the trail remains on the north side of Sugarloaf Creek. Step across a pleasant side stream about a mile from the junction and continue the pleasant descent, past a junction with a trail to Rowell Meadow, to aspen- and willow-lined Comanche Meadow. Near the far end of the clearing, a short path leads to campsites (bear box) and access to Sugarloaf Creek.

The descent continues from Comanche Meadow through lush foliage to the crossing of a stream draining Williams Meadow. From there, pass into the markedly drier surroundings of a Jeffrey pine forest, which still reveals evidence of the extensive 1974 fire. Pass through a drift fence and drop into Sugarloaf Valley, with fine views through scattered trees and over clumps of manzanita to Sugarloaf, the prominent hump of granite for which the valley is named. Reach a junction marked simply BEAR BOX, where a short path leads to a shady campsites (and, as promised, a bear box) and a hitching post near a small stream.

Cross a side stream and proceed on gently graded and dusty tread to a ford of Sugarloaf Creek, the lowest point of the journey. Plan on a wet ford here, even if the water is low. A couple marginal campsites are located above the far side of the creek.

Climb through dense forest and across minor rivulets toward tumbling Ferguson Creek. Reach the top of a manzanita-covered and pine-dotted moraine at the lip of Roaring River canyon with fine views of Palmer Mountain, Sphinx Crest, and peaks of the Great Western Divide. The river lives up to its name with a tumultuous roar that reverberates up the wall of the canyon.

Drop to the floor of the canyon, pass through a drift fence, and begin the steady climb up the drainage, at times right next to frothy Roaring River tumbling down the boulder-strewn canyon. Just beyond another drift fence, you hop across a side stream and reach the grassy clearing of Scaffold Meadow, followed by a T-junction near the Roaring River Ranger Station. Up either trail are numerous campsites (bear boxes) near the river.

Take the footbridge across Roaring River and make a steep then moderate climb through a light, mixed forest into Deadman Canyon, where more gently graded trail leads to campsites just before the ford of Deadman Canyon creek. Beyond the creek, pass through a pleasant, wildflower-covered meadow amid good views of the granite cliffs and walls of the canyon. Proceed through alternating stands of mixed forest and pockets of meadow, where tiny quaking aspens testify to the frequent avalanches that roar down the hillsides. Reach a long meadow, where the creek glides sinuously through grasses and flowers. At the near end of the meadow is a use trail that branches away to campsites, and at this junction is the gravesite for which the canyon is named. A deteriorating sign reads: HERE REPOSES ALFRED MONIERE, SHEEPHERDER, MOUNTAIN MAN, 18— TO 1887. As the story goes, Moniere took ill and passed away before his associate could make the round-trip to Fresno for help. Whether or not the tale is true, Deadman Canyon is one of the most magnificent burial plots in the Sierra.

Beyond the gravesite, you ford the creek again and continue upstream on a mild ascent through boulders, shrubs, and flowers to a picturesque area where the creek spills across a series of slabs. Pass through a drift fence and continue climbing through lush foliage to where the grade eases near a stand of lodge-poles and firs. Beyond the trees, you enter the extensive grasslands of Ranger Meadow, where the steep canyon walls and the peaks at the head of the canyon combine to create a stunning scene across the flower-bedecked meadow.

At the far end of Ranger Meadow, a moderate climb through lodgepole pines leads to the crossing of a lushly lined tributary and then continues across rocky slopes dotted with heather to a ford of the vigorous main channel of Deadman Canyon creek. From there, a moderate to moderately steep climb leads through a rock garden and past a drift fence to the lip of Upper Ranger Meadow. Just off the trail in a grove of pines on the right are two good campsites. With extra time, you could follow a steep use trail southwest from the camp area up to Big Bird Lake.

Gently graded trail proceeds through Upper Ranger Meadow, followed by increasingly steeper, switchbacking tread near the head of the canyon. After crossing the creek, the trail veers southwest to ascend a talus-and-boulder-filled cirque and zigzags up to Elizabeth Pass, where the views are remarkable.

Although the 2100-foot ascent is behind you, a more difficult challenge awaits as you cross from Kings Canyon into Sequoia and begin the 3300-foot, knee-wrenching descent to the Tamarack Lake junction. Unless the Park Service does some much-needed maintenance on the trail below the pass, you will most likely have to descend poor tread through eroded gullies and extensive wash-outs. Numerous cairns help guide you, although the general route down the gla-cier-scoured terrain is relatively straightforward. The upper part of the descent has fine views of Moose and Lost lakes, while a profusion of wildflowers grace the lower slopes. Farther down, dramatic views of Lion Rock, Mt. Stewart, and Eagle Scout Peak issue a siren call luring backpackers to the mountainous terrain surrounding Tamarack and Hamilton lakes. The descent finally eases near the Tamarack Lake Trail junction, where a couple campsites can be found a short distance up this path in a grove of trees near Lone Pine Creek.

Head south to make a short, mild descent to another junction, and veer right (southwest) to climb steeply on the Over the Hill Trail. Open areas along this ascent offer stunning views of the rugged terrain surrounding Lone Pine Canyon and up the Hamilton Creek drainage. The grade eases on a traverse of the brow of the slope, and then you descend through thickening forest on the way to a junction with the High Sierra Trail. A ranger station and Bearpaw High Sierra Camp lie about 200 yards east, while the lateral trail to Bearpaw Meadow Camp-ground, a heavily shaded backpackers camp with piped water, bear boxes, and outhouse, is about the same distance to the right (west).

Take the famed High Sierra Trail southwest and make a switchbacking de-scent through sugar pines and firs to a bridge over Buck Creek. Ascend the mostly open slopes of Buck Canyon and then curve around to a twin-branched tributary with good campsites (bear box). Beyond, a long, rolling traverse leads across the north slope of the Middle Fork Kaweah River canyon, crossing several refreshing brooks along the way. Through periodic gaps in the forest, you have excellent views of the canyon, Little Blue Dome, Sugarbowl Dome, and Castle Rocks. Past the junction with the Sevenmile Hill Trail, the trail climbs steeply northwest through thick stands of white fir and incense cedar, past Mehrten Creek, and continues through Jeffrey pine forest and patches of manzanita across two more branches of the stream. Eventually, the grade eases where the trail bends to the west and follows an ascending traverse back over the creek and some rills to a series of switchbacks leading up to a junction with the Alta Trail. Campsites at Mehrten Meadow lie a quarter mile to the east.

Turn west at the junction and follow the Alta Trail down a series of short switchbacks, cross a spring-fed rivulet, and then proceed across a south-facing, open hillside, enjoying views of the Middle Fork Kaweah River canyon along the way. After a mile of hiking, you reach Panther Gap and a junction with the Lakes Trail.

Follow the Lakes Trail, roughly paralleling Woolverton Creek, first northwest and then west, on a mild to moderate descent to a pair of T-junctions. From the first junction, a trail heads southeast to arc around Long Meadow, while from the second junction, a path heads south toward the Woolverton Trailhead. Continue straight ahead at both junctions, following signs for Lodgepole. As the descending trail bends south and the roar of Woolverton Creek fills the air, the trail merges with an old roadbed and then continues to the Lodgepole Trailhead.

PREVENT YOUR SLEEPING BAG FROM BECOMING A SUPERFUND SITE

After several trips your sleeping bag's brightly colored fabric will likely become muted by a film of dirt and human by-products. You can minimize the eventual descent of your bag into filth hell in a couple ways. At camp in the morning, turn your bag inside out on a large boulder or slab to allow the sun and fresh air to refresh it while you attend to chores. A sleeping bag liner is another great way to keep your bag clean. Although it's one more thing to throw in your pack, the extra comfort a liner provides is well worth the weight; plus washing a liner is a lot easier than washing a bag.

While airing your bag out and using a liner substantially postpone the need to launder it, prolonged use insures that, at some point, the bag must be cleaned—a fact that became abundantly clear to me after repeated use of my favorite goose down bag. Although both down and synthetic sleeping bags can be laundered, you must be careful to follow the manufacturers' instructions. If you send it out to be laundered, ask your local outdoor store for a recommendation.

BUILD-UP AND WIND-DOWN TIPS ·

A limited selection of lodges on the western side of the parks offers cushy accommodation for acclimatizing before a backcountry trip. From south to north, facilities include **Wuksachi Village** (888-252-5757), **Stony Creek Lodge** (866-522-6966), **Montecito Lake Resort** (800-227-9900), and **Grant Grove Cabins** and **John Muir Lodge** (866-522-6966). Two National Park Service campgrounds, **Lodgepole** and **Dorst Creek**, provide a less expensive way to get a jump on your trip (877-444-6777). Nearby Forest Service campgrounds include **Stony Creek**, **Upper Stony Creek**, **Buck Rock**, **Big Meadows**, **Tenmile**, **Landslide**, **Hume Lake**, and **Princess** (877-444-6777). There are also plenty of places to shower, wash clothes, get information, shop, mail letters, or simply lounge in **Lodgepole**.

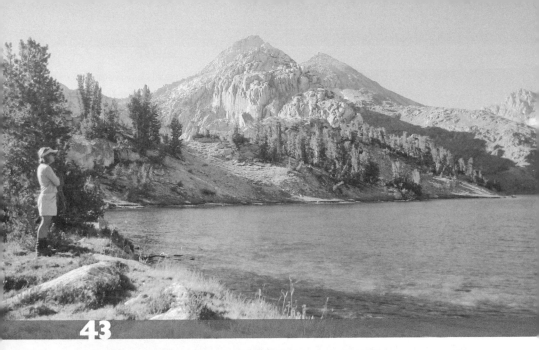

43

RAE LAKES LOOP

Mike White

MILES: 39.0
RECOMMENDED DAYS: 4–7
ELEVATION GAIN/LOSS: 3880´/3880´
TYPE OF TRIP: Loop
DIFFICULTY: Moderately strenuous
SOLITUDE: Moderately populated
LOCATION: Sequoia-Kings Canyon national parks
MAPS: USGS 7.5-min. *The Sphinx* and *Mt. Clarence King*
BEST SEASON: Late summer through early fall

PERMITS

A wilderness permit is required for entry into the backcountry of Sequoia and Kings Canyon National Parks. Trailhead quotas are in effect from about the end of May to the end of September, and approximately 75 percent of the daily trailhead quota is available by advanced reservation between March 1 and September 15. Get a permit application from the park website (www.nps.gov/seki) and submit the completed form by mail (Sequoia and Kings Canyon National Parks, Wilderness Permit Reservations, 47050 Generals Highway #60, Three Rivers, CA, 93271) or fax (559-565-4239). A $15, nonrefundable fee is assessed per reservation and can be made by credit card, check, or money order.

Photo: A hiker admires the scenery around one of the lakes in Sixty Lakes Basin.

TAKE THIS TRIP

Without a doubt, the Rae Lakes Loop is one of the most popular backcountry trips in Sequoia and Kings Canyon. For those who don't mind the company, the area offers some classic High Sierra scenery featuring crystalline, subalpine lakes that reflect an array of glacier-sculpted domes and jagged peaks. Beginning in the majestic setting of Kings Canyon, the route visits two major Sierra creeks (Woods and Bubbs), a significant waterfall (Mist Falls), and two beautiful meadows (Castle Domes and Lower Vidette). It also crosses a major Sierra pass (Glen Pass).

Those fortunate to have extra time can visit Sixty Lakes Basin. It's also possible to reverse the route or find alternative campsites—especially near Baxter Lakes, Dragon Lake, Sixty Lakes Basin, and East Creek—that are less crowded than the ones along this popular loop route. Cross-country enthusiasts will have even more options for secluded camping.

Applicants will receive a reservation confirmation by mail, which must then be turned into the nearest issue station to your departure trailhead in order to obtain the actual wilderness permit. Confirmation or pick up of your permit must occur before 9 AM on the departure day, otherwise the permit is cancelled and becomes available to other parties on a walk-in basis. Free walk-in permits may be obtained after 1 PM on the day before departure, and unclaimed reserved permits become available after 9 AM on the day of departure. Fees are charged for entrance into the park as well ($10 for a 7-day pass, $30 for an Annual Park Pass to Sequoia and Kings Canyon, and $80 for an America the Beautiful Pass that provides year-long access to all national parks and recreation areas).

CHALLENGES · · · · · · · · · · · · · · · · · · ·

Gas is not available within Kings Canyon National Park, so make sure you have enough gas to get into and out of the area. Campfires are banned in several places along this route, so plan on using a stove. Bears are active throughout Kings Canyon National Park, and bear canisters are required on the Rae Lakes Loop. Due to the area's popularity, one-night camping limits apply to Dollar, Arrowhead, Rae, and Charlotte lakes.

HOW TO GET THERE · · · · · · · · · · · · · · ·

From Fresno, follow Highway 180 east into Kings Canyon National Park, pass through Grant Grove, and continue to the overnight parking lot at Roads End, 5 miles past Cedar Grove.

TRIP DESCRIPTION · · · · · · · · · · · · · · ·

From the ranger station, a wide path heads east up the canyon of South Fork Kings River through a shady, mixed forest to a bridged crossing of Copper Creek.

Beyond the crossing, the trees thin for a while, allowing filtered views of the towering granite walls of the canyon before the trail reenters a dense forest of ponderosa pines, sugar pines, white firs, and alders. After almost 2 miles, you reach a Y-junction with the Paradise Valley Trail.

Veer left (northeast) at the junction and continue upstream along the river, past delightful pools and tumbling cascades with periodic views of Buck Peak, the Sphinx, and Avalanche Peak. Eventually, you hear the thundering roar of Mist Falls and reach a short lateral to a viewpoint near the base of the falls.

From Mist Falls, continue upstream on a moderate climb past a picturesque stretch of the river, which dances vigorously over granite slabs before tumbling into a sculpted pool. The trail weaves around large boulders and ascends rock-stepped switchbacks before the grade eases at the lower end of Paradise Valley. Beneath a forest of red firs, lodgepole pines, Jeffrey pines, aspens, and junipers, you reach the backpackers camp at Lower Paradise Valley, which has designated campsites, bear boxes, and a pit toilet. Proceed from there on a gentle stroll alongside the sedate river for 1.5 miles to the camp area of Middle Paradise Valley (designated sites and bear boxes).

Continue upstream on gently graded trail through alternating stands of mixed conifers and clearings with good views of the steep-walled canyon. After a stretch of moderate climbing, nearly level walking leads past a flower-filled meadow on the way to Upper Paradise Valley camp (designated sites, bear boxes). Immediately past the camp, a series of logs allows a straightforward crossing of the river just upstream from its confluence with Woods Creek. In early season, this crossing may be difficult.

After a half mile of gentle ascent away from the creek, the trail approaches the stream and starts a moderate climb up the steep-walled valley. Where avalanches have swept the slopes clear of trees, you have fine views of the granite canyon walls and the domes above. Cross over a pair of tributaries before emerging into Castle Domes Meadow, with campsites (bear box) near the east end. Beyond the meadow, gently graded trail heads east through a lodgepole pine forest toward a junction with the famed John Muir Trail. Just up the hillside, about 150 yards north of the junction is an open-air pit toilet.

Turn right onto the JMT and soon arrive at Woods Creek Crossing. Fortunately, a suspension bridge built in 1988 offers an attractive alternative to the otherwise difficult ford of this roaring creek. Across the lively bridge are a number of overused, shady campsites with bear boxes and fire rings, although most of the firewood is picked over by midsummer.

Beyond Woods Creek Crossing, the trail curves around the north end of King Spur and begins a moderate climb up the lightly forested canyon of South Fork Woods Creek. Well above creek level, the trail crosses a rushing stream draining Lake 3144 and climbs exposed, rocky terrain on the way to a boggy meadow. From there, you pass through a drift fence, ascend a rocky ridge, and pass a pair of campsites near the crossing of the willow- and wildflower-lined stream from Sixty Lakes Basin. A mile-long climb from the stream leads to a junction with the Baxter Pass Trail just north of Dollar Lake.

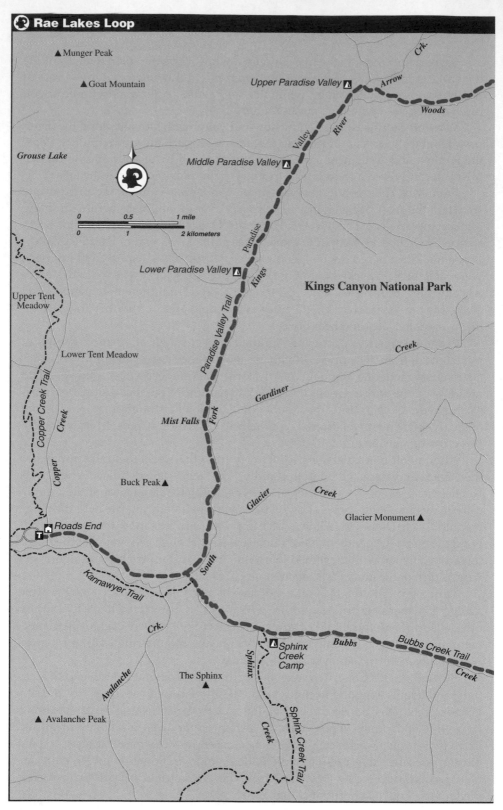

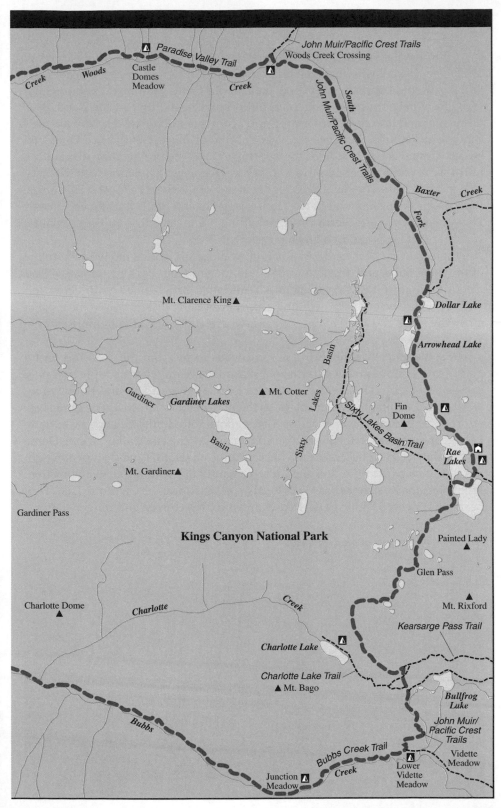

Paradise Valley Trail

Creek   Woods   Castle Domes Meadow   Creek

John Muir/Pacific Crest Trails
Woods Creek Crossing

John Muir/Pacific Crest Trails

South   Fork

Baxter   Creek

Mt. Clarence King ▲

Dollar Lake

Arrowhead Lake

Basin

Gardiner   Gardiner Lakes   ▲ Mt. Cotter

Lakes

Sixty Lakes Basin Trail

Fin Dome ▲

Basin

Sixty

Rae Lakes

Mt. Gardiner ▲

Gardiner Pass

Kings Canyon National Park

Painted Lady ▲

Glen Pass

Charlotte Dome ▲   Charlotte   Creek

Mt. Rixford ▲

Kearsarge Pass Trail

Charlotte Lake

Charlotte Lake Trail
▲ Mt. Bago

Bullfrog Lake

John Muir/ Pacific Crest Trails

Bubbs

Bubbs Creek Trail

Vidette Meadow

Junction Meadow   Creek

Lower Vidette Meadow

Continue the ascent with ever-improving scenery, including fine views of Fin Dome. Head past a small waterfall and across the creek to Arrowhead Lake, where a use trail near the north end leads to campsites (bear box). A short climb through widely scattered lodgepole pines leads to the first of the Rae Lakes. Campsites and bear boxes are nearby and also at the middle lake, where a ranger cabin is tucked into the pines above the northeast shore. Gently ascending trail passes around the east side of the two lower lakes before bending around the north shore of the upper lake to a ford of the stream and a junction with the Sixty Lakes Basin Trail. The Rae Lakes region is one of the Sierra's most scenic areas, with the peaks of monolithic Fin Dome, jagged King Spur, multihued Painted Lady, and the rugged Sierra Crest providing a fine backdrop to the sparkling, island-dotted lakes and rich green meadows.

From the Sixty Lakes Basin junction, walk south, above the west shoreline of the upper lake, and begin the stiff climb toward Glen Pass. Switchbacks lead through diminishing vegetation to a tarn-dotted bench filled with acres and acres of rock. The ongoing, winding ascent eventually brings you to the crest of a narrow ridge and the 11,978-foot pass, where you have a final glimpse of the Rae Lakes basin.

A serpentine, switchbacking descent leads away from the pass and past a pair of rockbound, greenish tarns to a seasonal stream with a couple marginal campsites nearby. The descent continues through more rocks and boulders toward more hospitable terrain below, as the path bends southeast. The grade eases on a descending traverse across a lodgepole-dotted hillside above Charlotte Lake. Through gaps in the pines, you enjoy views of the lake and Charlotte Dome farther down Charlotte Creek canyon. Continue on the JMT, past a junction with a trail to Kearsarge Pass, and then reach a sandy flat with a four-way junction: From here, the Kearsarge Pass Trail heads northeast, and the Charlotte Lake Trail heads northwest 0.8 mile to the lake (campsites, bear boxes, and ranger station).

The stunning scenery of the Rae Lakes

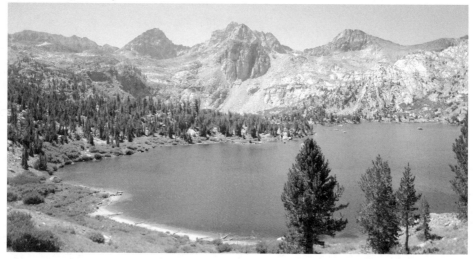

Follow the JMT east over a low rise, and then descend tight switchbacks through dense forest to the Bullfrog Lake junction (no camping). Continue the descent across the Bullfrog Lake's outlet and down to Lower Vidette Meadow and a junction with the Bubbs Creek Trail.

Following signed directions for Cedar Grove, you leave the JMT and head west on a short descent to the north edge of expansive Lower Vidette Meadow, with excellent campsites (bear box) nestled beneath lodgepole pines along the meadow's fringe. A more pronounced descent leads away from the meadow, following the now tumbling creek down the gorge. Hop across numerous freshets along a protracted descent to the grassy, fern-filled, and wildflower-covered clearing of Junction Meadow and a three-way junction with a trail to East Lake and Lake Reflection. Campsites can be found a short distance up this trail on either side of the Bubbs Creek ford, or farther down the Bubbs Creek Trail, past a horse camp near the west edge of the meadow.

Head west, away from Junction Meadow, and follow a moderate descent alongside turbulent Bubbs Creek through white fir forest. After a couple miles, the creek mellows, and you follow gently graded trail through a grove of aspens with a groundcover of ferns on the way to a log crossing of Charlotte Creek. Nearby, a short path leads to campsites along Bubbs Creek. The gentle grade continues for a while beyond the crossing, as you hop over a trio of side streams and stroll through shoulder-high ferns. Once the creek resumes its tumultuous course, you make a moderate descent down Bubbs Creek canyon for the next several miles to Sphinx Creek Camp (bear boxes) and a junction of the Sphinx Creek Trail.

Proceed straight ahead (west-northwest) at the junction and continue down Bubbs Creek canyon to the top of a series of switchbacks that drop down the steep east wall to the floor of Kings Canyon. Along the way, deciduous trees start to appear amid the conifers, and open stretches of chaparral-covered slopes offer fine views of the canyon and the Sphinx. At the bottom, stroll across the floor of the canyon to a series of short, wood bridges over braided Bubbs Creek and reach a junction with the Kannawyer Loop Trail. Proceed ahead (north) a short distance to a bridge across South Fork Kings River, and close the loop at a junction on the far side with the Paradise Creek Trail. From there, turn left (west) and retrace your steps 1.9 miles to the trailhead.

BUILD-UP AND WIND-DOWN TIPS

Backpackers can shower off the backcountry grit and grime at the coin-operated **Showers and Laundromat** in **Cedar Grove**. Additional services include a visitor center, campgrounds, and a pack station. The **Cedar Grove Lodge** offers backpackers the opportunity to spend a night in relative comfort (reservations recommended: 866-522-6966 or www.sequoia-kingscanyon.com), grab a bite in the snack bar before or after a trip, or pick up supplies and souvenirs at the market/gift store. **Kings Canyon Lodge**, located 17 miles from Cedar Grove, offers cabin rentals, dining, and not-so-cheap gasoline (559-335-2405).

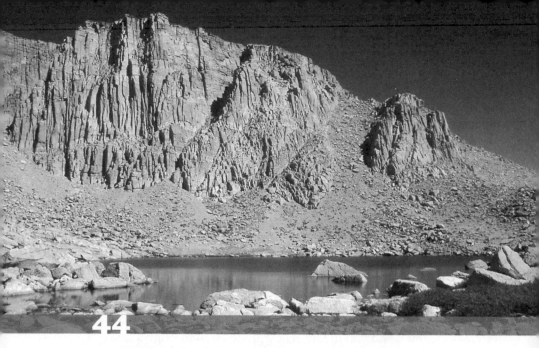

44

COTTONWOOD LAKES TO UPPER ROCK CREEK LOOP

Mike White

> **MILES:** 27.0
> **RECOMMENDED DAYS:** 4–7
> **ELEVATION GAIN/LOSS:** 4550´/4550´
> **TYPE OF TRIP:** Loop or point-to-point
> **DIFFICULTY:** Moderate
> **SOLITUDE:** Moderate solitude
> **LOCATION:** Sequoia-Kings Canyon National Park, Golden Trout and
> John Muir Wilderness Areas
> **MAPS:** USGS 7.5-min. *Cirque Peak, Mt. Whitney,* and *Johnson Peak*
> **BEST SEASON:** Late summer through early fall

PERMITS

Overnight stays in the John Muir Wilderness, Golden Trout Wilderness, and Sequoia National Park require a wilderness permit, and daily trailhead quotas are in effect. Permits can be obtained at Inyo National Forest facilities at Mono Basin Scenic Area visitor center, Mammoth Lakes visitor center, White Mountain ranger station in Bishop, or the Eastern Sierra Interagency visitor center south of Lone Pine. Sixty percent of the reservations are available in advance, anytime from six months to two days before your trip.

Photo: High Lake from the New Army Pass Trail

Download an application from the Inyo National Forest website (www.fs.fed.us.r5/inyo), and mail the completed application to the Wilderness Permit Reservation Office at 351 Pacu Lane Suite 200, Bishop, CA 93514; fax it to 760-873-2484; or call the Wilderness Permit Reservation Line at 760-873-2483. A $5 per-person fee is required, paid for by credit card, cash, check, or money order. The remaining 40 percent of the daily quota is available for walk-in permits, which can be obtained after 11 AM the day before departure. Unclaimed advanced reservations will be made available for walk-in permits after 9 AM on the day of departure.

CHALLENGES

Campfires are banned in several places along this route, so plan to use a stove. Bears are active throughout Sequoia National Park and the surrounding National Forest, and although bear canisters are not required, they are highly recommended. In lieu of canisters, use the bear boxes at locations noted in the trip description. Bear-bagging food has proved to be largely ineffectual.

HOW TO GET THERE

Rather than parking a car at each trailhead, make this a loop trip by walking the mere 1.5 miles between the Cottonwood Lakes and Horseshoe Meadows trailheads.

Cottonwood Lakes Trailhead: Take U.S. Highway 395 to the small town of Lone Pine and turn west onto Whitney Portal Road. Proceed 3 miles and turn left onto Horseshoe Meadow Road. After 18 miles, turn right at a signed junction for Cottonwood Lakes, and continue past the walk-in campground to the trailhead parking area (vault toilet, running water).

Horseshoe Meadow Trailhead: Follow directions above, except proceed straight ahead at the Cottonwood Lakes junction.

TAKE THIS TRIP

Magnificent terrain near the southeastern boundary of Sequoia National Park beckons backpackers to enjoy a host of pursuits—from fishing for golden trout, to climbing Mt. Langley or Cirque Peak, to exploring the rugged beauty of Miter Basin, to simply enjoying this 27-mile loop's bevy of lakes, two alpine passes, and several picturesque meadows.

It's possible to reverse this trip or to shorten it to a 24-mile loop by backtracking from Lower Soldier Lake on the New Army Pass Trail to the lateral heading south to the junction of the Cottonwood Pass Trail northeast of Siberian Outpost.

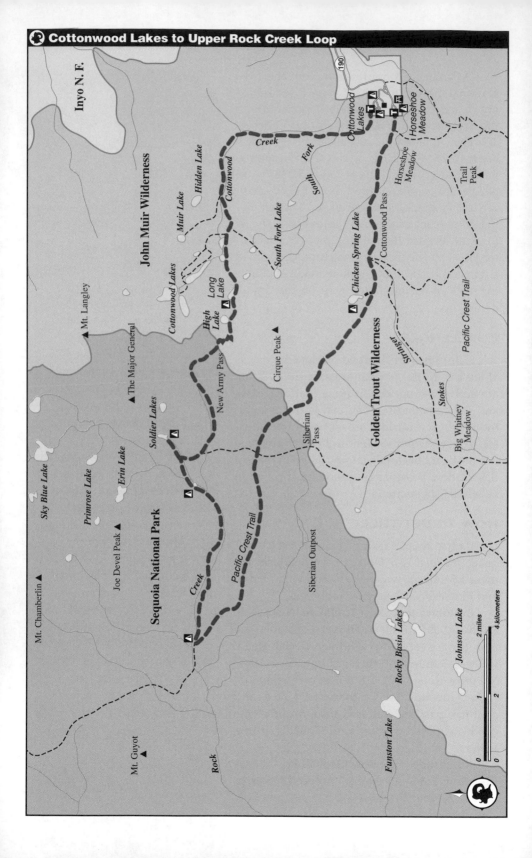

Inyo N. F.

John Muir Wilderness

Sequoia National Park

Golden Trout Wilderness

Mt. Chamberlin ▲

Sky Blue Lake

Primrose Lake

Joe Devel Peak ▲

Erin Lake

Soldier Lakes

Mt. Langley ▲

The Major General ▲

Cottonwood Lakes

High Lake

Long Lake

New Army Pass

Cirque Peak ▲

Muir Lake

Hidden Lake

Cottonwood Creek

South Fork Lake

South Fork

Cottonwood Creek

Chicken Spring Lake

Cottonwood Pass

Horseshoe Meadow

Trail Peak ▲

190

Cottonwood Lakes

Horseshoe Meadow

Pacific Crest Trail

Siberian Pass

Siberian Outpost

Pacific Crest Trail

Rock Creek

Mt. Guyot ▲

Funston Lake

Rocky Basin Lakes

Johnson Lake

Big Whitney Meadow

Stokes

Stringer

0   1   2 miles

0   2   4 kilometers

The trailhead is 0.5 mile farther, at the end of Horseshoe Meadow Road (vault toilet, running water).

TRIP DESCRIPTION

The Cottonwood Lakes Trail begins somewhat auspiciously as a short, brick-lined path near a restroom building. Beyond the trailhead signboard, gently graded, sandy tread leads west, slightly uphill and into Golden Trout Wilderness. Pass a spur on the left to the Cottonwood Lakes Pack Station and follow nearly level trail toward a crossing of South Fork Cottonwood Creek. Climb gently through scattered pines, meeting and then following the main branch of Cottonwood Creek up a broad valley. Cross the boundary between the Golden Trout and John Muir wildernesses beneath steep cliffs on the left and across from the wood structures of the privately owned Golden Trout Camp in a meadow on the right. Beyond the boundary, the trail curves west on a more moderate ascent up the narrowing canyon. Cross a beveled log over Cottonwood Creek and then make your way through light forest while continuing to head upstream along the meadow-lined creek. Just after the ford of a tributary, reach a Y-junction between the Cottonwood Lakes Trail on the right and the New Army Pass Trail on the left, 3.3 miles from the trailhead.

Veering left on the New Army Pass Trail, you soon cross the creek and then climb moderately for a little over a mile to a junction with the South Fork Lakes Trail. Continue west on the New Army Pass Trail, climbing over a forested moraine to the edge of a large meadow and a junction with a lateral north to a connection with the Cottonwood Lakes Trail. Proceed ahead, skirting Cottonwood Lake 1 and 2 before leaving the meadow behind and climbing shortly to a desolate-looking area covered with large granite boulders. Eventually, you leave the boulder field and follow mildly graded trail around a lightly forested hillside. Below, a stream rushes down toward the westernmost South Fork Lake, and a faint use trail leads across the stream and down to campsites situated between this lake and Long Lake above. A moderate climb takes you up to the south shore of Long Lake. The best campsites are found beneath a stand of pines along the southeast shore, with a few less-protected sites above the north shore.

From the east side of Long Lake, the trail begins a steep climb toward High Lake and the pass beyond. Past timberline, you weave up rocky switchbacks to the lake, where the scarce campsites are exposed to the elements. Rocky switchbacks continue up the cirque headwall to New Army Pass (at 12,315 feet), with superb views of the lakes below and the Cottonwood Creek drainage.

From the pass, a moderate descent across barren slopes of coarse granite eventually leads to more hospitable terrain, where the trail meets and then follows a tributary of Rock Creek through boulder-sprinkled meadows rimmed by rocky cliffs and ridges. Stunted pines start to appear, and shortly thereafter, the trail skirts flower-filled meadows and passes through a scattered-to-light forest of foxtail and lodgepole pines on the way to a junction with a lateral south to a union with the Pacific Crest Trail.

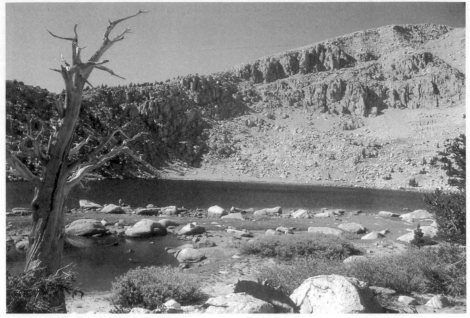

Chicken Spring Lake

Veer right (west) and travel past a thin strip of meadow to a lateral leading to pine-shaded campsites (bear box) on a low rise above the outlet from Soldier Lakes. A short distance farther, you boulder hop the outlet and reach a junction with the trail up to the lower lake. Turn right and head northeast through scattered pines, following the edge of a narrow, flower-covered meadow to the southern tip of Lower Soldier Lake. While a boot-beaten path continues along the west shore, you must cross the outlet just below the lake on some well-placed rocks and logs in order to access the shady campsites on the east side. Dramatically framed by the towering walls of the Major General to the northeast, serene Lower Soldier Lake is visible in a scenic cirque. Anglers should find fishing for the resident golden trout to be a sufficient challenge. The remote upper lake is just a short, cross-country jaunt to the east. For a nice layover day, follow a use trail north then northeast along upper Rock Creek to Sky Blue Lake in Miter Basin. If you have even more time and are an experienced cross-country traveler, continue over Crabtree Pass (Class 2) to Crabtree Lakes and return to the Rock Creek Trail via the Pacific Crest Trail.

Return from Lower Soldier Lake to the Rock Creek Trail and continue downstream (southwest) through a thickening forest of lodgepole pines. A short, steep descent down a narrow gully along a riotous section of the creek passes a campsite just below the edge of a broad meadow, where the use trail mentioned above heads toward Miter Basin. Gently graded trail leads around the fringe of the meadow to a ford of the creek, and then passes a large pond and campsites (bear box) in a grove of pines. Reenter lodgepole pine forest beyond the meadow and pass through a drift fence. A moderate descent resumes, and the trail veers away from the creek for a while. Soon, the trail again draws near to the stream, which dances over slabs and cascades over boulders between meadow- and willow-lined banks. Cross Rock Creek on a pair of logs and continue downstream to a picturesque meadow with a number of lodgepole-shaded campsites along its fringe. A short, forested descent leads to a junction with the PCT.

Turn left (southeast) and follow the PCT above small meadows to the start of several switchbacks on a moderate climb out of Rock Creek canyon. After a mile or so, the grade eventually eases where the trail follows a broad ridge through a lodgepole and foxtail pine forest to the north of Siberian Outpost. Pass a little-used trail headed south to Siberian Pass and then make a short, mild climb to a three-way junction with a northbound lateral to the New Army Pass Trail. Veer right (southeast) to remain on the PCT and climb through lodgepole pines; here you have good views of Siberian Outpost, Mt. Kaweah, and the Great Western Divide. On loose, sandy tread you reach the inauspicious boundary between Sequoia National Park and Golden Trout Wilderness on a minor ridge west of Cirque Peak. Contour above a meadow with a seasonal tarn, and then make a long traverse across slopes at the head of Golden Trout Creek canyon, while enjoying good views of Big Whitney Meadow and the Great Western Divide. A short, moderate descent leads to a junction with the short use trail that follows the seasonal outlet northwest to Chicken Spring Lake. The lake is situated in a rugged granite cirque, and the shoreline is dotted with weather-beaten foxtail pines. Good campsites can be found in sandy patches around a bay on the south side, near the outlet, and in the scattered pines above the west shore.

Return down the outlet to the PCT and head east on an easy traverse to a junction with the Cottonwood Lakes Trail and a lesser-used path to Big Whitney Meadow. Turn left (east) and make the very short climb to Cottonwood Pass (at approximately 11,200 feet), with good views of the Inyo and Panamint ranges to the east and the Great Western Divide to the west.

Switchbacks lead down from the pass across a steep, rock-strewn hillside to a small meadow, where the grade eases considerably. Proceed on gently graded trail to a couple of stream crossings. Near the second crossing, a use trail leads to an old, dilapidated cabin (no camping). Continue through moderate forest cover along the northern fringe of expansive Horseshoe Meadow. Just after a junction with trails heading south to Trail Pass and north to the pack station, you exit the Golden Trout Wilderness, and soon reach the Horseshoe Meadows Trailhead. Unless other arrangements have been made, someone will have to make the 1.5-mile trek down the Horseshoe Meadows Road and up the Cottonwood Lakes Road back to the Cottonwood Lakes Trailhead to retrieve a vehicle.

BUILD-UP AND WIND-DOWN TIPS

Lone Pine offers a handful of restaurants serving fare ranging from burgers and pizza to steaks and seafood. There are also a few budget motels in this tiny town.

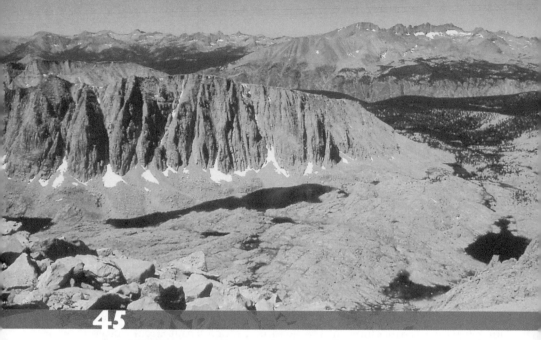

45

HORSESHOE MEADOW TO WHITNEY PORTAL

Mike White

MILES: 36.0
RECOMMENDED DAYS: 5–7
ELEVATION GAIN/LOSS: 7405´/8885´
TYPE OF TRIP: Point-to-point
DIFFICULTY: Moderately strenuous
LOCATION: Sequoia-Kings Canyon national parks and Golden Trout and John Muir Wilderness Areas
SOLITUDE: Moderately populated
MAPS: USGS 7.5-min. *Cirque Peak, Johnson Peak, Mt. Whitney,* and *Mt. Langley*
BEST SEASON: Late summer through early fall

PERMITS

Overnight stays in the John Muir Wilderness, Golden Trout Wilderness, and Sequoia-Kings Canyon national parks require a wilderness permit, and daily trailhead quotas are in effect. Permits can be obtained at Inyo National Forest facilities at Mono Basin Scenic Area visitor center, Mammoth Lakes visitor center, White Mountain ranger station in Bishop, or the Eastern Sierra Interagency visitor center south of Lone Pine. Sixty percent of the reservations are available

Photo: The westward view from Trail Crest

in advance, anytime from six months to two days before your trip.

Download an application from the Inyo National Forest website (www.fs.fed.us.r5/inyo), and mail the completed application to the Wilderness Permit Reservation Office at 351 Pacu Lane Suite 200, Bishop, CA 93514; fax it to 760-873-2484; or call the Wilderness Permit Reservation Line at 760-873-2483. A $5 per-person fee is required, paid for by credit card, cash, check, or money order. The remaining 40 percent of the daily quota is available for walk-in permits, which can be obtained after 11 AM the day before departure. Unclaimed advanced reservations will be made available for walk-in permits after 9 AM on the day of departure.

CHALLENGES

Campfires are banned in several places along this route, so plan on using a stove. Bears are active throughout Sequoia National Park and surrounding national forest lands, and bear canisters are required on the Mt. Whitney Trail. As of 2007, all human waste must be packed out of the Mt. Whitney area; pack-out kits are available at the visitor center in Lone Pine and the Crabtree ranger station, and they may be disposed of at the human-waste receptacle at Whitney Portal.

HOW TO GET THERE

This point-to-point trip is one of the more easily managed shuttles in the High Sierra, as both the put-in and take-out trailheads are accessed from the town of Lone Pine.

Horseshoe Meadow Trailhead: Take U.S. Highway 395 to the small town of Lone Pine and turn west onto Whitney Portal Road. Proceed 3 miles and turn left onto Horseshoe Meadow Road. After 18 miles, continue straight ahead at the Cottonwood Lakes junction, reaching the trailhead in another half mile at the end of Horseshoe Meadow Road (vault toilet, running water).

TAKE THIS TRIP

If you happen to be one of the many unlucky backpackers who don't score a permit to bag the coveted Mt. Whitney via the traditional route, you haven't lost your chance to climb up this highest of peaks in the continental United States. This route provides a longer alternative with the bonus of some of the southern Sierra's most striking scenery. High-alpine basins, rushing creeks, crystalline lakes, and serene forests are present in abundance—not to mention the chance to legally stand atop Mt. Whitney.

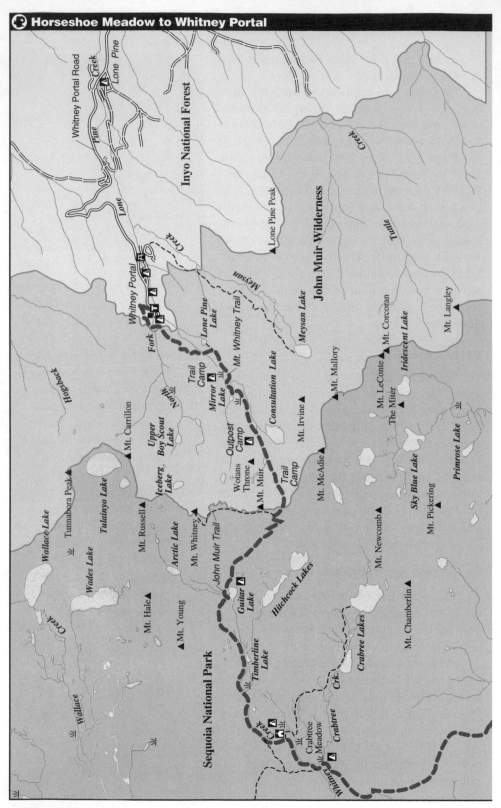

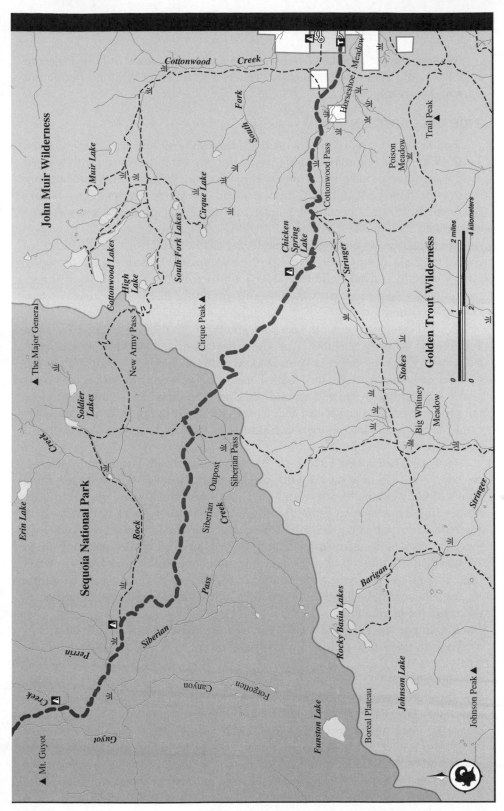

John Muir Wilderness

Cottonwood Creek

South Fork

Muir Lake

Cirque Lake

South Fork Lakes

Cottonwood Lakes

High Lake

New Army Pass

Cirque Peak ▲

Horseshoe Meadow

Trail Peak ▲

Cottonwood Pass

Poison Meadow

Chicken Spring Lake

Stringer

Golden Trout Wilderness

Stokes

Big Whitney Meadow

▲ The Major General

Soldier Lakes

Siberian Pass

Outpost

Siberian Pass

Erin Lake

Creek

Rock

Sequoia National Park

Siberian Creek

Perrin

Siberian Pass

Guyot Pass

Forgotten Canyon

Funston Lake

Boreal Plateau

Johnson Lake

Rocky Basin Lakes

Barigan

Stringer

Johnson Peak ▲

▲ Mt. Guyot

2 miles

0

1

2

4 kilometers

0

2

Whitney Portal: Take U.S. Highway 395 to the small town of Lone Pine and turn west onto Whitney Portal Road. Proceed 13 miles to Whitney Portal and park in the overnight lot.

TRIP DESCRIPTION

Follow gently graded trail west from the trailhead and across the Golden Trout Wilderness boundary. Pass a junction with a trail heading south toward Trail Pass and a second junction a very short distance farther with a trail heading north toward the pack station. Continue ahead (west) from the junction, skirting the northern fringe of expansive Horseshoe Meadow. Hop across a stream to a use trail on the far side that leads shortly to a dilapidated cabin. The trail soon re-crosses the stream and begins a moderate ascent away from the meadow, incorporating a series of switchbacks up a rock-strewn hillside. The zigzagging path eventually reaches Cottonwood Pass, with excellent views behind of Horseshoe Meadow and the distant Inyo Mountains and ahead of the Great Western Divide's southern extremity.

A short distance beyond the pass is a junction with the Pacific Crest Trail and a trail to Big Whitney Meadow. Turn right (north) and follow the PCT on an easy traverse to Chicken Spring Lake's seasonal outlet, where a use trail follows the outlet upstream a short distance to the lakeshore. Tucked into a cirque, the lake is nearly surrounded by rugged granite cliffs, and the shoreline is dotted with foxtail pines; several old snags add character to the surroundings. Sandy campsites can be found near a bay on the south side, near the outlet and beneath scattered pines above the west shore.

From Chicken Spring Lake, retrace your steps to the PCT and continue north on a moderate ascent to the crest of a ridge west of the lake, where you have fine views of Big Whitney Meadow and the Great Western Divide. Follow a mildly descending traverse away from the ridge, and eventually skirt a meadow with a seasonal tarn. Circle the base of some cliffs before making a short climb to an excellent vista of desolate Siberian Outpost, Mt. Kaweah, peaks along the Great Western Divide, and a part of the Sierra Crest above Rock Creek. A short stroll from there leads you across the boundary of Sequoia National Park. Continue the traverse across the lightly forested hillside to a junction with the infrequently used trail to Siberian Pass.

Remain on the PCT and head west, toward Rock Creek, initially on a mild ascent, and then on a gentle to moderate descent to a junction with the New Army Pass Trail.

Heading west, you make a winding, moderate descent away from the junction through alternating sections of forest and flower- and fern-covered meadows. Pass a lateral to the Rock Creek ranger station and soon come to some shady campsites just before a ford of Lower Rock Creek.

Past the ford, you begin a moderately steep, switchbacking climb up the north wall of Rock Creek canyon through a light forest of lodgepole pines. The grade eases on the way to a crossing of Guyot Creek (campsites). Make sure you acquire water here, as the next 4.5 miles are dry. Gently graded trail leads across Guyot Flat's wide, sandy basin, and then makes an undulating traverse toward the south lip of Whitney Creek canyon, followed by a steep, switchbacking descent to the canyon floor. A gentle stroll over rocky terrain brings you to Lower Crabtree Meadow and campsites with bear boxes near the ford of Whitney Creek. Just beyond the crossing is a junction with a connecting trail to the John Muir Trail.

Leaving the PCT, turn right (north-northwest) and make a gentle, half-mile ascent along the north bank of Whitney Creek to the lush environs of Upper Crabtree Meadow. Near the far end of the meadow, just before a crossing of the creek, the unmarked Crabtree Lakes Trail branches east. Beyond the ford, a lateral provides access to campsites (bear box) and the Crabtree ranger station (pick up a waste pack-out kit). Cross back over the creek to the north bank and intersect the John Muir Trail, with additional campsites nearby.

Follow the JMT along the north side of Whitney Creek through scattered foxtail and lodgepole pines to picturesque Timberline Lake. Although closed to campers for several decades, the lake is worth a visit, especially to a vantage point on the south shore, where the hulk of Mt. Whitney is reflected in the surface. Beyond Timberline Lake, the steady ascent continues as you leave the trees behind and pass through an open basin laden with granite slabs and benches. Ascend over a flat-topped ridge to Guitar Lake and proceed past a pair of tarns— the last reliable water sources prior to the stiff climb to Trail Crest. Campsites may be found in sandy patches near Guitar Lake and the tarns.

As the ascent grows steeper, Hitchcock Lakes appear to the south, luring off-trail enthusiasts to more remote campsites beneath the precipitous north face of Mt. Hitchcock. A series of long-legged switchbacks leads up the steep west face of the Sierra Crest on a steady, 1500-foot climb to the Mt. Whitney Trail junction. On a typical summer day, you will see a bounty of colorful backpacks against a rock wall, temporarily left behind by hopeful Whitney peakbaggers. Feel free to add your backpack to the pile and carry a small daypack with valuables and necessities on the 2-mile climb to the summit.

From the junction, make a short climb southeast up to Trail Crest. From there, follow the Mt. Whitney Trail down the east side of the peak, through Trail Camp, past Mirror Lake, and through Outpost Camp to the trailhead at Whitney Portal.

BUILD-UP AND WIND-DOWN TIPS

After five to seven days on the trail, you will be pleased to taste real food (even if it is only hamburgers and milkshakes) again at the **Whitney Portal Store**. If you need a more varied menu, head to the tiny town of **Lone Pine**, which has a handful of restaurants serving fare ranging from burgers and pizza to steaks and seafood. It also has a few budget motels if you need a pillow for the night.

46

SOUTH LAKE TO NORTH LAKE

Mike White

MILES: 56.5
RECOMMENDED DAYS: 5–7
ELEVATION GAIN/LOSS: 9240´/9790´
TYPE OF TRIP: Point-to-point
DIFFICULTY: Strenuous
SOLITUDE: Moderately populated
LOCATION: Sequoia-Kings Canyon national parks and
John Muir Wilderness
MAPS: USGS 7.5-min. *Mt. Thompson, North Palisade, Mt. Goddard,*
Mt. Henry, Mt. Hilgard, Mt. Darwin, and *Mt. Tom*
BEST SEASON: Late summer through early fall

PERMITS

Overnight stays in the John Muir Wilderness and Kings Canyon National Park require a wilderness permit, and daily trailhead quotas are in effect from May 1 to October 1. Permits can be obtained at Inyo National Forest facilities at Mono Basin Scenic Area visitor center, Mammoth Lakes visitor center, White Mountain ranger station in Bishop, or the Eastern Sierra interagency visitor center south of Lone Pine. Sixty percent of the reservations are available in advance, anytime from six months to two days before your trip.

Photo: Lower Golden Trout Lake, one of the many beautiful lakes in Humphreys Basin

Download an application from the Inyo National Forest website (www.fs.fed.us.r5/ inyo), and mail the completed application to the Wilderness Permit Reservation Office at 351 Pacu Lane Suite 200, Bishop, CA 93514; fax it to 760-873-2484; or call the Wilderness Permit Reservation Line at 760-873-2483. A $5 per-person fee is required, paid for by credit card, cash, check, or money order. The remaining 40 percent of the daily quota is available for walk-in permits, which can be obtained after 11 AM the day before departure. Unclaimed advanced reservations will be made available for walk-in permits after 9 AM on the day of departure.

CHALLENGES

Campfires are banned in several places along this route, so plan on using a stove. Bears are active throughout Kings Canyon National Park and surrounding national forest lands, and bear canisters are required on the Bishop Pass Trail.

HOW TO GET THERE

South Lake Trailhead: From U.S. Highway 395 in the center of Bishop, turn west on Line Drive, which becomes South Lake Road (Highway 168) at the city limits, and proceed 15 miles to a junction. Turn left and drive another 6.75 miles on South Lake Road to the overnight parking lot at the end of the road near South Lake (vault toilets). If this lot is full, which frequently is the case, you must backtrack 1.3 miles to the overflow parking area below Parchers Resort. A footpath connects the upper and lower parking areas.

North Lake Trailhead: From U.S. Highway 395 in the center of Bishop, turn west on Line Drive, which becomes South Lake Road (Highway 168) at the city limits, and proceed past the South Lake junction for 3 miles to a right turn on the road to North Lake. Take this

TAKE THIS TRIP

Many backpackers view the South Lake to North Lake loop as one of the supreme backpacks in the High Sierra—it offers a visit to three incomparable alpine basins, Dusy, Evolution, and Humphreys; and three scenic canyons, LeConte, Evolution, and Goddard. In addition, you'll experience a bevy of picturesque lakes, rollicking streams, serene forests, and flower-bedecked meadows.

The short distance between the two trailheads allows for a fairly straightforward shuttle. This trip also can be reversed, exchanging the steep climb on poor tread up Piute Canyon for the similarly steep ascent on better tread from LeConte Canyon to Dusy Basin.

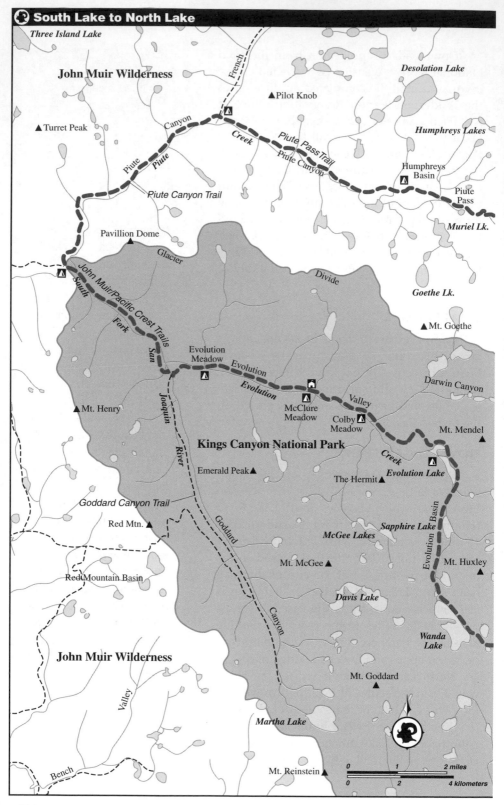

Three Island Lake

John Muir Wilderness

French

▲Pilot Knob

Desolation Lake

▲ Turret Peak

Canyon

Creek

Piute Pass Trail

Humphreys Lakes

Piute

Piute

Piute Canyon

Humphreys
Basin

Piute
Pass

Piute Canyon Trail

Muriel Lk.

Pavillion Dome ▲

Glacier

Divide

Goethe Lk.

John Muir/Pacific Crest Trails

South

▲ Mt. Goethe

Fork

San

Evolution
Meadow

Evolution

Darwin Canyon

Evolution

Joaquin

Valley

▲ Mt. Henry

McClure
Meadow

Colby
Meadow

Mt. Mendel
▲

River

Kings Canyon National Park

Emerald Peak ▲

The Hermit ▲

Creek

Evolution Lake

Goddard Canyon Trail

Goddard

Sapphire Lake

Red Mtn. ▲

McGee Lakes

Evolution Basin

Mt. Huxley
▲

Red Mountain Basin

Mt. McGee ▲

Canyon

Davis Lake

*Wanda
Lake*

John Muir Wilderness

Valley

Mt. Goddard
▲

Bench

Martha Lake

0   1   2 miles

0   2   4 kilometers

Mt. Reinstein ▲

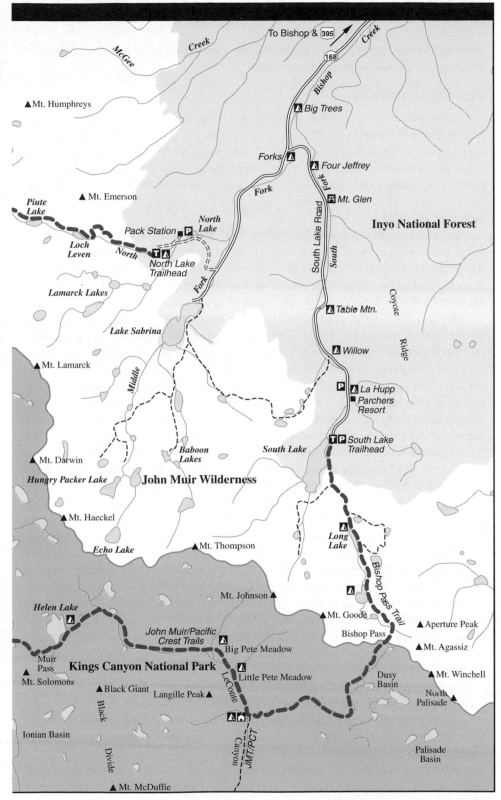

To Bishop & 395

Inyo National Forest

McGee Creek

Bishop Creek

▲ Mt. Humphreys

Big Trees

Forks

Four Jeffrey

Fork

South Fork

Mt. Glen

▲ Mt. Emerson

Piute Lake

North Lake

South Lake Road

South

Pack Station

Loch Leven

North Lake Trailhead

North Fork

Fork

Lamarck Lakes

Lake Sabrina

Middle

Table Mtn.

Coyote Ridge

Willow

La Hupp

▲ Mt. Lamarck

Parchers Resort

Baboon Lakes

South Lake Trailhead

South Lake

John Muir Wilderness

Hungry Packer Lake

▲ Mt. Darwin

▲ Mt. Haeckel

Echo Lake

▲ Mt. Thompson

Long Lake

Bishop Pass Trail

Mt. Johnson ▲

▲ Aperture Peak

Helen Lake

▲ Mt. Goode

Bishop Pass

▲ Mt. Agassiz

John Muir/Pacific Crest Trails

Big Pete Meadow

Muir Pass

Kings Canyon National Park

LeConte

Little Pete Meadow

Dusy Basin

▲ Mt. Winchell

Mt. Solomons

▲ Black Giant

Langille Peak ▲

North Palisade ▲

Ionian Basin

Black

Divide

Canyon

JMT/PCT

Palisade Basin

▲ Mt. McDuffie

narrow dirt road 1.6 miles to a turnoff to the overnight parking lot (vault toilets) between the pack station and North Lake.

TRIP DESCRIPTION

After a very brief descent through lush vegetation, the Bishop Pass Trail climbs above the east shore of South Lake, crosses into the John Muir Wilderness, and reaches a junction with a trail to Treasure Lakes. Continue ahead (southwest) to the crossing of a small, flower-lined stream, and past a faint, unmarked path to the Marie Lakes. Just beyond this, you cross over another creek and then climb a series of short switchbacks over rocky terrain to the lower Chocolate Lakes Trail junction.

Continue south along the Bishop Pass Trail to the north shore of aptly named Long Lake, whose crystal-blue waters are surrounded by green meadows, granite boulders, and scattered conifers. Overused campsites abound around this popular destination, especially on a knoll near the south end of the lake. Near the far (south) end of the lake is the upper junction with the Chocolate Lakes Trail.

Beyond Long Lake, cross the inlet from Ruwau Lake and climb through a light forest of whitebark pines. Through small, grassy meadows, rock fields, and patches of wildflowers, you ascend to Spearhead Lake, a picturesque body of water backdropped by the spine of the Inconsolable Range. Isolated Margaret Lake is a straightforward, 0.4-mile, cross-country jaunt to the southwest. A half-mile climb leads up a rocky slope and past tumbling cascades to the lovely Timberline Tarns, where little-used campsites will tempt overnighters. From the tarns, a short climb heads up to island-dotted, austere Saddlerock Lake, nestled into a glacier-scoured basin near the foot of the northeast buttress of towering Mt. Goode. Backpackers interested in camping at nearby Bishop Lake should follow a use trail south from Saddlerock Lake and over a low rise. Continuing, you climb above timberline and enter the alpine zone, passing through rocky terrain on a winding climb to 11,972-foot Bishop Pass and the boundary of Kings Canyon National Park. The striking view to the west includes verdant, tarn-dotted Dusy Basin backdropped by rugged Giraud and Columbine peaks, and the deep chasm of LeConte Canyon is framed by the Black Divide. Flanking the pass to the north, Mt. Agassiz beckons energetic peakbaggers toward its summit.

From the pass, descend on sandy tread to some switchbacks, where a short use trail leads to a fine viewpoint, and continue downhill through welcome patches of green meadow dotted with wildflowers and bisected by sparkling rivulets. Along the descent, you enjoy the stunning scenery of Dusy Basin's meadows and tarns, which are dramatically framed by the craggy Palisades, Isosceles, and Columbine peaks. About 1.5 miles from the pass, a use trail branches east toward the uppermost tarn (at approximately 11,350 feet) in the basin, near where you could camp for the night. Alternatively, you can continue farther into the basin for more secluded sites. Another 0.75 mile down the Bishop Pass Trail, a second use trail leads to additional tarns and campsites.

Wherever you end up camping, Dusy Basin is an exquisite location, with small pockets of luxuriant meadow and sparkling granite slabs bordering azure

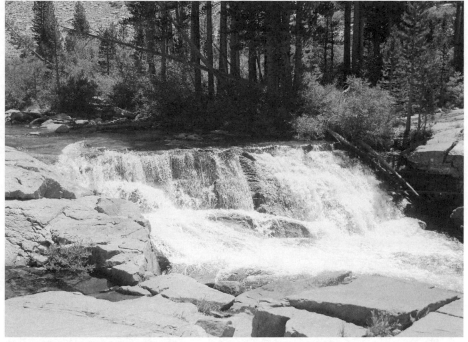

Dramatic cascade on Piute Creek

tarns and crystalline streams. The ragged spires of nearby peaks pierce the rarified air, and the precipitous faces and knife-edged ridges provide stimulating challenges for the hardiest of mountaineers. The delicate alpine vegetation is fragile, so limit campsites to sandy areas only and, while traveling in the basin, avoid trampling this vegetation wherever possible. Dusy Basin is truly a magical place and many extra days could be filled exploring its nooks and crannies. At least one layover day should be used for an off-trail ramble east over Knapsack Pass into Palisade Basin.

Continue the descent along the Bishop Pass Trail through increasing numbers of whitebark pines. Interspersed between granite slabs and boulders, pockets of meadow are graced by clumps of willow, patches of heather, and an assortment of wildflowers, including shooting star, penstemon, Indian paintbrush, aster, cinquefoil, pennyroyal, columbine, and buttercup. Follow the sparkling Dusy Branch downstream on its lively dance toward a union with Middle Fork Kings River, reaching the edge of the basin and a staggering view into the deep declivity of LeConte Canyon. With a nearly constant view of the imposing granite wall on the far side, you embark on the steep, switchbacking descent toward the canyon floor. Zigzag down the east wall of the canyon to the wood bridge across Dusy Branch, and continue the plunging descent to a lightly forested bench with a number of fine campsites along the creek. Proceed through scattered to light lodgepole pine forest, interrupted briefly by an open stretch of chaparral that offers an imposing view of the canyon and gigantic Langille Peak. As the end of the descent approaches, the forest closes in again and you reach a junction with the John Muir Trail. Campsites are near the junction on either side of the LeConte Canyon ranger station.

Turn right and proceed north on the JMT on a mild, then moderate grade through light lodgepole pine forest. The towering mass of 12,018-foot Langille Peak constantly looms over you to the left. A prolific display of wildflowers lines the trail, including corn lily, fireweed, wallflower, penstemon, larkspur, penny-royal, goldenrod, shooting star, heather, monkeyflower, and tiger lily. The ascent eases at Little Pete Meadow, where the river meanders through the sloping, grass-covered clearing bordered by sagebrush and scattered groves of lodge-pole pines and mountain hemlocks. A number of shady campsites can be found around the fringe of the meadow.

Scenic Piute Canyon

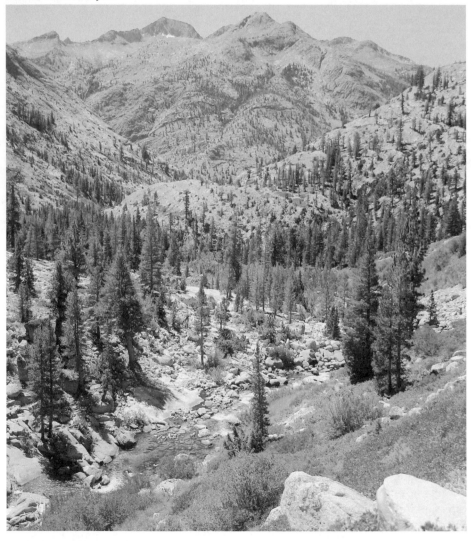

Beyond the meadow, the climb resumes through open terrain, with fine views of the canyon and the now cascading river. After crossing a pair of side streams, you drop into a lush wildflower garden intermixed with young aspens. Pass through a drift fence, and climb through scattered pines to Big Pete Meadow and a number of fine campsites.

Toward the far (west) end of the meadow, hop over streams and pass through an area damaged by an avalanche, where massive Langille Peak continues to dominate the view. Pass more campsites, as the trail closely follows the course of the river in and out of the shade from a light forest. A moderate to moderately steep climb follows between walls of granite, which can make the area seem like an oven during the heat of the day. Above a talus slope, the trail skirts the side of the canyon and climbs above granite slabs to a fine view of a waterfall on the turbulent Middle Fork. Continue across a luxuriant, seep-watered hillside amid a bounty of wildflowers to a series of rocky switchbacks leading above the falls and into a small, picturesque basin filled with verdant meadows, delightful tarns, and intermittent stands of conifers.

Cross a small stream and make a short climb to shady campsites near the trail. Another set of switchbacks leads to views of a pond-filled basin, where primitive campsites are scattered around the shorelines. After crossing the dwindling Middle Fork, wander around a number of rock humps to the largest tarn below Helen Lake, where overnighters can set up camp on a rock shelf above the south shore, or on a hillside to the southwest, amid widely scattered trees. Leaving the last of the whitebark pines, you cross back over the Middle Fork and climb over slabs to a crossing of the meadow-lined outlet of the tarn immediately below Helen Lake. The winding climb continues through rocky terrain, past a short use trail leading to a view-filled campsite on a forested knoll, the last decent place to pitch a tent on this side of Muir Pass. Keep climbing, generally following the outlet to Helen Lake (at 11,617 feet), which was named for one of John Muir's two daughters. The austere lake possesses a stark beauty, but backpackers searching for a viable campsite will be disappointed by the tiny, marginal sites in this rocky basin near the convergence of the Black and Goddard divides.

Follow the JMT around the south shore, past some tarns, and make a steady, winding climb toward 11,955-foot Muir Pass. Visitors will revel in the extraordinary views from this notch in the Goddard Divide, although your immediate attention may be captivated by the interesting manmade structure nearby. The Muir Hut was erected by the Sierra Club and dedicated in 1933 as a memorial to their founder and most notable member—John Muir. Due primarily to human waste concerns, camping is not allowed anywhere in the immediate vicinity, except for emergencies.

The descent from Muir Pass begins moderately and then eases across the head of the canyon holding Evolution Basin. Less than a mile from the pass, the trail reaches lonely Lake McDermand, passing the west shore on the way to giant Wanda Lake, which was named for Muir's other daughter. Spartan campsites near the outlet appear devoid of life at first, but the dramatic views of such notable peaks as Huxley, Spencer, Darwin, Mendel, and Goddard, and the Goddard

Divide more than compensate for the austere surroundings. A mild descent continues along the course of Evolution Creek, and you ford the stream before continuing past the next unnamed gem in the chain of lakes. Enter the glacier-polished basin of Sapphire Lake and drop to campsites near the north end.

Proceeding through the deep cleft of the canyon, make a short descent to the last lake in the chain, Evolution. The JMT follows the east side of the large lake, which is tucked into a long, narrow chasm at the north end of Evolution Basin and is towered over by the hulks of 13,831-foot Mt. Darwin and 13,710-foot Mt. Mendel. Verdant strips of meadow soften the otherwise granite surroundings of Evolution Lake, providing a less hostile environment than that around the upper lakes. Near the north side, the trail crests a low rise and swings around the north end of a large cove to a small, slightly elevated peninsula, where you'll find a number of view-filled campsites. Additional sites may be found amid the scattered groves of pines on the hillside north of the lake and near the outlet on the northwest side. The slender Evolution Basin, graced with a string of jeweled lakes and rimmed by a procession of magnificent peaks, provides some of the most glorious scenery in the High Sierra.

From Evolution Lake, follow sandy tread past small tarns and over granite slabs to switchbacks that lead through thickening lodgepole pine forest down into Evolution Valley. Nearing the floor of the canyon, the trail passes a thundering waterfall on the creek that drains Darwin Bench.

Proceed down the valley on gently graded trail through stands of scattered pines, across small pockets of meadow, and beside granite slabs and boulders to Colby Meadow, which has pleasant campsites along its fringe. Continuing on the JMT, you cross a couple of side streams before arriving at McClure Meadow, the largest of the meadows in Evolution Valley. Numerous campsites are scattered around the edge of the expansive meadow, some offering picturesque views of Evolution Creek sinuously coursing through the meadowlands. The McClure

THE CHALLENGE OF OBTAINING ACCURATE INFORMATION FROM GOVERNMENT AGENCIES

As the budgets of federal agencies charged with overseeing the backcountry become more inadequate, fewer and fewer rangers are available to set foot outside their offices. When contacting the U.S. Forest Service by phone, don't expect the person answering to have any valuable backcountry information—rather ask them to direct you to a backcountry ranger or wilderness specialist. Consider yourself very fortunate if a particular office has an employee in such a position and that person happens to be available when you call. You will mostly likely have to wait for a Forest Service employee to return your call, so don't wait until the last minute before inquiring. Although you should be careful to evaluate your sources, you could also always try surfing online for postings by other backpackers who have recently hiked the particular trail you're interested in.

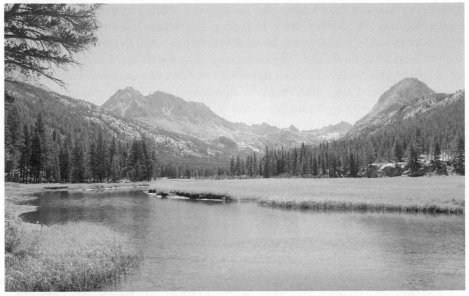

Pastoral McClure Meadow

Meadow ranger station sits on a low rise just north of the trail. Beyond the cabin, nearly level trail continues past more campsites to the far end of the meadow.

For the next couple of miles, the trail weaves in and out of forest cover and crosses a trio of streams draining the Glacier Divide above on the way to Evolution Meadow. The trail travels a fair distance away from the clearing, passing sheltered campsites on the way. At the far end of the meadow, you cross a twin-channeled stream and then curve south toward a ford of Evolution Creek. Except in early season, the crossing should not be difficult, although you should expect to get your feet wet in the process.

Beyond the ford, a short stretch of gently graded trail leads along the south bank to where the creek suddenly begins a raucous plunge toward the canyon below, tumbling over slabs and careening around boulders on its way to South Fork San Joaquin River. The course of the trail nearly matches the fall of the creek, with its zigzagging descent of the exposed, west-facing wall. You will, however, get nice views of the canyon and river below. The welcome shade from aspens, lodgepole pines, and incense cedars greets you at the canyon floor, where a short stroll leads to a bridge over the river and a junction with the Goddard Canyon Trail. A bounty of well-used, shady campsites lines both sides of the river.

Turn downstream (northwest) and follow the river through mixed forest to a crossing of the stream draining the canyon east of Mt. Henry. Continue through alternating sections of forest and open slopes covered with sagebrush, currant, and an assortment of wildflowers. Just before a bridge over the river, a spur trail leads to campsites in a dense grove of pines above the south bank.

Downstream from the crossing, the canyon narrows, propelling the river through a slim, rocky chasm. Continue alongside the raging river until more placid waters appear about 1 mile from the bridge. Just beyond a crossing of a tributary, you reach Aspen Meadow—which is actually more of an aspen grove than a meadow—with a few sheltered campsites nearby.

Away from Aspen Meadow, head downstream through open, rocky terrain, around John Muir Rock, and then veer away from the river through widely scattered conifers to a lightly forested flat with a number of campsites. Exiting Kings Canyon National Park, you cross a bridge over Piute Creek and immediately reach a junction with the Piute Pass Trail.

Leaving the JMT, you turn right (north) and follow the Piute Pass Trail, initially close to tumbling Piute Creek. Farther on, the trail climbs steeply above creek level on poor tread across open, chaparral-covered slopes, which makes the stiff ascent seem unusually hot on a warm summer day. To add insult to injury, the trail occasionally loses precious elevation that must be regained on the way up the canyon. The only advantage to this arrangement is the stunning view of the canyon and the highly fractured Pavilion Dome and associated, unnamed domes along the west end of Glacier Divide. Just beyond Turret Creek, the trail bends east, fords West Pinnacles Creek, and then climbs moderately steeply northeast beneath the welcome shade from a lodgepole pine forest. Nearing Hutchinson Meadow, you reach a junction with the Pine Creek Pass Trail, which has several campsites in the vicinity. Although spacious and shady, most of these campsites are heavily used by horse packers, which tend to generate copious amounts of horse dung and accompanying horse flies. Unless the stiff climb has tuckered you out, press on to the much more scenic Humphreys Basin for a campsite.

Away from the junction, the trail makes several fords of the braided creek draining French Canyon before resuming a moderate climb up Piute Creek Canyon. Through midseason, a fine wildflower display accompanies your ascent through slowly diminishing forest cover on the way to expansive Humphreys Basin. Once you reach the sweeping, flower-sprinkled basin, the options for campsites are virtually unlimited, at least for those who don't mind leaving the security of a maintained trail. Other than a 500-foot ban around Lower Golden Trout Lake, camping is available near any of the numerous lakes and unnamed tarns sprinkled across the basin. The massive hulk of nearly 14,000-foot Mt. Humphreys above the east edge of the basin dominates the landscape. Extra layover days can be spent exploring the far reaches of the basin. Heading up the trail, you pass a junction with a fairly distinct trail to Desolation Lake and then a faint use trail to Humphreys Lakes before climbing above Summit Lake to 11,423-foot Piute Pass.

From the pass, head down North Fork Bishop Creek, past Piute Lake, Loch Leven, and a handful of unnamed tarns and ponds. Beyond Loch Leven, the trail traverses the north wall of the canyon and then switchbacks below Piute Crags on a descent into a thickening forest of lodgepole pines. Cross the creek on a pair of log bridges and proceed downstream into North Lake Campground and the end of single-track trail. From there, take the campground access road and the spur road to the overnight parking area near North Lake.

BUILD-UP AND WIND-DOWN TIPS ·

Both trailheads begin at high elevations, so camping the night before your trip at one of the nearby **Forest Service campgrounds** would be wise, especially if you have just traveled here from sea level.

Resorts in the area include **Parchers Resort** (760-873-4177; www.parchersresort.net), about 1.5 miles below the dam along the South Lake Road, and **Cardinal Village Resort** (760-873-4789; www.cardinalvillageresort.com), in the community of Aspendell. The town of **Bishop** offers several choices for lodging, dining, and acquiring supplies.

High Sierra Transportation (760-872-1111) is a fully licensed and insured company providing transportation services to trailheads and airports.

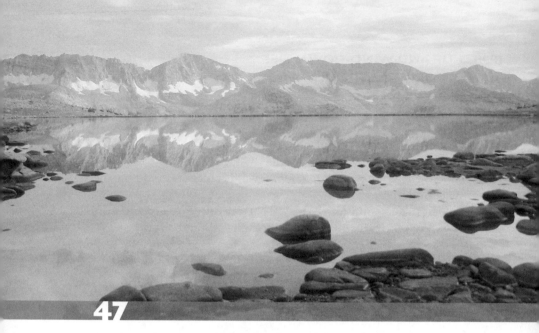

NORTH LAKE TO HUMPHREYS BASIN LOOP

Mike White

MILES: 27.0
RECOMMENDED DAYS: 4–6
ELEVATION GAIN/LOSS: 5150´/5150´
TYPE OF TRIP: Loop
DIFFICULTY: Strenuous
SOLITUDE: Moderately populated
LOCATION: Sequoia-Kings Canyon national parks and
    John Muir Wilderness
MAPS: USGS 7.5-min. *Mt. Darwin* and *Mt. Tom*
BEST SEASON: Late summer through early fall

PERMITS

Overnight stays in the John Muir Wilderness and Kings Canyon National Park require a wilderness permit, and daily trailhead quotas are in effect from May 1 to October 1. Permits can be obtained at Inyo National Forest facilities at Mono Basin Scenic Area visitor center, Mammoth Lakes visitor center, White Mountain ranger station in Bishop, or the Eastern Sierra interagency visitor center south of Lone Pine. Sixty percent of the reservations are available in advance, anytime from six months to two days before your trip.

Photo: *Mesa Lake backdropped by the Glacier Divide*

Download an application from the Inyo National Forest website (www.fs.fed.us.r5/inyo), and mail the completed application to the Wilderness Permit Reservation Office at 351 Pacu Lane Suite 200, Bishop, CA 93514; fax it to 760-873-2484; or call the Wilderness Permit Reservation Line at 760-873-2483. A $5 per-person fee is required, paid for by credit card, cash, check, or money order. The remaining 40 percent of the daily quota is available for walk-in permits, which can be obtained after 11 AM the day before departure. Unclaimed advanced reservations will be made available for walk-in permits after 9 AM on the day of departure.

CHALLENGES

Campfires are banned in several places along this route, so plan on using a stove. Bears are active throughout Kings Canyon National Park and surrounding national forest lands, and bear canisters are highly recommended. Due to overuse, camping is banned within 500 feet of Lower Golden Trout Lake.

HOW TO GET THERE

From U.S. Highway 395 in the center of Bishop, turn west onto Line Drive, which becomes South Lake Road (Highway 168) at the city limits. Proceed 3 miles past the South Lake junction to the right-hand turn to North Lake. Continue 1.6 miles on this narrow dirt road to a turnoff to the overnight parking lot (vault toilets) between the pack station and North Lake.

TRIP DESCRIPTION

Begin your journey by walking the road from the overnight parking area 0.7 mile west to the trailhead in North Lake Campground. From there, follow the single-track Piute Pass Trail west through aspen stands, lodgepole pine forest, and patches of meadow into the John Muir Wilderness. Beyond two bridged

TAKE THIS TRIP

The scenic features of the first part of this trip provide enough incentive for a visit: You will climb along a robust stream with a picturesque waterfall through flower-covered meadows and past a string of lakes to a view-filled pass. However, the supreme climax of this journey lies just beyond the pass, at one of the High Sierra's most picturesque locales, Humphreys Basin, an alpine wonderland with a bounty of scenic lakes and tarns. Bordered by rugged peaks of the Glacier Divide and the Sierra Crest, the large basin is a cross-country enthusiast's paradise, with easy off-trail travel available in virtually every direction. You could spend a week here without visiting every beautiful nook and cranny.

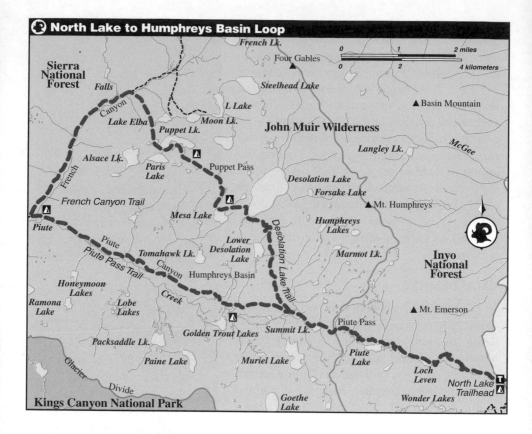

North Lake to Humphreys Basin Loop

crossings of North Fork Bishop Creek, switchbacks lead you well above the canyon floor to a long, ascending traverse, with fine views of a waterfall plunging steeply out of the basin above, as well as Mt. Emerson and the Piute Crags to the north. Rock steps and more switchbacks follow, leading up the narrowing canyon through a diminishing pine forest. Cresting the headwall, you reach Loch Leven and some marginal campsites scattered around the shore, 3 miles from the parking area. Midway along the north shore, a use trail on the right leads to a horse packer camp.

Leaving Loch Leven, a short, moderate climb leads through scattered lodgepole and whitebark pines past a pair of small ponds and up to the east shore of Piute Lake, which is surrounded by meadows, patches of willow, and scattered groves of whitebark pines. Campsites close to the trail are badly overused—search for other sites scattered farther around the lakeshore. Overnighters looking for more secluded camping can head northeast 0.3-mile cross-country to rockbound Emerson Lake.

Follow the trail northwest toward timberline, and ascend over granite slabs to pass through meadowlands watered by refreshing brooks and tiny ponds. A final traverse brings you to 11,423-foot Piute Pass, where your stiff climb is rewarded by a sweeping view across the broad expanse of lake-dotted Humphreys

Basin to the rugged Glacier Divide, the dramatic summit of Mt. Humphreys, Pilot Knob, and the deep cleft of the South Fork San Joaquin River canyon. If decision-making is not your strong suit, you'll surely be in trouble at Humphreys Basin, as myriad lakes tempt travelers in virtually every direction.

If Muriel Lake is your goal, leave the trail near the pass and traverse cross-country southwest and then west over open slopes to the lake (at 11,336 feet). Otherwise, remain on the Piute Pass Trail, following long-legged switchbacks on a descent high above Summit Lake to a crossing of the outlet from Humphreys Lakes. Here, a faint use trail climbs alongside the stream toward secluded terrain around Marmot and Humphreys lakes. A short distance farther is a junction with the trail to Desolation Lake.

Leaving the Piute Pass Trail, you turn right (north) and follow the Desolation Lake Trail on a mild climb across open, rolling terrain composed of granite and interspersed with alpine meadows. Pass well above Lower Desolation Lake and then wind your way through rock humps toward the south shore of much larger Desolation Lake, situated near the edge of Humphreys Basin below the towering Sierra Crest. Cross Desolation Lake's outlet and work your way shortly around the west shore before climbing west over a low ridge and then descending to lovely Mesa Lake, where a few campsites are spread around the shoreline on patches of granite sand. Widely scattered clumps of wind-battered and gnarled

A sweeping view from Puppet Pass

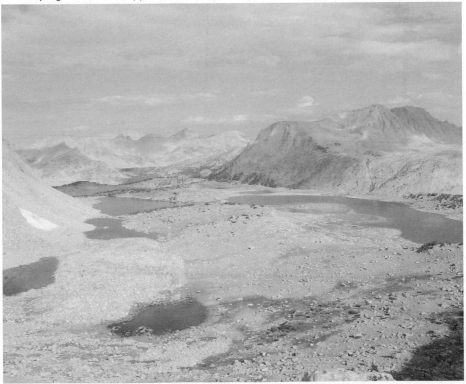

whitebark pines, the trademark conifer of the Sierra alpine zone, are sprinkled on the hillside north of the lake, adding a touch of character to the otherwise low-growing vegetation. From the north shore, you have an unobstructed view across the water to the spectacular Glacier Divide, which forms the northern boundary of Kings Canyon National Park. No trail and only three moderately difficult cross-country routes breach this nearly impenetrable wall.

Travel to the lake's northwest shore, and then make a 0.4-mile climb along the lushly lined inlet through alpine tundra and granite talus to a couple tarns near the head of a tiny basin. Continue ascending north, then northwest along the rivulet to a nearly level patch of alpine tundra, where you make the easy climb to 11,800-foot Puppet Pass. The view from the pass includes the picturesque bench below, which is sprinkled with a cluster of shimmering lakes. Just beyond the bench is the broad vale of French Canyon, towered over by the impressive profile of Seven Gables. Numerous other summits pierce the skyline, including Merriam and Royce peaks directly northwest, and Bear Creek Spire farther north.

Drop from the pass across talus to Roget Lake and continue across meadowlands to the north shore of Puppet Lake. Sprinkled around the shoreline are several campsites—more than enough for the few overnight visitors the area receives. A base camp at Puppet Lake provides a fine launching point for cross-country excursions to the other lakes in the vicinity, as well as more far-flung destinations such as Royce Lakes, Merriam Lake, or Bear Lakes.

Circle the west side of Puppet Lake and drop down a steep slope to the west shore of Lake Elba. Stroll across gentle meadowlands to the edge of the canyon, a

GREASING THE WHEELS OF THE WILDERNESS PERMIT SYSTEM

Many trips into the Sierra Nevada that require wilderness permits for overnight stays are under a strict quota system limiting the number of daily departures from trailheads. Consequently, for more popular areas, ill-prepared backpackers may be left scrambling to find open space at another trailhead. Highly organized backpackers can apply for reservations. If you're more spur-of-the-moment, however, you can increase your odds at landing a permit for a desired trailhead (with the exception of trips into the Mt. Whitney Zone, which usually requires winning a lottery held for this area's permits).

Some governing agencies post the availability, or lack thereof, of permits on their websites, allowing potential backpackers to see how many permits are still available before showing up at a ranger station. Since the highest demand for permits usually occurs for trips beginning on Fridays or Saturdays, consider embarking on another day if possible. Walk-in permits typically become available by late morning the day before a trip would begin, so arriving at a ranger station shortly before that time may be advantageous. Finally, reducing your party size to the smallest number increases your chances.

fine place to enjoy the vista of the awesome cascade tumbling down from Royce Lakes over the rock face on the far side of French Canyon. As you begin the descent into the canyon, you pass through mostly open terrain carpeted with willows and flower-covered patches of meadow, followed by a thickening forest of lodgepole pines. Boulder hop across the stream on the floor of the canyon and immediately come to the dirt tread of the Pine Creek Pass Trail.

Turn left (southwest) and head downstream beneath the towering granite wall on the north side of the canyon, through meadowlands thick with clumps of willow, patches of heather, and a profusion of wildflowers through midseason. Hop across the braided stream from Royce Lakes and continue the mild descent of French Canyon through stands of lodgepole pines alternating with stretches of open meadow. Along the way, you pass an occasional, infrequently used campsite tucked into the trees between the trail and the creek. Cross the stream from Merriam Lake and another creek that drains an unnamed tarn about a mile later before dropping more steeply through lodgepole pines to a junction with the Piute Pass Trail near Hutchinson Meadow; there are several campsites in the vicinity. Although spacious and shady, most of these campsites are heavily used by horse packers, and this tends to generate copious amounts of horse dung and accompanying horse flies.

The trail heads east from the junction and makes several fords of the braided creek draining French Canyon before climbing moderately up Piute Creek Canyon. Through midseason, a fine wildflower display accompanies your ascent through slowly diminishing forest cover on the way back to expansive Humphreys Basin. Once you reach the sweeping, flower-sprinkled basin, the options for campsites are virtually unlimited, at least for those who don't mind leaving the security of a maintained trail. Other than a 500-foot ban around Lower Golden Trout Lake, camping is available near any of the numerous lakes and unnamed tarns sprinkled across the basin. Upper Golden Trout Lake has a number of scenic campsites a relatively short distance from the Piute Pass Trail. The massive hulk of nearly 14,000-foot Mt. Humphreys above the east edge of the basin dominates the landscape. Extra layover days can easily be spent exploring the far reaches of the basin.

Heading up the Piute Pass Trail, you eventually reach the junction with the Desolation Lake Trail. Turn left (north) to retrace your steps to the parking area near North Lake.

BUILD-UP AND WIND-DOWN TIPS

Since this trail begins at a high elevation, camping the night before your trip at one of the nearby **Forest Service campgrounds** is wise, especially if you arrive here from sea level. Resorts in the area include **Parchers Resort** (760-873-4177; www.parchersresort.net), about 1.5 miles below the dam along the South Lake Road, and **Cardinal Village Resort** (760-873-4789; www.cardinalvillageresort.com), in the community of Aspendell. The town of **Bishop** offers several choices for lodging, dining, and acquiring supplies.

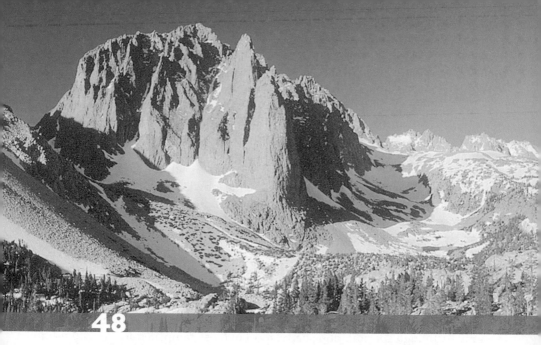

48

NORTH FORK BIG PINE CREEK LOOP

Andy Selters

MILES: 16.0
RECOMMENDED DAYS: 3
ELEVATION GAIN/LOSS: 3600´/3600´
TYPE OF TRIP: Loop
DIFFICULTY: Moderately strenuous
SOLITUDE: Crowded
LOCATION: John Muir Wilderness, Inyo National Forest
MAPS: USGS 7.5-min. *Coyote Flat*, *Split Mountain*, and *North Palisade*
BEST SEASON: Summer

PERMITS

A wilderness permit is required for all overnight visits in the John Muir Wilderness. The quota in place typically fills up at least a couple of weeks in advance for Friday and Saturday departures during mid-season. Contact Inyo National Forest, 351 Pacu Lane Suite 200, Bishop, CA 93514, 760-873-2400 or 760-873-2538 (TTY). Permits can be reserved until two days before departure ($5 per person), or on a first-come, first-served basis (no charge) starting the afternoon before your departure at White Mountain Ranger Station, 798 North Main Street, Bishop, CA 93514, 760-873-2500 or 760-873-2501 (TTY). For more information about

Photo: Temple Crag and the Palisades from Second Lake

getting a permit, visit http://www.fs.fed.us/r5/inyo/recreation/wild/howto.shtml.

CHALLENGES

This is one of the most highly renowned backpacks in the Eastern Sierra, and if you want to take it during the peak weekend, do *not* expect to be alone, either on the trail or in getting a permit. The higher lakes actually see relatively fewer campers, however. Campfires are prohibited in this basin, but camp stoves are permitted. For people arriving from low elevations, the somewhat stout hike up to camp above 10,000 feet can bring on mountain sickness. For those coming from sea level, a night before the trip at 7500 feet in one of the U.S. Forest Service campgrounds up the canyon can give valuable acclimatization to the relatively high altitude here, and make for easier, more enjoyable hiking.

HOW TO GET THERE

From the center of Big Pine on U.S. Highway 395, the road west up Big Pine Creek begins as Crocker Street. Just out of town the road climbs steeply into Big Pine Creek's canyon. Once in the forest zone it passes a couple of U.S. Forest Service campgrounds and ends at the trailhead 11.6 miles from Highway 395. Dayhikers can park here at the road's end if there is space. Overnight hikers can drop off their packs here, but they must park their cars 0.6 mile below the trailhead in the large lot provided.

TRIP DESCRIPTION

The hike starts behind the locked gate at the road's end, beside rushing Big Pine Creek and below some private summer cabins. Walk past the cabins, follow TRAIL signs pointing uphill past a couple access paths, and then climb a pair of short switchbacks. The second takes you across a bridge over the North Fork, right below crashing First Falls. Beyond the

TAKE THIS TRIP

At the head of Big Pine Creek soars the longest spine of 13,000- to 14,000-foot peaks in the Lower 48, the legendary Palisades. At every turn the North Fork Trail reveals new perspectives on these splintery crests, all while touring nine inviting lakes. The largest glaciers in the Sierra gather in the benches below the peaks, completing the setting for an alpine tableau unmatched in California.

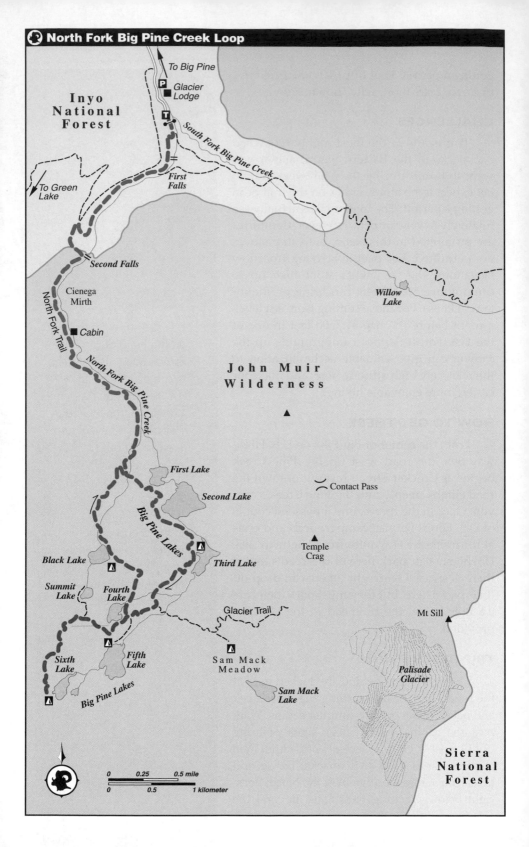

To Big Pine

P

Glacier
Lodge

T

Inyo
National
Forest

South Fork Big Pine Creek

First
Falls

To Green
Lake

Second Falls

Cienega
Mirth

North Fork Trail

Cabin

North Fork Big Pine Creek

John Muir
Wilderness

▲

Willow
Lake

First Lake

Second Lake

Contact Pass

Big Pine Lakes

Black Lake

Third Lake

Temple
Crag
▲

Summit
Lake

Fourth
Lake

Glacier Trail

Mt Sill ▲

Sixth
Lake

Fifth
Lake

Sam Mack
Meadow

Sam Mack
Lake

Palisade
Glacier

Big Pine Lakes

Sierra
National
Forest

0   0.25   0.5 mile

0   0.5   1 kilometer

streamside birches you come to where the trail up the Big Pine Creek's south fork continues traversing, and where you resume switchbacking uphill. Already the first great mountain vista appears above the South Fork canyon, with Middle Palisade poking over a ridge, and the "Twilight Pillar" of Norman Clyde Peak dominating the skyline.

In the shade of Jeffrey pines and aspens, climb to a bench, or an old roadbed. Hikers once drove this road to a high trailhead below Second Falls. But in September 1982 a tropical storm drenched this canyon with an estimated 6 inches of rainfall in one night, flooding the road below First Falls. Just up-canyon on this path another bridge takes you back across the creek, and on the other side you see a picnic site, a former campground. Here you can take a spur trail up to a path that comes directly from the overnighter's parking lot, but the main route turns up-canyon on sandy footing and leaves the shade of cottonwoods and Jeffrey pines. In midsummer, an early start makes the ensuing stretch of sunny climbing more pleasant.

With a couple of gentle switchbacks, turn uphill among manzanita and tobacco brush and then angle up to a triple intersection. Here the route to the upper Baker Creek drainage and Green Lake continues angling east-southeast up this moraine; the stock and overnighter's trail from below Glacier Lodge arrives here from the southeast; your route up cuts back and continues climbing west toward Second Falls. The last uphill chug rounds the steep corner near the falls then you return to shade next to the churning creek.

Now the trail cruises through an aspen grove and the sylvan flats known as Cienega Mirth. Lush undergrowth, including head-high larkspurs, contrast with the sun-baked slopes of your earlier climb. To the left you pass a cabin built as a summer retreat by actor Lon Chaney in the 1920s. The U.S. Forest Service eventually took over the cabin and now uses it to house their wilderness ranger. Beyond here easy walking continues through some moist glades rich in shooting star, tiger lily, and columbine. With a couple of slight rises you reach a dry meadow and your first view of some of the towering ramparts ahead—the flying buttresses of Temple Crag. Although this citadel stands below the Sierra crest and doesn't quite reach 13,000 feet, its Gothic battlements are the most impressive in the area. As you rise a little more, the tip of the highest peak in the region also comes into view, the North Palisade.

Next you hop across a tributary, swerve around a rise, reford the tributary, and return into woods. Here you meet the path descending from Black Lake, the return leg of the loop. Keep left and again cross the stream you've been following to resume a steady but gentle, winding climb under lodgepole pines and past outcrops to a slope above First Lake. A little farther southwest you pass a couple of woodsy campsites and ascend through a granite portal to an overlook of Second Lake, the largest in the group. Both here and at Third Lake, Temple Crag really commands the terrain.

The trail continues rising gradually past shady cliffs to Third Lake. Small campsites on the north, east, and south rim of this lake basin probably get more use than any others in the area. Whether you camp or rest here, the grand view includes a couple interesting features. In summer Third Lake has a milky aqua hue because the water is rich in superfine silt, rock ground into a fine powder by the Palisade Glacier out of sight above. Another curiosity here is the contrast between Temple Crag's dark granodiorite, studded with inclusions, and the blond granite of the massive hill to its east. The notch between them, where the two distinct rock types meet, is known as Contact Pass. The darker rock of the Palisades is part of an older pluton; millions of years ago the lighter-toned granite intruded around it.

From Third Lake you curve north, weave up a few short switchbacks, cruise to a small meadow, and cross a freshet issuing from Fourth Lake. Just beyond this ford the Glacier Trail forks to the southwest. For those ready to hike high and hard, this trail takes you up to the foot of the Palisades (see side trip). The North Fork Trail curves north and gently climbs to a three-way split. The left pathway rounds a ridge to Fifth Lake, where fine campsites, decent fishing and more great panoramas await, just 0.2 mile away. The right fork is the trail to Black Lake (described later in this trip), the leg back toward the trailhead. Continue straight ahead and wind past campsites near the west shore of Fourth Lake, the lake with the most relaxing view—good for anyone ready for a break from the stimulation of awesome peaks. Just beyond Fourth Lake, the trail comes to another fork.

SIDE TRIP: PALISADE GLACIER

This tough path climbs nearly 2000 feet in a steep couple of miles but is a must-do pilgrimage for anyone who thrills at the highest peaks of the High Sierra. From the North Fork Trail 1.0 mile past Third Lake, the Glacier Trail descends southwest to cross the main creek and start a steep, rocky climb. After gaining about 600 feet the grade pauses at Sam Mack Meadow, a timber line hollow with a couple of campsites. From here the rough path climbs steeply east in tight switchbacks up the adjacent ridge. Once atop this ridgeline, you should be able to trace a route southwest through the krummholz and barren rocks along its crest.

To get the full view you've been waiting for, you must continue another half mile along this low spine up to nearly 12,500 feet. But there you're ensconced in the most alpine amphitheater in the Sierra—the cirque of the Palisade Glacier. Reigning center is the third highest peak in California, the North Palisade with its icy couloirs, proud buttresses, and distinctive high snowfield; to the left juts the big thumb of Mt. Sill, and to the right splintery crests extend through Starlight and Thunderbolt peaks. The Palisade Glacier fans out below you. To return, retrace your steps back to the North Fork Trail.

The left branch here is the direct, unmaintained, and unsigned path to Sixth Lake. It heads up along a swale and makes a couple small switchbacks to a spur overlooking Fifth Lake. From a sign there this route is just a foot-worn rocky way heading northwest up and around a knob and then a short stroll to Sixth Lake.

Back at the fork, take the right branch northeast and quickly meet the canyon's final junction, with the 0.2-mile spur to tiny Summit Lake. Keep left on the signed HORSE PATH for Sixth Lake, climbing gently toward treeline on the west side of a small meadow. Near the base of the long rock slope ahead veer west over a spur and then gain a final 250 feet to the ridge above Sixth Lake. This high-est section of rough trail through spindly whitebark pines has some of the best panoramas of the trip, in a sense more spectacular than the closer scene at the top of the Glacier Trail. From the top of the ridge a brief rocky descent finishes the North Fork Trail near the north shore of Sixth Lake. Seventh Lake lies at tree line, a short walk west. The best camping near these highest lakes may be on the low rise between them.

Sixth and Seventh lakes are sites where California Department of Fish & Game (CDFG) is attempting to reestablish the mountain yellow-legged frog. In recent years biologists have found that this frog, once common in most of the higher Sierra lakes, has become fairly rare, and it's become clear that the primary reason for their decline is the widespread introduction of trout, which eat the tadpoles. Starting in 1999, CDFG has netted out the alien trout, with the expecta-tion that the frogs will recolonize the lakes from the tiny adjacent ponds where a few have hung on. The department's failure to fully involve the public in this decision has upset some, but most people, including many fishermen, are happy to see native fauna returned to some high lakes where the fishing has not been so great anyway.

For the return loop, hike back down to the wooded intersection for the Fifth Lake turnoff near the southwest shore of Fourth Lake. Take the eastbound trail here to cross Fourth Lake's outlet. Next you climb slightly around a ridge and then descend northeast to Black Lake. Although less popular, this lake makes an excellent base, as fine campsites await above the trail here, deep water may offer the best fishing in the area, and a short scramble up the slope north of the lake presents a view as grand as any in this basin.

East from Black Lake the trail continues descending, crossing the outlet stream and then breaking out of the lodgepole forest to another Palisade pan-orama. Next some long switchbacks gradually descend open slopes with sage-brush, mountain mahogany, and whitebark and lodgepole pine (a hot climb on a midsummer afternoon). The descent runs to the return junction with the primary North Fork Trail, 4.4 miles from the trailhead. At the triple junction a couple of miles from the road's end, most backpackers continue walking east-southeast on the trail that gradually descends the long slope. This path contours above the road's end, traverses just above the pack station, and goes directly to the overnighter's parking lot.

BUILD-UP AND WIND-DOWN TIPS

Wilson's Eastside Sports in Bishop (12 miles north of Big Pine) is well stocked with anything for the backpacker and climber, and their staff has experience and knowledge not usually found in urban-based stores. Anyone interested in climb-ing the Palisades might want to hire a guide through the **Sierra Mountain Center** or **Sierra Mountain Guides**, also in Bishop.

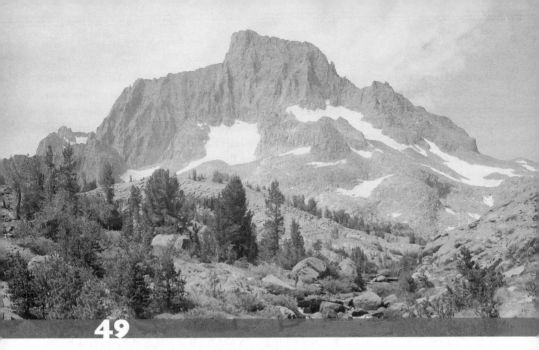

49

AGNEW MEADOWS TO DEVILS POSTPILE

Mike White

MILES: 24.0
RECOMMENDED DAYS: 4–6
ELEVATION GAIN/LOSS: 4360´/5120´
TYPE OF TRIP: Point-to-point
DIFFICULTY: Strenuous
SOLITUDE: Crowded
LOCATION: Ansel Adams Wilderness
MAPS: USGS 7.5-min. *Mammoth Mountain* and *Mount Ritter*
BEST SEASON: Late summer through early fall

PERMITS

A wilderness permit is required for each party entering the backcountry of Ansel Adams Wilderness, and trailhead quotas are in effect from May 1 to October 1. Sixty percent of the daily trailhead quota is available by reservation anytime between six months and two days before your departure date. To apply for a permit, download an application from the Inyo National Forest website (www.fs.fed.us.r5/inyo) and submit the completed form and applicable fees to: Wilderness Permit Reservation Office, 351 Pacu Lane Suite 200, Bishop, CA 93514. You

Photo: The impressive profile of Banner Peak is a frequent landmark on this loop.

TAKE THIS TRIP

This trip represents the best and the worst of the High Sierra. The best entails picturesque alpine lakes, such as Thousand Island, Garnet, Minaret, and Ediza, and spectacular mountain scenery from the Ritter Range, which includes such notable summits as Mt. Ritter and Banner Peak, as well as the string of arêtes known as the Minarets. The worst includes battling fellow backpackers for a limited number of wilderness permits, traffic congestion in Reds Meadow Valley, and camping bans due to previous overuse.

Negotiating an icy snowfield may be necessary before midseason, and climbing a short section of Class 3 rock below Iceberg Lake will be necessary in order to successfully complete the loop. If you'd rather avoid the cross-country section of the route between Ediza and Minaret lakes, hike back down Shadow Creek from Lake Ediza and continue past Shadow Lake to a bridge over Middle Fork San Joaquin River and a junction with the River Trail. Head downstream along the River Trail, following signs at all junctions for Agnew Meadows. Be prepared for a half-mile climb from the bottom of the valley across an open hillside to easier terrain near the meadows.

can also fax in the form (760-873-2484) or call the Wilderness Permit Reservation Line (760-873-2483).

With a reservation, permits can be obtained at Inyo National Forest facilities at Mono Basin Scenic Area visitor center, Mammoth Lakes visitor center, White Mountain ranger station in Bishop, or the eastern Sierra interagency visitor center south of Lone Pine. A $5 per-person fee is required, paid for by credit card, cash, check, or money order. The remaining 40 percent of the daily quota is available for walk-in permits, which can be obtained after 11 AM the day before departure. Unclaimed advanced reservations will be made available for walk-in permits after 9 AM on the day of departure.

CHALLENGES ·

As mentioned above, this is a popular trip, which means it can be difficult to secure a permit. Also, campfires are banned in several places along this route, so plan on using a stove. Bears are active throughout this area, and bear canisters are required. Due to overuse, camping is banned at Shadow Lake and within a quarter mile of the outlets of Thousand Island and Garnet lakes.

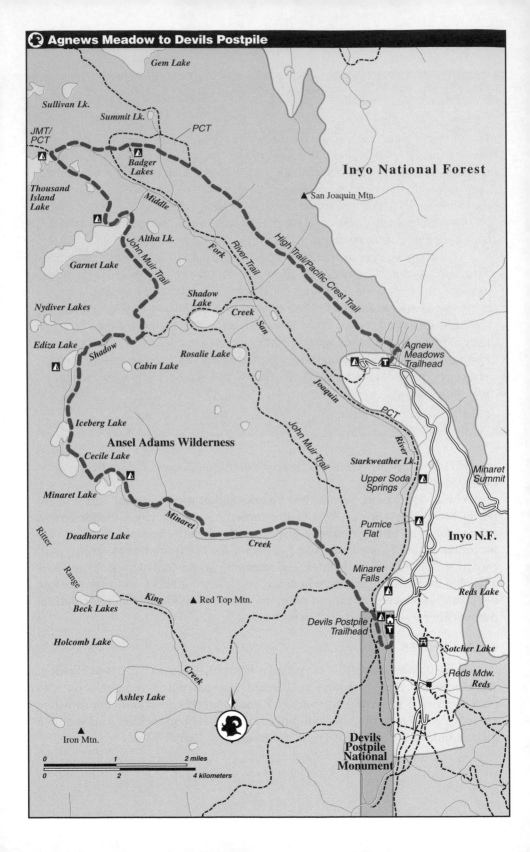

Gem Lake

Sullivan Lk.

Summit Lk.

PCT

JMT/ PCT

Badger Lakes

Inyo National Forest

▲ San Joaquin Mtn.

Thousand Island Lake

Middle

Altha Lk.

John Muir Trail

Fork

River Trail

High Trail/Pacific Crest Trail

Garnet Lake

Nydiver Lakes

Shadow Lake

Creek

San

Ediza Lake

Shadow

Cabin Lake

Rosalie Lake

Agnew Meadows Trailhead

Joaquin

PCT

Iceberg Lake

Ansel Adams Wilderness

John Muir Trail

River

Cecile Lake

Starkweather Lk.

Minaret Summit

Minaret Lake

Minaret

Upper Soda Springs

Ritter

Deadhorse Lake

Creek

Pumice Flat

Inyo N.F.

Range

Minaret Falls

King

▲ Red Top Mtn.

Reds Lake

Beck Lakes

Holcomb Lake

Creek

Devils Postpile Trailhead

Sotcher Lake

Ashley Lake

Reds Mdw.
Reds

▲ Iron Mtn.

Devils Postpile National Monument

0   1   2 miles

0   2   4 kilometers

HOW TO GET THERE

From U.S. Highway 395, take the Mammoth Lakes exit and follow Highway 203 west toward town. The Mammoth ranger station is on the right, 2.4 miles from 395, and you can pick up your wilderness permit here. Continue another 1.4 miles to the second traffic light and veer right on Minaret Road. Proceed 4.2 more miles to the large parking area for Mammoth Mountain Ski Area.

There is a $7 per-person fee for traveling beyond Minaret Summit. Unless you arrive before or after hours, or have an exemption, you must park in the ski area lot and ride the Reds Meadow shuttle bus into Reds Meadow Valley. Bus service usually runs through the summer season, with exact opening and closing dates dependent on weather conditions. The buses run daily from around 7:15 AM to 8:30 PM every 30 minutes (more frequently when necessary). Tickets can be purchased at the shuttle bus terminal at Mammoth Mountain Main Lodge Gondola Building (730-934-2289).

Agnew Meadows Trailhead: Take the Reds Meadow shuttle bus to the first stop, at Agnew Meadows, 2.7 miles from Minaret Summit, and walk the campground access road 0.3 mile to the trailhead.

Devils Postpile Trailhead: The trip ends at bus stop #6, Devils Postpile, 7 miles from Minaret Summit.

TRIP DESCRIPTION

From the bus stop, follow the access road toward Agnew Meadows Campground to the trailhead just past the pack station. Following signed directions northwest for the High Trail/Pacific Crest Trail, make a short, mild to moderate climb to a twin-log bridge over a stream, and then follow switchbacks through a red fir forest onto an open slope and into the John Muir Wilderness. Along the climb, views start to open up of Mammoth Mountain and the impressive Ritter Range. At the top of the switchbacks, the trail begins a long, ascending traverse beneath the ridge leading to the summit of San Joaquin Mountain, crossing several lushly lined brooks spilling down the hillside along the way. Wildflowers along these streams include delphinium, yarrow, cow parsnip, leopard lily, paintbrush, lupine, shooting star, larkspur, columbine, penstemon, scarlet gilia, and monkeyflower. Scattered to light forest obscures the views for a while, until you reach a stunning vista point near the 3-mile mark, directly across from the deep cleft of Shadow Creek canyon, with shimmering Shadow Lake attracting your gaze.

Continue the steady ascent across open slopes that offer continuous views across the Middle Fork San Joaquin River canyon to the serrated peaks of the Ritter Range. Hop across a number of flower-lined streams and proceed to where a series of descending switchbacks interrupts the climb. The ascending traverse resumes shortly, leading across more streams on the way to a junction, where the High Trail and Pacific Crest Trail diverge. A dry campsite is near the junction.

Turn left (northwest) and follow the High Trail on gently descending tread through a light forest of lodgepole pines to a creek crossing. Beyond the creek, the trail climbs briefly to a junction with the Pacific Crest Trail and a lateral to the River Trail. Following signed directions for Thousand Island Lake, proceed generally west on a mild to moderate climb that leads 0.3 mile to an unmarked junction with a path heading southeast to Badger Lakes. If you got a late start, or feel too tired to reach Thousand Island Lake, pleasant campsites around the largest Badger Lake provide an overnight alternative.

A pleasant stroll west across the basin of Badger Lakes is followed by a moderate climb over a low ridge to a junction with a trail to Clark Lakes. Continue ahead (west) to the top of a rock rib, and then make a short, winding descent to a junction with the River Trail, which heads south. Heading northwest, within earshot of the Middle Fork San Joaquin River's upper reaches, follow rising tread through scattered lodgepoles, and then switchback up a gully to a view of Banner Peak. From there, a gentle stroll through granite humps leads to a junction of the John Muir Trail, near the meadow-lined outlet at the northeast shore of large Thousand Island Lake, which has a picturesque backdrop of the craggy summits of Banner Peak and the rest of the Ritter Range. Camping is banned within a quarter mile of the outlet, as shown on an area map posted next to the trail. Legal campsites are spread along the northwest shore and seem to improve in quality and serenity the farther away from the JMT you go.

A backpacker negotiates a creek crossing.

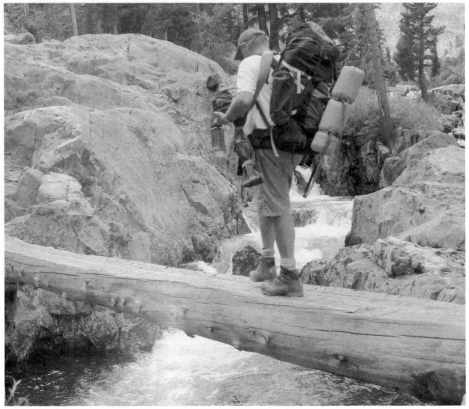

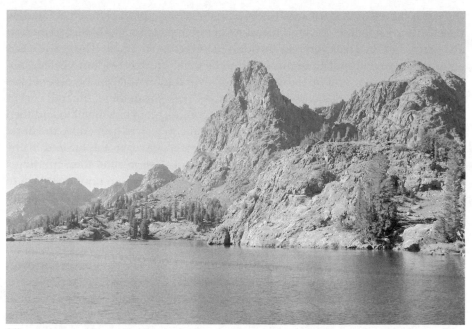

Minaret Lake makes a fine campsite.

Leaving Thousand Island Lake, head south on the JMT, crossing the two-log bridge over the lake's outlet. From here, you make a short, winding climb over a low ridge and down into the Emerald Lake basin. Backpackers wishing to escape the crowds at Thousand Island Lake may be able to find more secluded camping around Emerald Lake. A short climb out of the basin leads to Ruby Lake, where potential campsites are much more limited, thanks to the steep terrain of the lake's bowl. At the far (southeast) end of the lake, you cross over the outlet and begin a stiff, switchbacking climb over the ridge separating Ruby and Garnet lakes. As you descend toward Garnet Lake, a rock outcropping provides a fine vista point of the lake, backdropped by the Ritter Range. There is an unmarked junction with a use trail to campsites on the north side of the lake. If you plan on camping at Garnet Lake, follow this trail, as campsites are virtually nonexistent on the south shore. The path drops rather stiffly before approaching the lake near a peninsula with a number of campsites. Additional campsites are scattered farther along the north shore.

Continuing on the JMT, a view-packed, switchbacking descent circles the lake's north end to a bridged crossing of the outlet before an equally stiff climb takes you out of the basin through scattered whitebark pines and mountain hemlocks to a saddle with a nearby swimming hole. A rocky, switchbacking descent leads to a grass-covered basin and alongside a nascent tributary of Shadow Creek, which the JMT follows all the way to its union with Shadow Creek. This protracted descent is met with an increasing forest cover of lodgepole pines, red firs, and western white pines. Where the trail bottoms out, reach a junction with the Ediza Lake Trail.

Turn right (southwest) and head upstream along a placid stretch of Shadow Creek around a willow-covered meadow before the trail starts a mild to moderate climb, and the creek tumbles through picturesque cataracts. The grade eases again, and you will spot an unmarked trail heading south to seldom-visited Cabin Lake. Continuing east up the canyon, hop over the stream from Nydiver Lakes and proceed to a bridged crossing of Shadow Creek. From there, the trail curves away from the creek for a short while before coming alongside it again and then ascending the narrow, rocky gorge to Ediza Lake, which is framed by the dark, jagged summits of the Ritter Range. You'll have to travel to the far end of the lake for campsites, crossing the meadow on the south shore, and then crossing a couple streams—one from Iceberg Lake, and another from an unnamed tarn to the west. Shady campsites can be found on the hillside above the second stream and along the southwest shore of the lake.

To leave Ediza Lake, look for the somewhat obscure start of the unmaintained trail to Iceberg Lake near Ediza's southeast point. The path climbs south steeply, and switchbacks occasionally, through overgrown willows on the lower slope and across sloping meadowlands above that are carpeted with pussypaws, lupine, and heather. The generally open terrain provides fine views of Banner Peak and Mt. Ritter along the way, as well as the black Volcanic Divide to the east. Continue climbing up poor, rocky tread to the outlet, and then follow the cascading stream to the northern tip of bleak-looking Iceberg Lake.

An ascending path continues across talus slopes on the east side of Iceberg Lake before climbing the steep slope on the south side of the basin up toward Cecile Lake. After years of average to above average snowfall, this north-facing slope maintains an icy snowfield well into summer and should be attempted only by experienced parties with the proper equipment.

A ducked route passes around the east side of Cecile Lake across a sea of talus. The lake offers an up-close view of Clyde Minaret rising steeply and dramatically above the surface. Proceed to a cliff (and the crux of this route) at the far southeast edge of the basin, where you have the option of downclimbing a 10-foot chimney with a chockstone near the top, or a 15-foot rock face with numerous holds just to the right of the chimney. By mountaineering standards, neither route is particularly difficult, but either way, you will have to make a short, Class 3 climb while carrying a backpack. Inexperienced parties should either pack a short stretch of climbing rope for the descent, or avoid the route altogether; rangers report that someone usually gets in trouble here at least once every season. (See "Take This Trip" on p. 329 for information about an alternate route.)

Once safely down this minor obstacle, follow a use trail down the canyon of the inlet to scenic Minaret Lake. Campsites may be found near where the stream enters the lake, farther around the lake on the south side, or on the north end, where a large peninsula nearly divides the lake in two. Clumps of mountain hemlock and patches of meadow surrounding Minaret Lake create a much more inviting ambiance than the environment at rockbound Cecile and Iceberg lakes. The supreme view of the towering arêtes of the Ritter Range, known as the

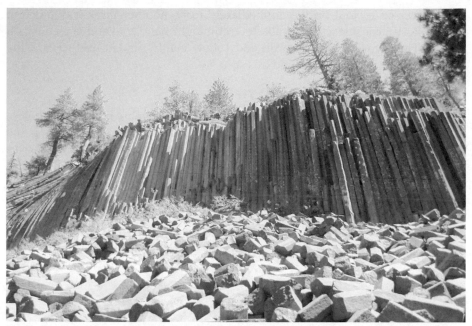

Devils Postpile is a must-see feature just off the main loop.

Minarets, enhances the alpine scene. From south to north, the prominent Minarets include Riegelhuth, Pridham, Kehrlein, Ken, and Clyde. Pridham Minaret offers unroped climbers a Class 2 route to the summit.

Take the shoreline trail around the north side of Minaret Lake and over a couple low rock humps to the west side. From there, switchbacks take you away southeast from the lake and down to Shadow Creek, which you follow through open, rocky terrain to a light forest of lodgepole pines and mountain hemlocks. A lengthy stretch of gently graded trail leads past some shady campsites alongside the creek before descending more steeply through an open area of granite, where Shadow Creek tumbles downslope in a series of picturesque cascades. Below the cascades, the trail continues the descent through a mixed forest of lodgepole pines, western white pines, red firs, and a diminishing number of mountain hemlocks. The grade eases near Johnson Meadow, where you reach a junction with the John Muir Trail.

Head south on the JMT, past Johnson Lake at the far end of the meadow, and then resume a moderate descent to a log crossing of Shadow Creek. Pass through a drift fence and reach a junction shortly afterward with the Beck Lakes Trail. Proceed downhill on the pumice tread of the JMT to a pair of switchbacks. Where the grade eases, cross the signed boundary between Inyo National Forest and Devils Postpile National Monument. Continue a short distance to the next junction, where the northbound Pacific Crest Trail veers left to follow the Middle Fork San Joaquin River upstream. Remaining on the JMT, you drop down to a log crossing of a rock-filled gully and travel around a meadow to a three-way junction. Following a sign to Devils Postpile, proceed ahead (east) to a crossing of the river on a stout bridge. Immediately reach another three-way junction (Devils Postpile is just a short walk down the right-hand trail and is well worth a visit). Here, you turn left (north) and follow gently graded trail toward the Devils Postpile ranger station and bus stop #6.

BUILD-UP AND WIND-DOWN TIPS •

The community of **Mammoth Lakes** offers an inordinate number of choices for food, lodging, and entertainment. One of the best breakfast haunts is the **Stove** (644 Old Mammoth Road; 760-934-2821). Unlike many of Mammoth's eateries, which are stuck into relatively new commercial complexes, the Stove occupies an old house that gives it a decidedly non-franchised character. If, however, after several days in the wilderness you're not quite ready to jump back into the frenzied activity of civilization in Mammoth Lakes, you could visit **Reds Meadow Campground** for a hot shower, or go a little farther to **Reds Meadow Resort** (800-292-7758) for a simple meal at the cafe or a cold one from the store.

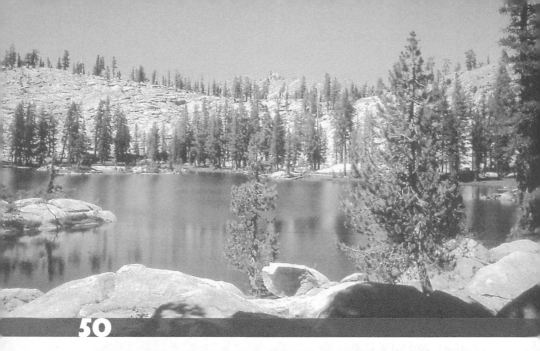

50

LILLIAN LAKE LOOP

Jeffrey P. Schaffer

MILES: 12.6 (another 7.2 with side trips)
RECOMMENDED DAYS: 2–3
ELEVATION GAIN/LOSS: 2440´/2440´
TYPE OF TRIP: Semiloop
DIFFICULTY: Easy
SOLITUDE: Moderately populated
LOCATION: Ansel Adams Wilderness, Sierra National Forest
MAP: USGS 7.5-min. *Timber Knob*
BEST SEASON: Midsummer

PERMITS

A wilderness permit is required year-round for all those spending the night in Ansel Adams Wilderness. Additionally, a quota system is in effect from late June through September 15, and up to two-thirds of the daily quota can be reserved in advance (on summer weekends the Lillian Lake Loop may reach its quota). For reservations, contact the Bass Lake Ranger District office, P.O. Box 10, North Fork, CA 93643, 559-877-2218. If you're driving through Oakhurst, get a permit at the Yosemite-Sierra Visitors Center, on Highway 41, 2.2 miles north of the Highway 49 junction. Alternatively, you can take your chances and drive up Forest Route 7 to the Clover Meadow Ranger Station and get one in person. To

Photo: Rainbow Lake

TAKE THIS TRIP

This loop passes three lakes, not bad for a 12.6-mile hike. However, if you have time, you should also visit Lady, Chittenden, Flat, and Rainbow, which add about 7.2 miles to the trip and 50 percent more elevation change. This country is just too beautiful to rush through, so take a leisurely three days to savor the country. Be sure to visit Rainbow Lake, one of the top Sierran lakes; you can't camp there, but spacious camping lies at Flat Lake just below it.

reach it, from the Road 5S05 junction continue 2.1 miles east on Forest Route 7 to the north end of Forest Route 81, or Minarets Road, ascending 52 paved miles north from the small community of North Fork. From this junction turn left and drive northeast 1.8 miles to the ranger station.

CHALLENGES

Most of this route is above 8000 feet, which means that you can expect lots of early-season snow. Even in an average snow year you're likely to find a few small patches of snow on the trail well into July. This is generally not a problem, but in early July there are enough patches that you could lose the trail.

HOW TO GET THERE

From the Highway 49 junction in Oakhurst, drive north on Highway 41 for 3.5 miles to a junction with Road 222, signed for Bass Lake. Follow this east 3.5 miles to a fork, veer left, and continue east 2.4 miles on Malum Ridge Road 274 to a junction with north-climbing Forest Route 7, or Beasore Road. (In case you need food or fuel at the last minute, immediately before this junction, south-dropping Beasore Road goes briefly to Pines Village, just above Bass Lake.) Forest Route 7 climbs 11.4 miles to an intersection at Cold Springs Summit, and then it winds 16.2 miles to Road 5S05 just 100 yards *after* Forest Route 7 crosses Ethelfreda Creek, which is about 0.5 mile past the Bowler Group Camp entrance. Ascend Road 5S05 2.3 miles to its end, complete with a large turnaround and parking lot.

TRIP DESCRIPTION

From the trailhead at 7530 feet in elevation, you start west up the Fernandez Trail, passing through a typical mid-elevation Sierran forest. After a gentle ascent 0.3 mile across slopes, you reach a small meadow, and from

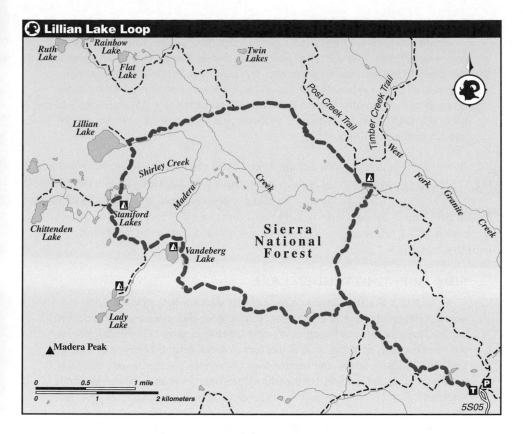

Lillian Lake Loop

Ruth Lake
Rainbow Lake
Flat Lake
Twin Lakes
Post Creek Trail
Timber Creek Trail
West
Lillian Lake
Shirley Creek
Madera Creek
Creek
Fork
Granite Creek
Chittenden Lake
Staniford Lakes
Sierra National Forest
Vandeberg Lake
Lady Lake
▲ Madera Peak

0   0.5   1 mile
0   1   2 kilometers

5S05

its west side an easily missed old trail meanders westward. Beyond the meadow your trail's gradient becomes moderate, and then you follow some short, steep switchbacks below a small, exfoliating "dome." Now entering Ansel Adams Wilderness, you have a steady 0.5-mile ascent to a near-crest junction and then briefly continue 0.2 mile up to a crest junction at 1.9 miles and 8320 feet. The Fernandez Trail continues right, but you branch left to begin the Lillian Loop Trail. For some, Vandeberg Lake, the first along the trail, is a worthy goal in itself, ideal for novice backpackers, dayhikers, or those with young children.

Heading west toward peaks and lakes, you start up the Lillian Loop Trail. This trail's first 2 miles are generally easy, and then the trail climbs almost 200 feet to a bedrock notch in a granitic crest and then makes a short descent almost to Vandeberg Lake at 8650 feet to a junction above Madera Creek at 4.3 miles. The right branch—for horses—descends north to Madera Creek and then circles counterclockwise to rejoin the left branch. We take the left branch, curving above fine campsites along the Vandeberg Lake's north shore. Where the trail branches reunite, you make a short climb to a junction at the edge of a lodgepole flat at 4.7 miles and 8800 feet.

SIDE TRIP: LADY LAKE

Here a southbound trail climbs gently to moderately 0.5 mile up to a large campsite on the north shore of Lady Lake at 8908 feet. On the east-shore moraine that juts into the lake, you'll find another fine campsite. This lake's irregular form, speckled with several boulder islands, makes it a particularly attractive lake, backdropped by metamorphic Madera Peak. Like all the lakes you might visit along this hike, Lady Lake has trout. Because it is shallow, it is a good lake for swimming from late July through mid-August.

Beyond the junction your Lillian Loop Trail crosses the lodgepole flat and then climbs a couple hundred feet up fairly open granitic slabs with a panorama from the Minarets south to the Mt. Goddard area in Kings Canyon National Park. You'll gain about 200 feet up to a ridge and then lose 200 feet down to a flat with a junction at 5.4 miles and 8790 feet—easily missed if it is not well-signed—the trail to Chittenden Lake.

SIDE TRIP: CHITTENDEN LAKE

Close to a Staniford Lakes creek, you can start a mile-long climb up to cliff-bound Chittenden Lake at 9182 feet. (If you miss this junction, you probably wouldn't be able to follow the obscure trail to that lake anyway.) Chittenden may be the most beautiful of all the lakes in this part of Ansel Adams Wilderness, though Lady and Rainbow lakes offer competition. Chittenden's water usually does not get warmer than the low 60s, but the lake's three bedrock islands may tempt some swimmers. Don't camp here, for there is precious little flat space.

Continuing on the Lillian Loop Trail, you go north only about 200 yards past the junction before you pass a waist-deep lakelet. Then after a similar distance you'll come to a trailside pond atop a broad granitic crest at 5.6 miles and 8790 feet.

SIDE TRIP: STANIFORD LAKES

In this vicinity you can leave the trail, and on your third optional excursion descend southeast briefly cross-country on low-angle slabs to the largest of the Staniford Lakes at 8708 feet. If any sizable lake along this route will warm up to the low 70s in midsummer, it will be this one—it's the best lake for swimming on this trip. The bulk of the lake is shallower than 5 feet, with a diving area, the only deep spot, along the west shore. Among the slabs you can find camp spots.

On the loop trail, you head north past more ponds, dip into a gully, and then head diagonally up a ridge with many glacier-polished slabs. You soon cross the ridge, quickly descend to Lillian Lake's outlet creek, and walk momentarily upstream to reach Lillian Lake at 6.2 miles and 8868 feet. Here is a lodgepole-shaded area that once comprised the largest campsite in this part of the wilderness. Since camping is prohibited within 400 feet of this northeast shore, be inventive and try elsewhere. The largest and deepest lake in the area, Lillian Lake is also the coldest (brisk swimming!), but it has a large trout population.

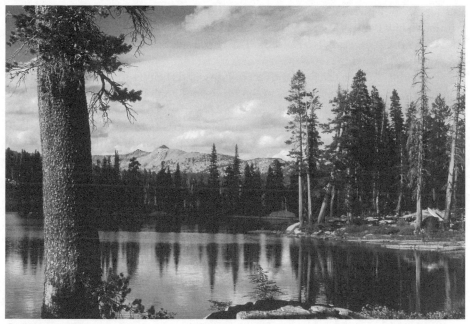

Staniford Lake

With your basic hike now half over, leave the lake's outlet and descend a forested mile east to a two-branched creek with easy fords. The Lillian Loop Trail ends in 0.3 mile, after a short, stiff climb over a gravelly knoll. Here, at a junction on a fairly open slope, you rejoin the Fernandez Trail at 7.4 miles, which you'll take back to the crest junction on which you started the loop. First, you might consider a side trip to Rainbow Lake.

SIDE TRIP: RAINBOW LAKE

Your fourth optional side trip ascends the Fernandez Trail 1 mile northwest up to a junction, from which the Rainbow Lake Trail first wanders 0.9 mile southwest up a ridge that is just north of Lillian Lake. On the ridge the trail becomes vague on bedrock slabs where it bends from southwest to northwest, and unsuspecting hikers may continue southwest down toward Lillian Lake, 400 feet below. If you are good at cross-country hiking, you can start from the northeast shore of that lake and hike up this "erroneous" route, and just beyond its ridge's crest locate the trail, saving about 2 miles of hiking. From the ridge the Rainbow Lake Trail then roller-coasters northwest 0.7 mile to the prized lake, where camping is prohibited within a quarter mile of the lakeshore. If you are interested, you can cross this multilobed lake by swimming from island to island.

From the junction of Lillian Loop and Fernandez trails, descend 0.3 mile east on the Fernandez Trail to a linear gully, follow it a short distance, and then drift over to the crest of a moraine, about 0.5 mile from the previous junction. Your route, which has been eastward, now turns southeast and follows the crest to its end, from where you soon engage a few short switchbacks near some junipers, get a good view of much of your basin's landscape, and then descend 0.5 mile to a junction at 9.0 miles and 7950 feet. A trail 70 yards north to a crest saddle forks into the Post Creek Trail (left) and the Timber Creek Trail (right), neither of which are worth taking.

From the junction the Fernandez Trail descends briefly to a gravelly flat along the north bank of Madera Creek at 9.3 miles and 7800 feet. This spacious flat is well suited for camping, and here you may see the former Walton Trail heading east; it used to cross Madera Creek about 250 yards below the Fernandez Trail ford and once provided an alternate route to your current trailhead. With that goal in mind, cross the creek and gain about 500 feet on the Fernandez Trail, your ridge ascent ending after a brief contour southeast to the crest junction with the start of the loop at 10.7 miles. From it retrace your steps back to the parking area at the end of Road 5S05 at 12.6 miles.

BUILD-UP AND WIND-DOWN TIPS ·

Unless you're backpacking with a group, you can't stay in Bowler Group Camp. The closest campground along Forest Route 7 is **Upper Chiquito**, about 1.0 mile east of the Globe Rock junction, but it's not as appealing as **Clover Meadow Campground**. To reach the latter, from the Road 5S05 junction continue 2.1 miles east on Forest Route 7 to a junction with entirely paved Forest Route 81, or Minarets Road. From the small community of North Fork, this is a long, winding road north, albeit a very scenic one. (If you're not in a hurry before or after your hike, it is worth taking.)

The route has three roadside campgrounds (plus others on lateral roads), and **Soda Springs** is the one farthest north, about 35 miles above North Fork and 17 miles before the junction with Forest Route 7. From this junction, take Road 5S30 northeast 1.8 miles to Clover Meadow Ranger Station, and get your permit there if you haven't gotten one earlier. To reach the primitive **Clover Meadow Campground**, which has only several sites, take the narrow road branching left from the ranger station. This road can be rutted and sometimes boggy. If the campground hasn't opened for the summer season, it's a good sign that you will find lots of snow along your hike.

NORTHERN SIERRA NEVADA

At 400 miles long, the Sierra Nevada is the longest and highest single-block range of mountains in the United States. Geographically, the Sierra Nevada range is generally divided into three sections: southern, central, and northern. For the purposes of this guide, the northern Sierra section also includes Yosemite National Park and vicinity, where the topography changes significantly. South of Sonora Pass is where the High Sierra truly begins, with some of Yosemite's mountains reaching heights of over 12,000 feet. Much more of the classic granite landscape is evident in the park, not only in Yosemite Valley but throughout the 1200 square miles of backcountry as well. The northern Sierra Nevada makes up about half that length, an area roughly 200 miles long, from the North Fork Feather River canyon southward to Yosemite National Park's south and southeastern boundaries.

Although much of the overlying rock in the northern Sierra is volcanic in nature, the underlying rock is part of the huge Sierra Nevada batholith, a composition of many granitic plutons, which are made up of intrusive igneous rock that crystallized beneath the earth's surface. This geologic distinction identifies the area as part of the Sierra Nevada, as opposed to including it with the southern Cascades, which are primarily volcanic in origin.

Around the North Fork Feather River canyon, the Sierra Nevada's crest lands are relatively low, the highest peaks rarely over 7000 feet, but the elevations increase southward. Around Donner Pass (Interstate 80), crest lands are mostly around 8000 feet, with the highest peaks exceeding 9000 feet. Around Lake Tahoe, crest lands are similarly high, but the highest peaks approach 11,000 feet. Finally, along Yosemite's crest lands, the canyon floors mostly are over 9000 feet and the peaks above them are mostly 11,000 to 12,000 feet, with two exceeding 13,000 feet.

Despite lacking the lofty grandeur of the southern Sierra, the northern Sierra is blessed with wonderful topography and beautiful scenery. One national park, several wilderness areas, a couple recreation areas, and a state park protect some of this stunning backcountry. Generally from south to north these areas include Yosemite National Park, Hoover Wilderness, Emigrant Wilderness, Carson-Iceberg Wilderness, Mokelumne Wilderness, Desolation Wilderness, Granite Chief Wilderness, Grouse Ridge Recreation Area, Lakes Basin Recreation Area, Plumas-Eureka State Park, and Bucks Lake Wilderness.

This section's south half, from Yosemite National Park north to Echo Summit (Highway 50), being higher, lacks the montane forests, and hence lacks the logging roads, while the north half has the roads, plus the urban developments in the Lake Tahoe Basin. Consequently, in this half the northern Sierra's recreational heritage is contained in small pockets of land surrounded by private land or public land crisscrossed by hundreds of miles of road, a fact easily confirmed by glancing at any U.S. Forest Service map.

YOSEMITE NATIONAL PARK

About 4 million people visit Yosemite National Park each year. The draw, of course, is Yosemite Valley, perhaps the world's most misinterpreted natural feature. Thought by John Muir to have been entirely excavated by glaciers, and thought by others later on to have been just greatly excavated by them, glacial erosion only minimally incised into the valley's walls. The valley is a very old feature, having evolved, after the last Sierra Nevada uplift, for at least 65 million years before any glacier ever reached it. Glaciers altered the valley's dimensions in two ways. First, each major glacier, which typically was about 1500 to 1000 feet thick, exerted pressure on the lower walls for thousands of years, and when each rapidly retreated, the pressure was suddenly released and a round of rapid exfoliation ensued. This process led to the accumulation of tremendous amounts of talus, such as you see today, some 15,000 years after the last glacier retreated. The valley, which already was wide due to mass wasting of its walls over tens of millions of years, became perhaps 10 percent wider due to the dozens of glaciations. Second, glaciers filled the valley with hundreds of feet of sediments, resulting in a broader, flat floor.

No other major canyon or valley in the Sierra Nevada is as steep-walled and flat-floored, making Yosemite Valley unique. Additionally, none has the valley's spectacular waterfalls, which may be its foremost draw. While most of the park's visitors marvel at the valley's waterfalls and monoliths, such as El Capitan and Half Dome, only a minority get off the road and into the park's wilderness, which comprises about 90 percent of the park. Like Sequoia and Kings Canyon National Parks, Yosemite National Park abounds in lakes, but ones that are arguably, if subjectively, better. They are reached with less elevation gain and closer to trailheads and, therefore, more accessible. Also most lie within montane and subalpine forests, much fewer in the cold, exposed alpine realm (the domain of many mountaineers, but not casual backpackers).

Of the dozens of fine backpack routes in the park, this book covers six, two out of Yosemite Valley and the others centered around Tuolumne Meadows. Trip 51, to Half Dome's summit, is an experience of a lifetime, and if you are in shape, you ought to consider doing it, since one day, perhaps soon, hikers may be banned from its summit. Trips 52 and 53 pass some of the Sierra's finest waterfalls and cascades, while Trips 54, 55, and 56 visit some admirable Sierran lakes.

HOOVER WILDERNESS

Hoover Wilderness is narrow and is, in effect, a buffer zone between Yosemite's Sierra crest and lower lands to the east. This zone almost coincides with a belt of metamorphic rocks, so this wilderness has a very different feel: deep, near-crest canyons painted in various earth hues of metamorphic rocks, which alternate with the grays of granitic rocks. The two trips offered in this wilderness are very different. Short, popular Trip 57 passes at least a dozen lakes of mostly metamorphic lands in as many miles, making it one of the top lake-blessed hikes in the Sierra. In contrast, lengthy, lightly traveled Trip 58, entirely across granitic terrain, has fewer lakes, but takes the backpacker through Yosemite National Park's most remote crest lands.

CARSON-ICEBERG WILDERNESS

Between Yosemite National Park and the Lake Tahoe Basin lie, from south to north, Emigrant, Carson-Iceberg, and Mokelumne wildernesses. Two trips in Carson-Iceberg Wilderness are included, despite the other two wildernesses having more lakes, because both are short enough that most beginning backpackers, or those with children, can handle them. One of these is to Sword and Lost lakes, among the warmest swimming (and diving) natural lakes in the range. In contrast, Emigrant Wilderness has lots of lakes, but most of the better lakes require a considerable hike to reach them. The best lakes in Mokelumne Wilderness are, like in Carson-Iceberg Wilderness, easy to reach, but these few are subalpine, and they tend to be windswept as well as chilly for swimming. Furthermore, they lack sufficient camp space to handle the weekend crowds. Because Carson-Iceberg Wilderness is lake-poor, many backpackers consider it unattractive and its many canyons tend to have very few hikers, making it a prime destination for seekers of solitude.

DESOLATION WILDERNESS, PLUMAS-EUREKA STATE PARK, AND BUCKS LAKE WILDERNESS

Three trips (61–63) described in this section travel through Desolation Wilderness, 63,960 acres of stunning backcountry near Lake Tahoe, composed of rich forests, granite and metamorphic peaks, and dozens of azure lakes. One of the most heavily visited wilderness areas in the U.S., Desolation is heavily regulated as well, with daily zone quotas, mandatory dayhiker registration, overnight wilderness permit fees, campfire bans, and parking fees at two of the more popular trailheads. Despite the regulation, a trip through Desolation Wilderness remains one of the northern Sierra's most coveted outdoor experiences.

North of the Tahoe area, Trip 64 passes through the combined lands of Lakes Basin Recreation Area and adjoining Plumas-Eureka State Park to four delightful lakes, some of only a handful of lakes backpackers are allowed to camp at in the area. The section concludes with a 20-mile loop through Bucks Lake Wilderness, a quiet tract of backcountry west of Quincy.

TAHOE RIM TRAIL

Located in two states, two mountain ranges, and three wilderness areas, the Tahoe Rim Trail (TRT) packs a lot of beauty and variety into only 165 miles: deep forests, sparkling mountain lakes, and mile after mile of spectacular views of Lake Tahoe. The TRT has eight trailheads, making it perfect for just a few hours, a few days, or a few weeks. Perhaps its best feature is that it encircles Lake Tahoe. Not only can you park your car and walk for two weeks and end up right where you started, but during the trip you can look across the lake and see where you have been and where you are going.

The trail was built and is maintained by the nonprofit Tahoe Rim Trail Association (TRTA), which runs a hiking program all summer and fall, including shuttle services, and is an excellent source for the latest trail information. If you hike the entire trail, you can become a member of the Tahoe Rim Trail 165 Mile Club.

51

HAPPY ISLES TO HALF DOME

Jeffrey P. Schaffer

MILES: 15.7
RECOMMENDED DAYS: 2
ELEVATION GAIN/LOSS: 5400´/5400´
TYPE OF TRIP: Semiloop
DIFFICULTY: Strenuous
SOLITUDE: Crowded
LOCATION: Yosemite National Park
MAP: USGS 7.5 min. *Yosemite Valley*
BEST SEASON: Summer

PERMITS ···

Pick up a wilderness permit at the Wilderness Center, located in the valley's Yosemite Village. You can also try calling them at 209-372-0740, but the reservation phone lines are often busy and so you may not get through. For general information about wilderness permits and the backcountry, call the center at 209-372-0745. You can also reserve a permit online at www.nps.gov/yose/wilderness. A $5 per person nonrefundable processing fee is charged for all reservation requests.

Photo: Tenaya Canyon and Clouds Rest from Half Dome

TAKE THIS TRIP

Half Dome may be the Sierra's most popular backcountry summit. It's no wonder that it attracts hikers worldwide. Where else do hikers use cables to hike/climb up to a summit? Additionally, this semiloop trip treats you to a close-up of two spectacular waterfalls, Vernal and Nevada. By camping in Little Yosemite Valley, you have a head start on the hordes of dayhikers, who typically impact the cables and crowd the summit in early and midafternoon.

CHALLENGES

This is safe for competent hikers, but the cables can be struck by lightning, and careless hikers occasionally fall to their deaths. Please don't bring children under 12 and no acrophobics!

HOW TO GET THERE

If you have a vehicle, you'll have to leave it at the backpackers' parking lot, which is about midway between Curry Village and Happy Isles. When you get your wilderness permit, you'll be told how to reach the lot. If you take the shuttle bus through the valley, your hike will begin at the Happy Isles shuttle-bus stop (stop 16), in southeastern Yosemite Valley. If you don't take a shuttle bus, then you'll have a half-mile walk, via trail or road, southeast to Happy Isles.

TRIP DESCRIPTION

From the shuttle-bus stop at 4020 feet in elevation you walk briefly east across an adjacent bridge and head south, soon reaching the start of the John Muir Trail. Soon the climb south steepens, and then you turn east and ascend a steep stretch before making a quick drop to the Vernal Fall bridge at 1.0 mile and 4440 feet. From it you see Vernal Fall, backdropped by Mt. Broderick (left) and Liberty Cap (right).

About 200 yards beyond the bridge you come to the start of your loop. Here the Mist Trail continues upriver while the John Muir Trail starts a switchbacking ascent to the right. You'll go up the Mist Trail and down the John Muir Trail.

Dressed for the upcoming mist, which can really soak you in June, start up the Mist Trail. The spray increases as you advance toward the fall, as you climb 300-plus steps to an alcove beneath an ominous overhang. A last set of stairs, protected by a railing, guides hikers to the brink of Vernal Fall at 1.6 miles and 5050

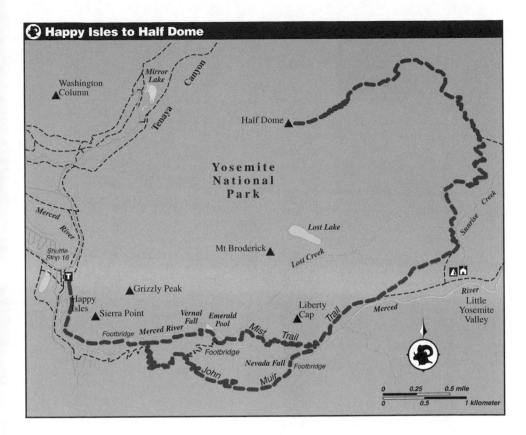

Happy Isles to Half Dome

Washington
▲Column

Mirror
Lake

Tenaya Canyon

Half Dome ▲

Yosemite National Park

Merced River

Shuttle
Stop 16

Lost Lake

Mt Broderick ▲

Lost Creek

Sunrise Creek

Happy
Isles

▲Grizzly Peak

▲Sierra Point

Vernal
Fall

Emerald
Pool

Liberty
Cap ▲

Trail

Merced

River
Little
Yosemite
Valley

Footbridge   Merced River

Mist   Trail

John   Muir

Footbridge

Nevada Fall   Footbridge

0   0.25   0.5 mile
0   0.5   1 kilometer

feet. Careless hikers have been swept to their deaths by slipping on slick rock or by swimming just above the brink in Emerald Pool.

Plunging into the upper end of chilly Emerald Pool is churning Silver Apron, and a bridge spanning its narrow gorge is your immediate goal. The trail leaves the pool's far (east) end (near some outhouses) and a nearby junction at 1.7 miles. From it a trail climbs almost a half mile to the John Muir Trail at Clark Point. You, however, curve left over to the Silver Apron bridge at 1.8 miles and 5140 feet. Beyond it you climb up to a broad bench and then toward Nevada Fall. Soon you commence a series of more than two dozen short switchbacks. The climb ends at the top of a gully where, on brushy slopes, you once again meet the John Muir Trail (there are more outhouses here) at 2.7 miles and 6000 feet.

From this junction you climb up the gully to its top and then quickly descend into forest cover and reach a fairly large swimming hole on the Merced River. Beneath conifers you continue northeast along the river's azalea-lined bank and then encounter a trail fork at 3.3 miles and 6120 feet. Take the right fork, which parallels the Merced River upstream to the Little Yosemite Valley's large back-packers' camp at 3.8 miles and 6130 feet, where you spend the night. It has bear-proof food storage boxes, outhouses, and a spur trail northeast over to a rangers' camp. Just north of that is a junction with the left-fork route.

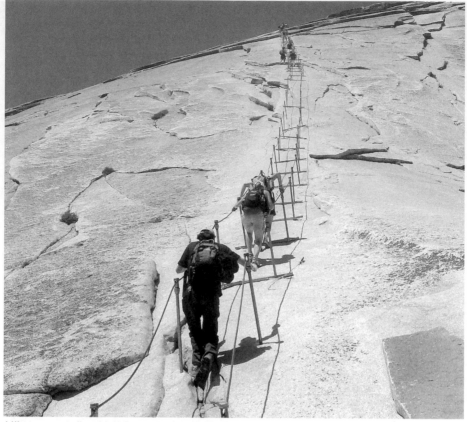

Hikers ascending Half Dome's notorious cables

From that junction you've not yet expended half the energy required to reach Half Dome's summit. Leave your backpack in the camp and with a day pack and adequate water, go 1.3 miles on a forested ascent up the John Muir Trail to a junction, where you branch left on the Half Dome Trail at 5.2 miles and 7010 feet. After about 0.7 mile the trail bends west just before reaching a saddle, which is worth the minor effort for a viewful rest stop.

In the next 0.5 mile, the trail first climbs through a forest and then Half Dome's northeast face comes into view before the trail tops a crest. Here you get a fine view of Clouds Rest and its satellites, the Quarter Domes. You now have a 0.3-mile traverse, which reveals more views, including Tenaya Canyon, Mt. Watkins, and Mt. Hoffmann before ending at the base of Half Dome's intimidating shoulder. Ascend short switchbacks up the shoulder to a ridge, where you are confronted with the dome's intimidating pair of cables. (Many hikers retreat—if you feel uncomfortable with them, you should as well.)

The cables too quickly steepen almost to a 45-degree angle. Looking down, you can see that you *don't* want to fall. Remember that even when thunderstorms are miles away, static electricity can build up here. Out of a seemingly fair-weather sky a charge can bolt down the cable, throwing your arms off it—or worse. If your hair starts standing on end, beat a hasty retreat. Eventually an easing gradient gives new incentive, and soon you are scrambling up to the broad summit of Half Dome at 7.3 miles and 8842 feet. Most hikers proceed to the dome's high point, located at the north end, from where they can view the dome's overhanging northwest point. Stout-hearted souls peer over the lip of this point for an adrenaline-charged view down the dome's 2000-foot-high northwest face, perhaps seeing climbers ascending it. From the broad summit you have a 360-degree panorama, including an aerial view down Yosemite Valley and up Tenaya Canyon past Clouds Rest.

To return, backtrack down to Little Yosemite Valley's camp at 11.3 miles and 6130 feet, pick up your backpack, and continue to backtrack to the junction northeast of Nevada Fall, at the top of the Mist Trail at 11.9 miles and 6000 feet. Rather than descend it, take the John Muir Trail over to the Nevada Fall bridge.

SIDE TRIP: BRINK OF NEVADA FALL

Just a few yards before the Nevada Fall bridge, you can strike northwest to find a short spur trail that drops to a viewpoint beside the fall's brink. This viewpoint's railing is seen from the fall's bridge, thereby giving you an idea where the trail ends. Don't stray along the cliff's edge and, as said earlier, respect the river—people have been swept over this fall too.

From the Nevada Fall bridge, strike southwest shortly to the Glacier Point-Panorama Trail at 12.3 miles and 5950 feet. Now begin a descent to Happy Isles, which starts with a high traverse that provides an ever-changing panorama of domelike Liberty Cap and broad-topped Mt. Broderick—both overridden by glaciers. As you progress west, Half Dome becomes prominent, its hulking mass vying for your attention. Eventually you descend to Clark Point at 13.4 miles and 5481 feet, where you meet a scenic connecting trail that switchbacks down to Emerald Pool.

Backpackers continue down the John Muir Trail, which curves south into a gully, switchbacks down to the base of spreading Panorama Cliff, and then switchbacks down a talus slope. Largely shaded, it reaches a junction with a horse trail to the valley's stables. Continue a brief minute more to a junction with the Mist Trail at 14.6 miles and 4510 feet, turn left, and quickly reach the Vernal Fall bridge, from which you retrace your steps down to Happy Isles.

BUILD-UP AND WIND-DOWN TIPS ·

It is difficult to find camping in or near Yosemite Valley, so plan to drive there on the day you'll start your hike. Wear good hiking shoes. Camping in Little Yosemite Valley, you won't need to carry a bearproof food canister because bearproof storage boxes are provided. Before mid-July when the Mist Trail can drench you, wear shorts and/or bring a lightweight rain parka. Be sure to bring a fresh pair of gloves to ascend the cables. After your hike, you might celebrate with pizza and beer at nearby **Curry Village**. Here you can also get showers (towels provided), which are great after a hot day on the trail.

52

HAPPY ISLES TO MERCED LAKE

Jeffrey P. Schaffer

MILES: 27.3

RECOMMENDED DAYS: 3

ELEVATION GAIN/LOSS: 4670'/4670'

TYPE OF TRIP: Semiloop

DIFFICULTY: Moderate

SOLITUDE: Moderately populated

LOCATION: Yosemite National Park

MAPS: USGS 7.5-min. *Half Dome* and *Merced Peak*

BEST SEASON: Midsummer

PERMITS ·

Pick up a wilderness permit at the Wilderness Center, located in the valley's Yosemite Village. You can also try calling them at 209-372-0740, but the reservation phone lines are often busy and so you may not get through. For general information about wilderness permits and the backcountry, call the center at 209-372-0745. You can also reserve a permit online at www.nps.gov/yose/wilderness. A $5 per person nonrefundable processing fee is charged for all reservation requests.

Photo: Merced Lake

CHALLENGES

The Mist Trail to the top of Vernal Fall is wet, especially before August, and a slip in the wrong place could be fatal. (Still, most tourists make it safely.)

HOW TO GET THERE

If you have a vehicle, you'll have to leave it at the backpackers' parking lot, which is about midway between Curry Village and Happy Isles. When you get your wilderness permit, you'll be told how to reach the lot. If you take the shuttle bus through the valley, your hike will begin at the Happy Isles shuttle-bus stop (stop 16), in southeastern Yosemite Valley. If you don't take a shuttle bus, then you'll have a half-mile walk, via trail or road, southeast to Happy Isles.

TRIP DESCRIPTION

From the shuttle-bus stop at 4020 feet in elevation you walk briefly east across an adjacent bridge and head south, soon reaching the start of the John Muir Trail. Soon the climb south steepens, and then you turn east and ascend a steep stretch before making a quick drop to the Vernal Fall bridge at 1.0 mile and 4440 feet. From it you see Vernal Fall, backdropped by Mt. Broderick (left) and Liberty Cap (right).

About 200 yards beyond the bridge you come to the start of your loop. Here the Mist Trail continues upriver while the John Muir Trail starts a switchbacking ascent to the right. You'll go up the Mist Trail and down the John Muir Trail.

Dressed for the upcoming mist, which can really soak you in June, start up the Mist Trail. The spray increases as you advance toward the fall, as you climb 300-plus steps to an alcove beneath an ominous overhang. A last set of stairs, protected by a railing, guides hikers to the brink of Vernal Fall at 1.6 miles and 5050 feet. Careless hikers have been swept to their

TAKE THIS TRIP

Mile for mile, this very popular ascent may be the most scenic one in the park. The first part goes up the famous (or infamous) Mist Trail—a steep, strenuous trail that sprays you with Vernal Fall's mist, which cools you on hot afternoons. Above Nevada Fall, climbing is quite minimal, and beyond Little Yosemite Valley and its crowds, the multi-stepped stretch to Merced Lake is lined with dramatic, towering, glacier-smoothed canyon walls. Over much of this distance you are accompanied by the musical sounds, if not the sight, of the Merced River, which alternates between quiet pools and dashing cascades.

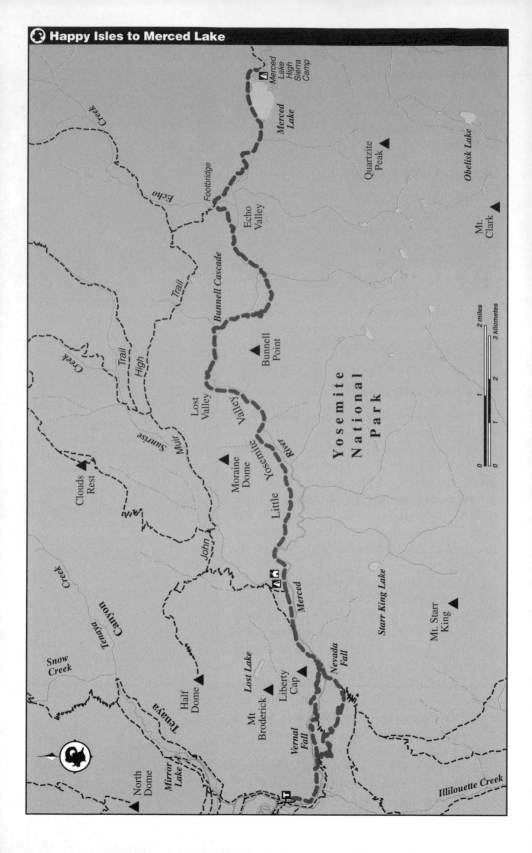

deaths by slipping on slick rock or by swimming just above the brink in Emerald Pool.

Plunging into the upper end of chilly Emerald Pool is churning Silver Apron, and a bridge spanning its narrow gorge is your immediate goal. The trail leaves the pool's far (east) end (near some outhouses) and a nearby junction at 1.7 miles. From it a trail climbs almost a half mile to the John Muir Trail at Clark Point. You, however, curve left over to the Silver Apron bridge at 1.8 miles and 5140 feet.

Vernal Fall and Liberty Cap

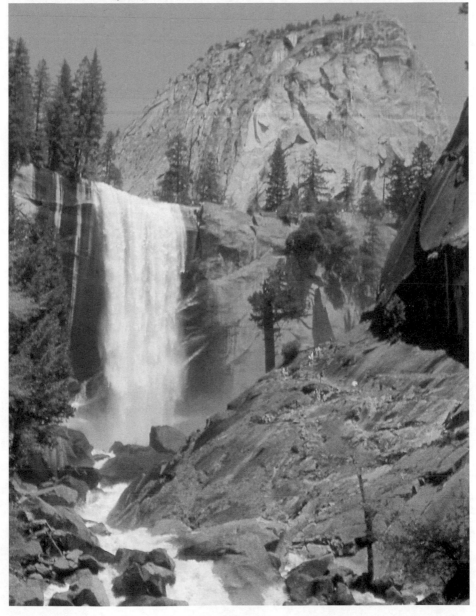

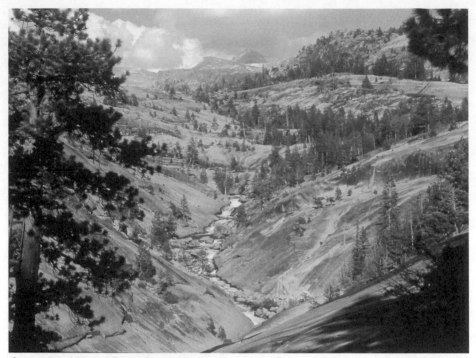

Cascading Merced River, from switchbacks east of Bunnell Point

Beyond it you climb up to a broad bench and then toward Nevada Fall. Soon you commence a series of more than two dozen short switchbacks. The climb ends at the top of a gully where, on brushy slopes, you once again meet the John Muir Trail (there are more outhouses here) at 2.7 miles and 6000 feet.

From this junction you climb up the gully to its top and then quickly descend into forest cover and reach a fairly large swimming hole on the Merced River. Beneath conifers you continue northeast along the river's azalea-lined bank and then quickly encounter a trail fork at 3.3 miles and 6120 feet. Take the right fork, which parallels the Merced River upstream to the Little Yosemite Valley's large backpackers camp at 3.8 miles and 6130 feet, where you spend your first night. It has bearproof food-storage boxes, outhouses, and a spur trail northeast over to a rangers' camp.

The next day, you embark on a shady 2-mile stroll, following the Merced Lake Trail through broad, flat-floored Little Yosemite Valley. The valley's east end is graced by the presence of a beautiful pool at the base of a Merced River cascade. Onward, you climb past the cascade and then head toward the 1900-foot-high Bunnell Point cliff. Rounding the base of a glacier-smoothed dome, unofficially called the Sugar Loaf, you enter shady Lost Valley. At the valley's east end, you switchback up past Bunnell Cascade, where the magnificent canyon scenery can easily distract you from the real danger of this exposed section of trail. Just beyond this heavily glaciated V-shaped gorge, the canyon floor widens a bit, and in this area you reach the first bridge over the Merced River at 8.5 miles.

Your up-canyon walk soon reaches a series of switchbacks that rise 400 feet above the river—a bypass route necessitated by another V-shaped gorge. The climb reaches its zenith amid a spring-fed profuse garden, bordered by aspens, which in midsummer supports a colorful array of various wildflowers. Beyond this glade you soon emerge onto a highly polished bedrock surface. Then you descend back into tree cover before emerging on a bedrock bench above the river's inner gorge. Traversing the bench, you come to a bend in the river and cross the second bridge over the Merced River at 10.4 miles and 6990 feet. Strolling east, you soon reach the west end of spacious Echo Valley, and proceed to its north edge, which has a junction with the Echo Valley/High Trail at 11.2 miles.

Now you immediately bridge Echo Creek, strike southeast through formerly burned, boggy Echo Valley, and climb about 0.75 mile east past some of the Merced River's pools and cascades to the outlet of Merced Lake at 12.6 miles and 7212 feet. Don't camp here, but rather head about 250 yards past the north shore to the spacious Merced Lake backpackers' camp at 13.1 miles. Complete with bearproof food-storage boxes, this is situated about 0.25 mile before the High Sierra camp. Because it's large and at a moderate elevation, nearby 80-foot-deep Merced Lake supports three species of trout: brook, brown, and rainbow.

After your stay at the lake, backtrack 9.3 miles to the junction with the John Muir Trail in Little Yosemite Valley at 22.4 miles and 6130 feet. Then backtrack some more to the junction northeast of Nevada Fall, at the top of the Mist Trail at 23.5 miles and 6000 feet. Rather than descend it, take the John Muir Trail over to the Nevada Fall bridge.

SIDE TRIP: BRINK OF NEVADA FALL

Just a few yards before the Nevada Fall bridge, you can strike northwest to find a short spur trail that drops to a viewpoint beside the fall's brink. This viewpoint's railing is seen from the fall's bridge, thereby giving you an idea where the trail ends. Don't stray along the cliff's edge and, as said earlier, respect the river—people have been swept over this fall too.

From the Nevada Fall bridge, strike southwest shortly to the Glacier Point-Panorama Trail at 23.9 miles and 5950 feet. Now begin a descent to Happy Isles, which starts with a high traverse that provides an ever-changing panorama of domelike Liberty Cap and broad-topped Mt. Broderick—both overridden by glaciers. As you progress west, Half Dome becomes prominent, its hulking mass vying for your attention. Eventually you descend to Clark Point at 25.0 miles and 5481 feet, where you meet a scenic connecting trail that switchbacks down to Emerald Pool.

Backpackers continue down the John Muir Trail, which curves south into a gully, switchbacks down to the base of spreading Panorama Cliff, and then switchbacks down a talus slope. Largely shaded, it reaches a junction with a horse trail to the valley's stables. Continue a brief minute more to a junction with the Mist Trail at 26.2 miles and 4510 feet, turn left, and quickly reach the Vernal Fall bridge, from which you retrace your steps down to Happy Isles.

BUILD-UP AND WIND-DOWN TIPS ·

It is difficult to find camping in or near Yosemite Valley, so plan to drive there on the day you'll start your hike. Wear good hiking shoes. Camping in Little Yosemite Valley, you won't need to carry a bearproof food canister because bearproof storage boxes are provided. Before mid-July when the Mist Trail can drench you, wear shorts and/or bring a lightweight rain parka. After your hike, you might celebrate with pizza and beer at nearby **Curry Village**. Here you can also get showers (towels provided), which are great after a hot day on the trail.

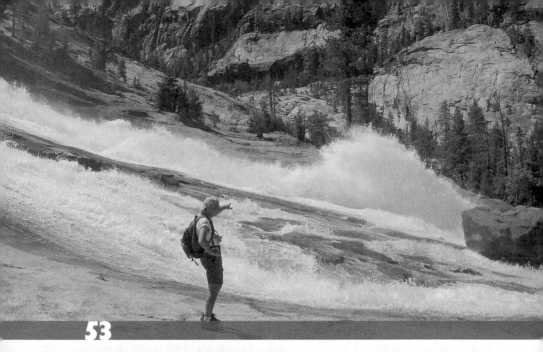

53

GLEN AULIN AND WATERWHEEL FALLS

Jeffrey P. Schaffer

MILES: 18.6
RECOMMENDED DAYS: 3
ELEVATION GAIN/LOSS: 5210´/5210´
TYPE OF TRIP: Out-and-back
DIFFICULTY: Moderate
SOLITUDE: Moderately populated
LOCATION: Yosemite National Park
MAPS: USGS 7.5-min. *Tioga Pass* and *Falls Ridge*
BEST SEASON: Early to midsummer

PERMITS

Pick up a wilderness permit at the Tuolumne Meadows wilderness-permit office by a backpackers' parking lot just east past the base of Lembert Dome. You reach this by taking the Tuolumne Meadows Lodge spur road momentarily south and then branching right into the parking lot. If you are descending from Tioga Pass, drive 6.4 miles southwest to the only left-branching road before reaching Tuolumne Meadows.

For reservations, you can try to call the Yosemite Valley Wilderness Center at 209-372-0740, but the phone lines are often busy and so you may not get through.

Photo: Waterwheel Falls

TAKE THIS TRIP

This popular hike to Glen Aulin is noted for the scenic pools, rapids, cascades, and falls it passes. Because the hike is virtually all downhill, it is ideal for hikers unaccustomed to high elevations. If you are hiking while the river is still swift, which usually is before mid-July, then it is worth your while to descend an additional 3.3 miles to Waterwheel Falls, the westernmost and most unique of the Tuolumne River's five major cascades.

For general information about wilderness permits and the backcountry, call the center at 209-372-0745. You can also reserve a permit online at www.nps.gov/yose/wilderness. A $5 per person nonrefundable processing fee is charged for all reservation requests.

CHALLENGES

Since there can be abundant hordes of mosquitoes before August, be sure to bring a tent and some insect repellent. Bears frequent this area, so be sure to use the bearproof storage boxes.

HOW TO GET THERE

The trailhead is located within eastern Tuolumne Meadows, which can be reached from all of Yosemite National Park's entrances. From the west, enter the park at the Big Oak Flat, Arch Rock (El Portal), or South Entrance (Wawona) entrance stations and drive to the west end of the Tioga Road up at Crane Flat. Take the road 39 miles east to a dirt road in eastern Tuolumne Meadows that starts west from the base of Lembert Dome, this junction located immediately north of the Tuolumne River.

From the east, start up Highway 120, just south of Lee Vining, and drive 12 miles west up to the Tioga Pass Entrance Station, and then continue another 6.8 miles down to the Lembert Dome parking area. (Just south of the river is the Tuolumne Meadows Campground, which is the area's only campground.) Alternatively, from the trailhead parking area, you can drive 0.3 mile west on the dirt road to a gate, from where the main road turns north, bound for the nearby stables; this extra driving saves you 0.3 mile of hiking each way.

TRIP DESCRIPTION

From the Lembert Dome parking area west of the Tioga Road at 8590 feet in elevation, walk west 0.3 mile along a dirt road to its bend north to horse stables, and then continue

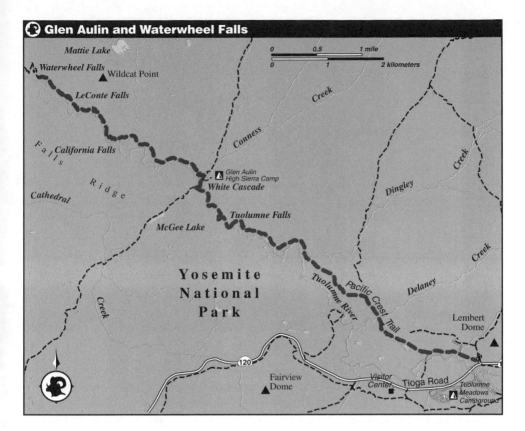

Glen Aulin and Waterwheel Falls

Mattie Lake

Waterwheel Falls
Wildcat Point

LeConte Falls

Creek

Conness

California Falls

Falls

Glen Aulin
High Sierra Camp
White Cascade

Ridge

Cathedral

Tuolumne Falls

McGee Lake

Dingley

Creek

Yosemite
National
Park

Tuolumne River

Pacific Crest Trail

Delaney

Creek

Creek

Lembert
Dome

120

Fairview
Dome

Visitor
Center   Tioga Road

Tuolumne
Meadows
Campground

west on a gated road that offers fine views south toward Unicorn Peak, Cathedral Peak, and some of the knobby Echo Peaks. After about a quarter mile you meet a trail to the stables, and about 200 yards past this junction you face a split. Keep right on the road, slightly uphill, and quickly encounter a trail, which you take to bubbling natural Soda Springs at 0.8 mile. From Soda Springs, you take a westbound, undulating trail, and in just under 1 mile descend to Delaney Creek, reached about 100 yards after a trail from the stables comes in on the right. In early season, look for a log to cross it; later on, boulder hopping will do. After 0.3 mile you reach the northbound Young Lakes Trail at 2.0 miles.

Continue westward on your rambling traverse, and after more winding through scattered lodgepole pines, the trail descends some bare granite slabs and enters a flat-floored forest. A mile's pleasant walking since the last junction brings one to the bank of the Tuolumne River, just before three branches of Dingley Creek, near the west end of the huge meadows. From here, the nearly level trail often runs along the river, and in these stretches by the stream, there are numerous glacier-smoothed granite slabs on which to take a break—or dip if the river's current is slow.

After a mile-long winding traverse, the trail leaves the last slabs to climb briefly up a granite outcrop to get around the river's gorge and then winds down

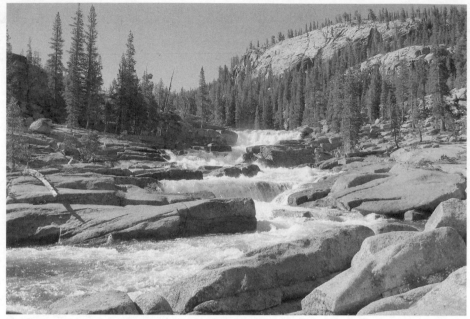

Tuolumne River cascades above White Cascade

eventually to a Tuolumne River bridge at 4.7 miles. As the river soon approaches nearby Tuolumne Falls, it flows down a series of sparkling rapids separated by large pools and wide sheets of water spread out across slightly inclined granite slopes. Beyond this beautiful stretch of river the trail descends, steeply at times, past Tuolumne Falls and White Cascade to a junction with the trail to May Lake at 5.8 miles and 7980 feet. From here it is only a few minutes' walk to Glen Aulin High Sierra Camp at 6.0 miles and 7870 feet, reached by crossing the river on a bridge below roaring White Cascade. During high runoff, you may have to wade just to reach this bridge! From the camp a short trail goes to Glen Aulin backpackers' camp, complete with bearproof food-storage boxes.

If you go no farther than the camp, your overall elevation gain and loss is about 2660 feet, which is similar to the 2550 feet you do when descending to and ascending from Waterwheel Falls. For this stretch, leave your backpack at the camp and dayhike to Waterwheel Falls and back. You begin on the westbound Tuolumne Canyon Trail, found only 15 yards beyond the spur trail across Conness Creek to Glen Aulin High Sierra Camp. This trail leaves the northbound Pacific Crest and Tahoe-Yosemite trails and climbs over a low knoll of metamorphic rock. From it you have an excellent view west down the flat-floored, steep-walled canyon. Leaving the low knoll, you switchback quickly down into Glen Aulin proper, and tread the gravelly flat floor of the glen for more than a mile. Then, on bedrock, you arrive at the brink of cascading California Falls at 7.6 miles and 7760 feet, perched at the base of a towering cliff. Be cautious around these falls and other falls downstream for the bedrock often is polished and slippery, even when dry.

Switchbacking down beside the cascade, you leave behind the glen's thick forest of predominantly lodgepole pines with associated red firs and descend past scattered Jeffrey pines and junipers and through lots of brush. At the base of the cascade you make a gentle descent north, and near the end of this short stretch parallel a long pool, which is a good spot to break for lunch or perhaps take a swim. However, stay away from the pool's outlet, where the Tuolumne River plunges over a brink. The trail parallels this second cascade as it generally descends through brush and open forest. On this descent, notice that red firs have yielded to white firs. Sugar pines also put in their first appearance as you reach the brink of broad LeConte Falls at 8.8 miles and 7100 feet, which cascades down fairly open granite slabs. On a flat-floored section of canyon, you reach the fifth and final cascade, extensive Waterwheel Falls at 9.3 miles and 6700 feet. This cascade gets its name from the curving sprays of water tossed into the air, which occur when the river is flowing with sufficient force. The cascade's classic views are from midway between its brink and its base. You'll probably spot a use trail out to this vicinity. On the slabs the falls descend, use extreme caution even where the rock is dry.

BUILD-UP AND WIND-DOWN TIPS ·

If getting a wilderness permit is stressful, so too is getting a campsite. The Tuolumne Meadows Campground simply cannot handle all who'd like to camp in it—skip camping, drive directly to the trailhead, and start hiking. If you camp at the **Glen Aulin High Sierra Camp** backpacker campground, you can store your food in their bearproof food-storage boxes. You can get food, drinks, and last-minute supplies at the **Tuolumne Meadows store**, just southwest of the campground.

54

HIGH SIERRA CAMPS LOOP, NORTHWEST PART

Jeffrey P. Schaffer

MILES: 17.6
RECOMMENDED DAYS: 3
ELEVATION GAIN/LOSS: 2620´/3000´
TYPE OF TRIP: Point-to-point
DIFFICULTY: Moderate
SOLITUDE: Moderately populated
LOCATION: Yosemite National Park
MAPS: USGS 7.5-min. *Tioga Pass, Falls Ridge,* and *Tenaya Lake*
BEST SEASON: Early to midsummer

PERMITS •

Pick up a wilderness permit at the Tuolumne Meadows wilderness-permit office by a backpackers' parking lot just east past the base of Lembert Dome. You reach this by taking the Tuolumne Meadows Lodge spur road momentarily south and then branch right into the parking lot. If you are descending from Tioga Pass, drive 6.4 miles southwest to the only left-branching road before reaching Tuolumne Meadows.

For reservations, you can phone the Yosemite Valley Wilderness Center at 209-372-0740, but the phone lines are often busy and so you may not get through.

Photo: Tuolumne River, Unicorn Peak, and Cathedral Peak from near Soda Springs

For general information about wilderness permits and the backcountry, call the center at 209-372-0745. You can also reserve a permit online at www.nps.gov/yose/wilderness. A $5 per person nonrefundable processing fee is charged for all reservation requests.

CHALLENGES ·

Since there can be abundant hordes of mosquitoes before August, be sure to bring a tent and insect repellent. Bears frequent the High Sierra Camps, so be sure to use the bear-proof storage boxes.

HOW TO GET THERE · · · · · · · · · · · · · ·

The trailhead is located within eastern Tuolumne Meadows, which can be reached from all of Yosemite National Park's entrances. From the west, enter the park at the Big Oak Flat, Arch Rock (El Portal), or South Entrance (Wawona) entrance stations and drive to the west end of the Tioga Road up at Crane Flat. Take the road 39 miles east to a dirt road in eastern Tuolumne Meadows that starts west from the base of Lembert Dome, this junction located immediately north of the Tuolumne River.

From the east, start up Highway 120, just south of Lee Vining, and drive 12 miles west up to the Tioga Pass Entrance Station, and then continue another 6.8 miles down to the Lembert Dome parking area. (Just south of the river is the Tuolumne Meadows Campground, which is the area's only campground.) Alternatively, from the trailhead parking area, you can drive 0.3 mile west on the dirt road to a gate, from where the main road turns north, bound for the nearby stables; this extra driving saves you 0.3 mile of hiking each way.

The route ends at the Tenaya Lake Trailhead, along the Tioga Road near the lake's southwest shore. It would be best if you park at the Tenaya Lake Trailhead and then take a free shuttle bus to the Tuolumne Meadows Trailhead. During the summer season, these

TAKE THIS TRIP

The High Sierra Camps Loop is very popular, since the 5 backcountry camps are spaced about 6 to 10 miles apart, ideal for most backpackers. The loop is broken into two parts because most hikers don't have six days free, and by being out fewer days, you will have a lighter pack. On your first day, when your pack is heaviest and you are perhaps are not in the best of shape, your hike, thankfully, is very easy.

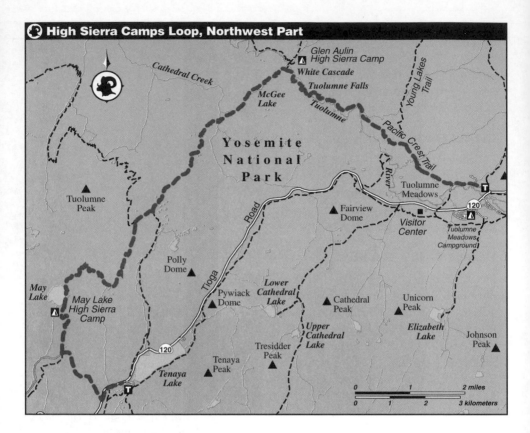

buses run about once an hour, plying between Olmsted Point and Tioga Pass and stopping at all the popular trailheads in-between.

TRIP DESCRIPTION· ·

From the Lembert Dome parking area west of the Tioga Road at 8590 feet walk west 0.3 mile along a dirt road to its bend north to horse stables, and then continue west on a gated road that offers fine views south toward Unicorn Peak, Cathedral Peak, and some of the knobby Echo Peaks. After about a quarter mile you meet a trail to the stables, and about 200 yards past this junction you face a split. Keep right on the road, slightly uphill, and quickly encounter a trail, which you take to bubbling natural Soda Springs 0.8 mile and 8600 feet. From Soda Springs, you take a westbound, undulating trail, and in just under 1 mile descend to Delaney Creek, reached about 100 yards after a trail from the stables comes in on the right. In early season, look for a log to cross it; later on, boulder hopping will do. After 0.3 mile you reach the northbound Young Lakes Trail at 2.0 miles.

Continue westward on your rambling traverse, and after more winding through scattered lodgepole pines, the trail descends some bare granite slabs and enters a flat-floored forest. A mile's pleasant walking since the last junction brings one to the bank of the Tuolumne River, just before three branches of Dingley Creek, near the west end of the huge meadows. From here, the nearly level trail often runs along the river, and in these stretches by the stream, there are numerous glacier-smoothed granite slabs on which to take a break—or dip if the river's current is slow.

After a mile-long winding traverse, the trail leaves the last slabs to climb briefly up a granite outcrop to get around the river's gorge and then winds down eventually to a Tuolumne River bridge at 4.7 miles. As the river soon approaches nearby Tuolumne Falls, it flows down a series of sparkling rapids separated by large pools and wide sheets of water spread out across slightly inclined granite slopes. Beyond this beautiful stretch of river the trail descends, steeply at times, past Tuolumne Falls and White Cascade to a junction with the trail to May Lake at 5.8 miles and 7980 feet. From here it is only a few minutes' walk to Glen Aulin High Sierra Camp at 6.0 miles and 7870 feet, reached by crossing the river on a bridge below roaring White Cascade. During high runoff, you may have to wade just to reach this bridge! From the camp a short trail goes to Glen Aulin backpackers' camp, complete with bearproof food-storage boxes.

The second day's hike is to the May Lake High Sierra Camp. From the junction immediately south of and above Glen Aulin's bridge across the Tuolumne River, you briefly curve northwest through a notch, and then your duff trail ascends gently southwest, soon crossing and recrossing McGee Lake's northeast-flowing outlet, which dries up by late summer. Where the trail levels off, McGee Lake, long, narrow, and bordered on the southwest by a granite cliff, comes into view through the lodgepole trees. In late summer the lake may dwindle to a stale pond. Beyond the lake your trail descends along its southwest-flowing outlet for 0.75 mile, and then you cross it. Soon you have a view northwest through the shallow Cathedral Creek canyon to hulking Falls Ridge, which Cathedral Creek has to detour around in order to join the Tuolumne River. After several minutes you reach Cathedral Creek, which can be a ford in early season but a boulder hop later on. Starting a moderate ascent beyond the creek, you soon reach a stand of tall, healthy red firs, and then, higher on the trail, have a good panorama, which is welcome after 3 miles of walking through moderate and dense forest. In the

May Lake

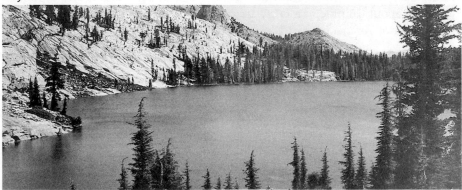

distant northeast stand Sheep Peak, North Peak, and Mt. Conness, while in the near north, Falls Ridge is a mountain of pinkish granite that contrasts with the white and gray granite of the other peaks.

The trail continues up a moderate slope on gravel and granite shelves, through a forest cover of hemlock, red fir, and lodgepole pines. After arriving at a branch of Cathedral Creek, you cross it and then continue for a half mile to a junction with the Murphy Creek Trail at 10.3 miles and 8700 feet, southbound down to Tenaya Lake. Just a half mile from this junction, you reach a junction with the Ten Lakes Trail at 10.9 miles, which climbs slopes beneath the very steep east face of Tuolumne Peak. Here you branch left and ascend briefly to a long, narrow, shallow, forested saddle beyond which large Tenaya Lake is visible in the south. After traversing somewhat open slopes, you momentarily come to a series of switchbacks. Progress up these is distinguished by the striking views of Mt. Conness, Mt. Dana, and the other peaks on the Sierra Crest and Yosemite border. The trail then passes through a little saddle just north of a glacier-smoothed peak, and ahead, suddenly, is another Yosemite landmark and the largest expanse of bare granite in the park, Clouds Rest, rising grandly in the south.

Now the trail descends gradually over fairly open granite to a forested flat and bends west above the north shore of Raisin Lake at 12.6 miles and 8870 feet, which is one of the warmest swimming holes in this area. Ahead, the trail continues beside a streambed and then swings west to cross three seasonal streams. Finally the trail makes a half-mile-long ascent steeply up to May Lake across a slope sparsely dotted with conifers. Views improve constantly, and presently you have a panorama of the peaks on the Sierra Crest from North Peak south to Mt. Gibbs. The Tioga Pass notch is clearly visible. In the west, Mt. Hoffmann dominates. From the top of this climb you swing south at the northeast corner of the lake and parallel its east shore to the May Lake High Sierra Camp at 14.4 miles and 9330 feet. From May Lake's southeast corner, you'll see a trail striking west, which has a backpackers' camp with bearproof food-storage boxes.

From here it's a mere 3.2 miles and virtually all downhill to the trailhead, first on the lake's short trail 1.2 miles south down to the May Lake Trailhead at 15.6 miles and 8846 feet. Here in Snow Flat along the old Tioga Road, you follow the road northeast for a few minutes to where it is blocked off and then descend the closed stretch of road southeast to the Tioga Road. Cross it and parallel it northeast about 0.6 mile to a fairly large trailhead parking area near the southwest corner of Tenaya Lake at 17.6 miles and 8160 feet.

BUILD-UP AND WIND-DOWN TIPS ·

If getting a wilderness permit is stressful, so too is getting a campsite. The Tuolumne Meadows Campground simply cannot handle all who'd like to camp in it—skip camping, drive directly to the trailhead, and start hiking. If you camp at the **Glen Aulin High Sierra Camp** backpacker campground, you can store your food in their bearproof food-storage boxes. You can get food, drinks, and last-minute supplies at the **Tuolumne Meadows store**, just southwest of the campground.

55

HIGH SIERRA CAMPS LOOP, SOUTHEAST PART

Jeffrey P. Schaffer

MILES: 32.5
RECOMMENDED DAYS: 4
ELEVATION GAIN/LOSS: 5930´/5550´
TYPE OF TRIP: Point-to-point
DIFFICULTY: Moderately strenuous
SOLITUDE: Moderately populated
LOCATION: Yosemite National Park
MAPS: USGS 7.5-min. *Tenaya Lake, Merced Peak, Vogelsang Peak,*
and *Tioga Pass*
BEST SEASON: Midsummer

PERMITS •

Pick up a wilderness permit at the Tuolumne Meadows wilderness-permit office by a backpackers' parking lot just east past the base of Lembert Dome. You reach this by taking the Tuolumne Meadows Lodge spur road momentarily south and then branching right into the parking lot. If you are descending from Tioga Pass, drive 6.4 miles southwest to the only left-branching road before reaching Tuolumne Meadows.

Photo: *Polly Dome rising above Tenaya Lake*

TAKE THIS TRIP

The High Sierra Camps
Loop is very popular, since
the 5 backcountry camps
are spaced about 6 to 10
miles apart, ideal for most
backpackers. The loop
is broken into two parts
because most hikers don't
have six days free, and by
being out fewer days, you
will have a lighter pack.
On your first day, when
your pack is heaviest and
you are perhaps are not
in the best of shape, you
have the shortest distance
to hike, just 5.8 miles to
Sunrise High Sierra Camp.

For reservations, you can phone the Yosemite Valley Wilderness Center at 209-372-0740, but the phone lines are often busy and so you may not get through. For general information about wilderness permits and the backcountry, call the center at 209-372-0745. You can also reserve a permit online at www.nps.gov/yose/wilderness. A $5 per person nonrefundable processing fee is charged for all reservation requests.

CHALLENGES

Since there can be abundant hordes of mosquitoes before August, be sure to bring a tent and insect repellent. Bears frequent the High Sierra Camps, so be sure to use the bear-proof storage boxes.

HOW TO GET THERE

The trailhead is located at a parking lot near the southwest corner of Tenaya Lake, which can be reached from all of Yosemite National Park's entrances. From the west, enter the park at the Big Oak Flat, Arch Rock (El Portal), or South Entrance (Wawona) entrance stations and drive to the west end of the Tioga Road up at Crane Flat. Then take the road 30 miles east to Tenaya Lake's trailhead parking lot. From the east, start up Highway 120, just south of Lee Vining, and drive 12 miles west up to the Tioga Pass Entrance Station, another 7 miles down to eastern Tuolumne Meadows near the Tuolumne River, and then 8.5 miles more to the parking lot.

You finish at a large backpackers' parking lot, complete with a small wilderness-permit office. You reach this on the Tioga Road in Tuolumne Meadows just east past the base of Lembert Dome, where you take the Tuolumne Meadows Lodge spur road momentarily south and then branch right into the parking lot. If you are descending from Tioga Pass, drive 6.4 miles southwest to the only left-branching road before reaching Tuolumne Meadows. It would be best if you park here and then take a

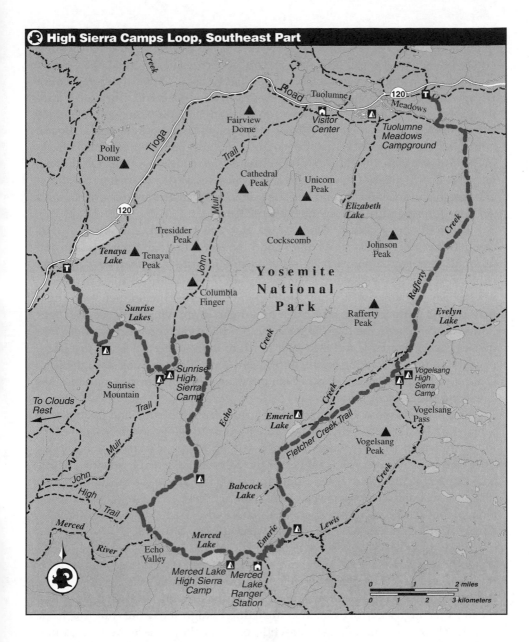

High Sierra Camps Loop, Southeast Part

free shuttle bus to the Tenaya Lake Trailhead. During the summer season, these buses run about once an hour, plying between Olmsted Point and Tioga Pass and stopping at all the popular trailheads in-between.

TRIP DESCRIPTION

From the trailhead parking area near the southwest corner of Tenaya Lake at 8160 feet, take a trail that heads east, and you soon cross the usually flowing outlet of Tenaya Lake. Just beyond this crossing you reach a junction with a trail that makes a loop around the lake. You veer right on a trail that heads south for 0.25 mile along Tenaya Creek. Then over the next 0.5 mile your trail ascends southeast in sparse forest over a little rise and drops to a ford of Mildred Lake's outlet, which, like the other streams, can dry up in late season. Onward the trail undulates, winds generally south, and then begins to climb in earnest through a thinning forest. As your trail rises above Tenaya Canyon, you pass several vantage points from which you can look back upon its polished granite walls, though you never see Tenaya Lake. To the east the canyon is bounded by Tenaya Peak; in the northwest are the cliffs of Mt. Hoffmann and Tuolumne Peak. On shaded, fairly steep switchbacks, you can rest and admire seasonally abundant wildflowers. Finally the switchbacks end and the trail levels as it arrives at a junction on a shallow, forested saddle at 2.9 miles and 9220 feet.

The trail ahead goes to Clouds Rest, but you turn left, and after 0.5 mile reach lower Sunrise Lake at 3.4 miles and 9166 feet. Climbing from this lake and its small campsites, you reach a crest in several minutes and then veer east and climb to upper Sunrise Lake at 4.0 miles and 9477 feet. With 1.8 miles remaining to your day's goal, leave it, climb south up a gully, cross it, and then soon climb up a second gully to the east side of a broad gap, from which you see the Clark Range head-on, piercing the southern sky. From the gap you descend south into denser cover, veer east, and then veer north to make a steep descent to a backpackers' camp. By walking briefly north from it you'll reach Sunrise High Sierra Camp at 5.8 miles and 9320 feet, which offers an inspiring sunrise over Matthes Crest and the Cathedral Range.

You begin the second day's hike by starting from the camp and treading the John Muir Trail 0.8 mile, first east and then north to the Echo Creek Trail at 6.6 miles, on which you will immediately ford Long Meadow's creek on boulders. This trail, which takes you 6.5 miles to the Merced Lake Trail, quickly switchbacks up to the top of a forested ridge, about 200 feet above the meadow. It then descends through a dense forest to a tributary of Echo Creek. Cross this, descend along it for 0.3 mile, recross it, and then momentarily reach the west bank of Echo Creek's Cathedral Fork, about 1.5 miles beyond Long Meadow.

From the trail beside the Cathedral Fork you have fine views of the creek's water gliding down a series of granite slabs, and then the trail veers away from the creek and descends gently above it for more than a mile. On this downgrade the trail crosses Long Meadow Creek, which has found an escape from that meadow through a gap between two small domes high above our trail. The route then levels out in a mile-long flat section of this valley where the wet ground yields wildflowers all summer but also many mosquitoes in the early season. Beyond this flat "park" the trail descends slopes that are more open, and eventually you can see across the valley the steep course of Echo Creek plunging down to its rendezvous with its western Cathedral Fork. By the Cathedral Fork your trail levels off and passes good campsites immediately before you take a bridge over Echo Creek.

Beyond the bridge, your trail leads down the forested valley and easily fords a tributary stream, staying well above the main creek. This pleasant, shaded descent soon becomes more open and steep, and it encounters juniper trees and Jeffrey pines as it drops to another bridge 1.3 miles from the first one. Beyond it, the trail rises slightly and the creek drops precipitously, so that you are soon far above it. Then the sandy tread swings west and diagonals down a brushy slope, with excellent views below of Echo Valley. On this slope you arrive at a junction with the High Trail at 13.1 miles and 7470 feet, which goes 3 miles west to a junction with the John Muir Trail.

Leaving the brush behind, you start southeast and drop 450 feet over 0.7 mile to the Merced Lake Trail junction in Echo Valley at 13.8 miles and 7010 feet. There is adequate camping here, but your goal is only 2.3 miles ahead, so head east, immediately bridging Echo Creek, pass through a burned-but-boggy area, and then climb east past the Merced River's largely unseen, but enjoyable, pools to Merced Lake's west shore. Don't camp here, but rather continue along the north shore for about a half mile and then east a quarter mile beyond it to Merced Lake High Sierra Camp at 16.1 miles and 7220 feet, which has an adjacent campground that you reach just before the camp.

While day three isn't the longest, it easily has the most elevation to gain, about 3150 feet, but your pack is lighter and you should be in better shape. You begin with an easy warm-up by hiking a level mile east to the Merced Lake Ranger Station and an adjacent trail junction at 17.0 miles and 7310 feet. From it you make a sustained climb 1.5 miles northeast up the Lewis Creek Trail to another trail junction at 18.2 miles and 8170 feet.

From the junction you branch left on the Fletcher Creek Trail, descending on short switchbacks to a bridge over Lewis Creek. Just 50 yards past it is a good campsite, and then the trail enters more-open slopes as it climbs moderately on a cobbled path. Just past a tributary 0.5 mile from Lewis Creek, you have fine views of Fletcher Creek chuting and cascading down from the notch at the base of the granite dome before it leaps off a ledge in free fall. At the notch your trail levels off and reaches the Babcock Lake Trail at 19.9 miles and 8890 feet, whose lake for most folks won't be worth the 3-mile round-trip effort.

Onward, the sandy Fletcher Creek Trail ascends steadily through a moderate forest cover, staying just east of Fletcher Creek. After 0.75 mile this route breaks out into the open and begins to rise more steeply via rocky switchbacks. From these you can see nearby the outlet stream of Emeric Lake in the north —though not the lake itself, which is behind a dome just to the right of the outlet's notch.

SIDE TRIP: EMERIC LAKE

If you wish to camp at Emeric Lake—and it's a fine place to do so, leave the trail here for a shortcut to it. First cross Fletcher Creek at a safe spot (do not attempt this in high water!), and then climb along the outlet creek's west side and camp above the lake's northwest shore. The next morning circle the head of the lake and find a trail at the base of the low granite ridge at the northeast corner of the lake. Follow this trail 0.5 mile northeast to a scissors junction in Fletcher Creek valley.

If you don't take the optional route to Emeric Lake, then take the equally long main route, which continues up the Fletcher Creek Trail into a long meadow guarded in the west by a highly polished knoll and presided over in the east by huge Vogelsang Peak. When you come to the scissors junction at 22.1 miles and 9400 feet near Emeric Lake, veer right and hike 2.3 miles northeast up to the Vogelsang High Sierra Camp at 24.4 miles and 10,140 feet. Backpackers use a designated camping area just to the northeast at Fletcher Lake.

Day four, your last day, is the easiest, since almost all of it is downhill or level. You begin by dropping slightly as you traverse 0.8 mile north across slopes to Tuolumne Pass at 25.2 miles and 9990 feet. From it is a large, linear meadow, and descending about 1.5 miles north through it, you have views north to the Sierra crest between Tioga Pass and Mt. Conness and views behind to cliffbound, dark-banded Fletcher Peak and Vogelsang Peak to the right of it. Where you leave the meadow, you have a 3.7-mile descent on the Rafferty Creek Trail. You go a viewless half mile down to a meadow, which is about a half mile long, but the trail stays just within the confines of a lodgepole pine forest. Beyond the meadow the trail descends its namesake creek for about 2.3 viewless miles to a junction with the combined John Muir and Pacific Crest Trail at 30.4 miles and 8720 feet.

Ahead, the route is almost flat. You traverse 0.7 mile west to a junction at 31.1 miles, leave the westbound trail, which goes 1 mile to Tuolumne Meadows Campground, and branch north. In about 70 yards you reach two bridges across branches of the Lyell Fork of the Tuolumne River. The meadows above these bridges are among the most delightful in all the Sierra, and anytime you happen to be staying all night at the lodge or nearby, the bridges are a wonderful place to spend the last hour before dinner, something you might consider for your hike out to your trailhead. Mts. Dana and Gibbs glow on the eastern horizon, catching the late sun, while trout dart along the wide Lyell Fork.

Past the second bridge the combined John Muir and Pacific Crest Trail leads over a slight rise and descends to a trail junction by the Dana Fork at 31.7 miles. Here a trail begins an ascent to the Gaylor Lakes. After a brief walk downstream you cross the Dana Fork on a bridge, and find a spur trail that goes shortly over to Tuolumne Meadows Lodge. You continue downstream 0.3 mile, paralleling the lodge's road, to where you see a large parking lot just across the spur road, but the recommended parking lot is just ahead, by the small wilderness-permit office, which is an additional 0.4 mile and at 8660 feet.

BUILD-UP AND WIND-DOWN TIPS ·

If getting a wilderness permit is stressful, so too is getting a campsite. The Tuolumne Meadows Campground simply cannot handle all who'd like to camp in it—skip camping, drive directly to the trailhead, and start hiking. If you camp at the **Glen Aulin High Sierra Camp** backpacker campground, you can store your food in their bearproof food-storage boxes. You can get food, drinks, and last-minute supplies at the **Tuolumne Meadows store**, just southwest of the campground.

56

TUOLUMNE MEADOWS TO EMERIC LAKE

Jeffrey P. Schaffer

MILES: 21.0
RECOMMENDED DAYS: 2–3
ELEVATION GAIN/LOSS: 2860´/2860´
TYPE OF TRIP: Out-and-back
DIFFICULTY: Moderate
SOLITUDE: Moderate solitude
LOCATION: Yosemite National Park
MAPS: USGS 7.5-min. *Tioga Pass, Vogelsang Peak,* and *Tenaya Lake*
BEST SEASON: Midsummer

PERMITS

Pick up a wilderness permit at the Tuolumne Meadows wilderness-permit office by a backpackers' parking lot just east past the base of Lembert Dome. You reach this by taking the Tuolumne Meadows Lodge spur road momentarily south and then branch right into the parking lot. If you are descending from Tioga Pass, drive 6.4 miles southwest to the only left-branching road before reaching Tuolumne Meadows.

For reservations, you can try to call the Yosemite Valley Wilderness Center at 209-372-0740, but the phone lines are often busy and so you may not get through.

Photo: Emeric Lake

For general information about wilderness permits and the backcountry, call the center at 209-372-0745. You can also reserve a permit online at www.nps.gov/yose/wilderness. A $5 per person nonrefundable processing fee is charged for all reservation requests.

CHALLENGES

If you choose to do this hike in two days, it is a little on the long side. Also, you'll need to carry a bearproof food canister.

HOW TO GET THERE

The trailhead is located in eastern Tuolumne Meadows, which can be reached from all of Yosemite National Park's entrances. From the west, enter the park at the Big Oak Flat, Arch Rock (El Portal), or South Entrance (Wawona) entrance stations and drive to the west end of the Tioga Road up at Crane Flat. Take the road 39 miles east to the base of Lembert Dome, just past the Tuolumne Meadows Campground and immediately north of the Tuolumne River, and continue 0.4 mile east to the Tuolumne Meadows Lodge spur road. From the east, start up Highway 120, just south of Lee Vining, and drive 12 miles up to the Tioga Pass Entrance Station, and then another 6.4 miles down to the spur road. Take the spur road 0.4 mile to a trailhead parking lot on your left; do not use the lodge's parking lot.

TRIP DESCRIPTION

Start on the combined John Muir and Pacific Crest Trail (JMT/PCT) at 8680 feet, which runs beside the Dana Fork of the Tuolumne River just yards south of the Tuolumne Meadows Lodge road. On the trail you hike briefly east up the Dana Fork to a junction with a spur trail at 0.3 mile that goes shortly to the west end of the lodge's parking lot. From this

TAKE THIS TRIP

Simply put, Emeric Lake is one of the best in the Sierra, not so low that it is ringed by trees and lacks views and not so high that it lacks trees that shelter you from occasional summer thunderstorms. Also, by being just off the High Sierra Camps Loop, the lake gets less use than if it were on it.

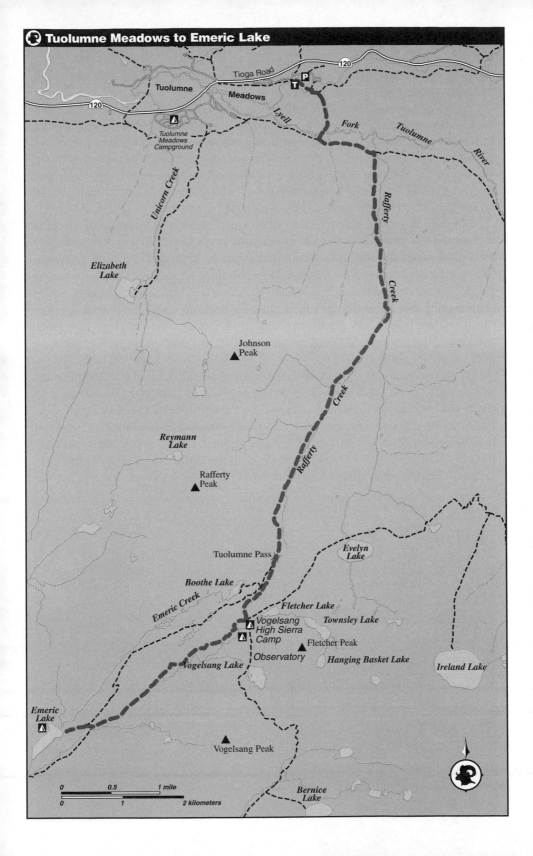

Tioga Road

120

P

T

Tuolumne

Meadows

Lyell

Fork

Tuolumne

River

120

Tuolumne
Meadows
Campground

Unicorn Creek

Rafferty

Creek

Elizabeth
Lake

Johnson
Peak

Creek

Reymann
Lake

Rafferty

Rafferty
Peak

Tuolumne Pass

Evelyn
Lake

Boothe Lake

Emeric Creek

Fletcher Lake

Townsley Lake

Vogelsang
High Sierra
Camp

Fletcher Peak

Ireland Lake

Observatory

Hanging Basket Lake

Vogelsang Lake

Emeric
Lake

Vogelsang Peak

Bernice
Lake

0	0.5	1 mile
0	1	2 kilometers

junction you bridge the Dana Fork and after a momentary walk upstream reach a junction with a trail to the Gaylor Lakes.

Veering right, the JMT/PCT leads over a slight rise and descends to the Lyell Fork, where there are two bridges. About 70 yards past the bridges you meet a trail at 1.0 mile that heads 1 mile west down the river to the Tuolumne Meadows Campground. Your route, the JMT/PCT, turns left (east) and skirts a long, lovely section of the meadow. Going through a dense forest cover of lodgepole pine, the route reaches a junction on the west bank of Rafferty Creek at 1.7 miles, from where the JMT/PCT continues its traverse east.

Your route, the Rafferty Creek Trail, turns right and immediately begins a climb whose grade is moderate as often as it is steep. Fairly well shaded by lodgepole pines, the climb eases well under a mile. Then, as the ascent decreases to a gentle grade, you pass through high, boulder-strewn meadows that offer good views eastward to reddish-brown Mt. Dana and Mt. Gibbs, and gray-white Mammoth Peak. Soon the trail dips close to Rafferty Creek, and after 2 miles of near-creek hiking, the gently climbing trail passes near the edge of a large meadow and continues its long, gentle ascent through a sparse forest of lodgepole pines.

In the next mile you cross several seasonal creeks, and, about 3.5 miles up the Rafferty Creek Trail, reach an even larger meadow. Through this you ascend easily up-canyon, having backward views north to the Sierra crest between Tioga Pass and Mt. Conness and views ahead to cliffbound, dark-banded Fletcher Peak and Vogelsang Peak to the right of it. After about 1.5 miles you reach Tuolumne Pass at 6.9 miles and 9990 feet, a major gap in the Cathedral Range. At the pass some lodgepole pines and a few whitebark pines diminish the force of winds

Clark Range reflected in Emeric Lake

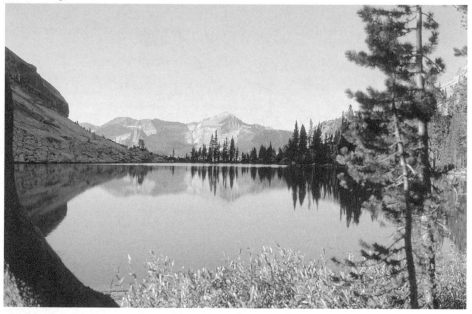

that often sweep through it. If you wanted to swim at any lake in the Vogelsang vicinity, you would take a trail that descends 0.5 mile to Boothe Lake. At 9850 feet elevation, it is the lowest of the lakes near Vogelsang High Sierra Camp. Still, the lake's temperatures are usually in the low 60s at best. Camping is forbidden at this lake.

To reach Vogelsang from the pass, keep to the main trail, which traverses across a moderately steep slope above Boothe Lake and its surrounding meadows. After about 0.8 mile your trail makes a short climb and reaches the tents of Vogelsang High Sierra Camp at 7.7 miles and 10,140 feet. Should you choose to take two days to reach Emeric Lake, you could camp at a designated camping area just to the northeast at Fletcher Lake, using bearproof food-storage boxes.

With Emeric Lake in mind, from the camp you descend 2.3 uneventful miles southwest, most of it along Fletcher Creek, to a scissors junction at 10.0 miles and 9400 feet. The High Sierra Camps Loop continues southwest down along the creek, but you, however, cross it and walk only 0.5 mile to the east shore of Emeric Lake, vaulting a low bedrock ridge between the junction and the lake at 10.5 miles. From about mid-July until early August swimming is quite pleasant, and the lake has granitic slabs that are great for drying off and warming up. To reach the lake's best campsites, traverse the lake's northeast shore and curve over to its northwest shore.

BUILD-UP AND WIND-DOWN TIPS ·

If getting a wilderness permit is stressful, so too is getting a campsite. The Tuolumne Meadows Campground simply cannot handle all who'd like to camp in it—skip camping, drive directly to the trailhead, and start hiking. Even if you start at noon, you should be able to reach Emeric Lake in six hours or less, well before sunset. You can get food, drinks, and last-minute supplies at the **Tuolumne Meadows store**, just southwest of the campground.

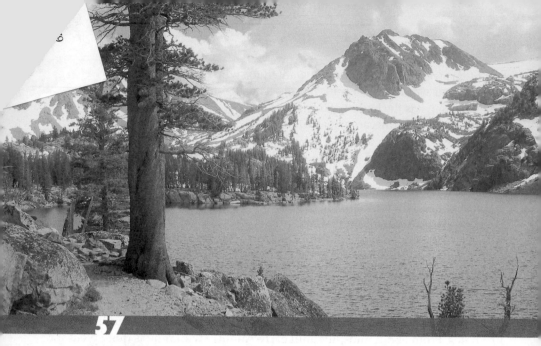

57

VIRGINIA LAKES BASIN TO GREEN CREEK

Jeffrey P. Schaffer

MILES: 11.9
RECOMMENDED DAYS: 2
ELEVATION GAIN/LOSS: 1720´/3550´
TYPE OF TRIP: Point-to-point
DIFFICULTY: Moderate
SOLITUDE: Moderate solitude
LOCATION: Hoover Wilderness, Yosemite National Park
MAP: USGS 7.5-min. *Dunderberg Peak*
BEST SEASON: Midsummer

PERMITS

In person, get your permit at the Bridgeport Ranger Station (760-932-7070); reservations are not necessary. It is on U.S. Highway 395 at the east end of Bridgeport, 1 mile east of the town's Twin Lakes Road junction.

CHALLENGES

Burro Pass and lands just below it lack shelter from the thunderstorms that occasionally hit the Sierra crest in mid- and late afternoon. Below, among trees, you are safe.

Photo: *East Lake and Epidote Peak*

HOW TO GET THERE • • • • • • • • • • • •

From Bridgeport along U.S. Highway 395, drive through the town to the Bridgeport Ranger Station, near its south edge. Continue about 12 miles south on Highway 395 to Conway Summit with its Virginia Lakes Road 021 junction, about 12 miles north of Lee Vining. On this broad, paved road you climb 4.5 miles west to a junction with broad, well-graded Dunderberg Meadow Road 020, which winds 9 miles north to a junction with Green Creek Road 142, the road up to your ending trailhead. Road 142 goes for about 5 miles to an obvious trailhead parking area, on the right, just before Green Creek Campground.

Your hike starts from the Virginia Lakes Trailhead, so from Road 020 you take Road 021 1.6 miles up to a trailhead at road's end, passing the Virginia Lakes Resort (with a cafe) on the left, and then Trumbull Lake Campground on the right. Rather than using two vehicles, consider bringing a mountain bike and hiding it near the ending trailhead, that is, if you think you'll be up to about a 15.5-mile ride back to the starting trailhead.

TRIP DESCRIPTION • • • • • • • • • • • • • • •

From the parking area at 9830 feet in elevation, the Blue Lake Trail traverses briefly west above Big Virginia Lake and then enters a stand of aspens. Soon you turn northeast, and ascend briefly to a junction with a horse trail branching right, east, down to Trumbull Lake and the pack station beyond it. Ahead, your trail quickly passes above two tarns and then reaches the Hoover Wilderness boundary. Here the trail forks, the left branch dropping slightly to 9886-foot Blue Lake. Moments later the two branches merge beside Blue Lake at 0.5 mile, then you veer up from it. At Blue Lake's western headwall your way climbs steeply, reaches an overlook, and then rounds talus to Moat Lake's outlet stream. Now the trail switchbacks southwest up a forested

TAKE THIS TRIP

The road up to the Virginia Lakes basin is paved, and for good reason: It attracts a lot of outdoor enthusiasts (hikers, equestrians, and anglers) because there is much to offer. Hiker options include spending a relatively short time exploring one or more of the Virginia Lakes, or, as in this trip, enjoying a moderate backpack to the Green Creek Trailhead, passing 10 lakes and several ponds along a mostly descending route.

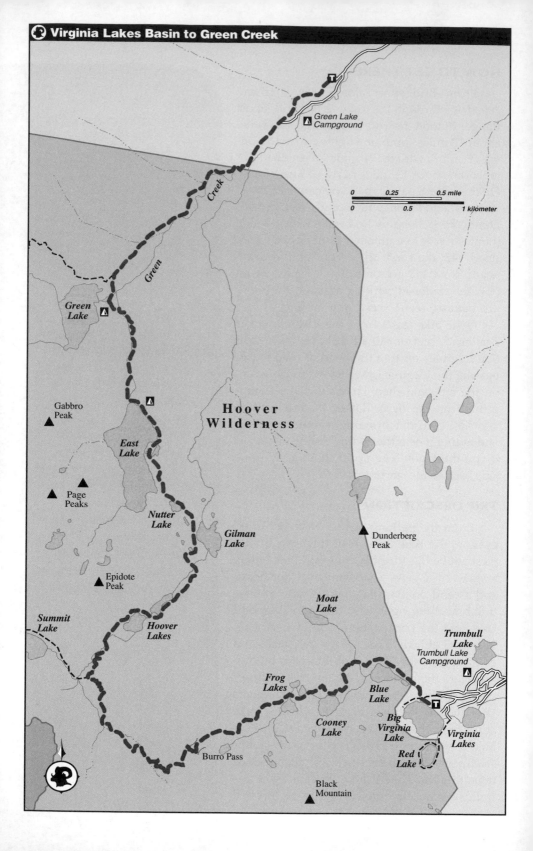

Green Lake
Campground

0   0.25   0.5 mile
0   0.5   1 kilometer

Green Creek

Green
Lake

Gabbro
Peak

**Hoover
Wilderness**

East
Lake

Page
Peaks

Nutter
Lake

Gilman
Lake

Dunderberg
Peak

Epidote
Peak

Moat
Lake

Summit
Lake

Hoover
Lakes

Trumbull
Lake
Trumbull Lake
Campground

Frog
Lakes

Blue
Lake

Cooney
Lake

Big
Virginia
Lake

Virginia
Lakes

Burro Pass

Red
Lake

Black
Mountain

hillside to arrive at the outlet of Cooney Lake at 1.2 miles and 10,070 feet. As you leave the lake, views open to your trip's high point as barren Burro Pass (a local name) saddles the western horizon, its metamorphosed tuffs looking cream-colored against the surrounding, darker, metamorphosed lavas, such as Black Mountain, to the south.

From Cooney Lake you ascend gently west into a rocky-meadowed draw, step across infant Virginia Creek, and find a second, rolling bench, harboring a clutch of small lakelets—the Frog Lakes—named for once numerous mountain yellow-legged frogs. You swing south of the meadowy, lowest Frog Lake—a mosquito haven before mid-August—and then ascend above some lush alpine turf to the highest lake. The next riser on your staircase ascent is steeper than those before and has even less tree cover. Finally, the trail resolves into switchbacks and then leaves the last whitebark pines behind for a true alpine ascent along the west wall of a cirque. Views across the Virginia Lakes basin continue to improve, and then after a burst of switchbacks you gain broad and relatively viewless Burro Pass at 2.8 miles and 11,120 feet. By walking north just a minute from the trail's high point, you can also view the Hoover Lakes at the base of Epidote Peak and, in the northwest, Summit Lake at the base of Camiaca Peak.

From the barren, windswept crest, you initially descend south, momentarily switchback northwest toward Summit Lake, and then take switchbacks down through a small, stark side canyon to a sloping subalpine bench, which gives your knees a rest. After about a 1.5-mile descent from Burro Pass, you arrive at a junction with the Summit Lake Trail, on a small bench at 4.3 miles and 10,100 feet.

From the junction you follow the Green Creek Trail northeast down past a tarn to an excellent overlook down-canyon to the Hoover Lakes, Dunderberg Peak, and light-granitic Kavanaugh Ridge above it. You drop to step north across East Fork Green Creek and then traverse talus above the west shore of upper Hoover Lake before walking along its north shore. At the northeast corner of upper Hoover Lake, you cross its wide rocky outlet stream. Lower Hoover Lake, just above which your trail traverses via talus, has in the past contained trout.

Blue Lake and Virginia Creek canyon

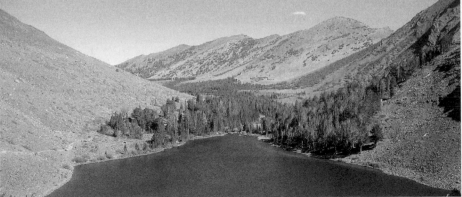

Below that lake, you drop easily over willowed benches and then circle above less-visited Gilman Lake to cross East Fork Green Creek in a stand of hemlocks and whitebark pines. The descent ends and the trail rises gently past outcrops of conglomerate rocks. You pass a short spur trail at 6.0 miles and 9580 feet to Gilman Lake, followed closely by small, green Nutter Lake. A short northwest climb from Nutter Lake on a mat-manzanita patched slope next presents a view of East Lake, largest of the Green Creek Lakes, spread 100 feet below you under Epidote Peak, Page Peaks, and Gabbro Peak. This is a large subalpine lake, fully 0.75 mile long, and the trail parallels its east side for most of its length. From the outlet south to the southeast shore there are scattered, usually small campsites on granite benches shaded mostly by whitebark pines. Finally you reach an extensive camping complex at East Lake's outlet. Fishing for rainbow trout is good here.

Your trail makes the first of three outlet creek crossings just below the lake, and then you descend to a moderate 500-foot drop in a relatively dense conifer forest and then the second crossing. In early season the creek can be swift, and a slip here will send you down its lethal, cascading course. With a more-moderate descent, you reach your third crossing, and soon the trail levels off, and you can branch left, west, toward Green Lake at 8.8 miles and 8940 feet and its adequate campsites. Being deep, the lake can be on the nippy side for some refreshing swimming followed by basking on slabs, but the relatively large volume and chilly temperatures make it ideal for a good-sized trout population. From the lake you have to cross Green Lake's outlet creek; early in the season it can be raging so you'll need to find a log or two to help you cross it. Once you get back on your trail, you make a brief jaunt 0.2 mile to a junction at 9.0 miles with a trail climbing 1.5 miles up to bleak West Lake.

From the junction the Green Creek Trail starts a descent, and you have a great view down the Green Creek canyon. Next, the trail descends through a swath of seasonally luxuriant wildflowers, and by mid-season, the display may be gone, but so will the water flowing down the trail. About 1.2 miles beyond the junction you leave the Hoover Wilderness in a forest dominated by lodgepole pines and aspens and descend a dozen short, rocky switchbacks to another view. You briefly drop for 0.1 mile down to a creek crossing and then make an easier descent 0.25 mile down a road from the Green Creek Campground. Take a trail branching left and pass above the campground to reach, in 0.6 mile, the parking area of the Green Creek Trailhead at 8030 feet.

BUILD-UP AND WIND-DOWN TIPS ·

Virginia Lakes Resort, just before the Virginia Lake Trailhead, has a cafe and small store, although if you are really hungry you'll probably want to eat at one of the establishments down in **Bridgeport**. From the west edge of that town, you could head south about 10 miles up to **Lower Twin Lake,** passing several campgrounds along the way. At the far end of Upper Twin Lake, about 13.5 miles from Bridgeport, is **Mono Village,** a private resort that also has a campground. These photogenic lakes appeal to those who like canoeing, kayaking, rafting, or fishing.

58

KERRICK CANYON AND MATTERHORN CANYON LOOP VIA BARNEY AND PEELER LAKES

Ben Schifrin

MILES: 53.6
RECOMMENDED DAYS: 5–7
ELEVATION GAIN/LOSS: 9300´/9300´
TYPE OF TRIP: Semiloop
DIFFICULTY: Moderately strenuous
SOLITUDE: Moderately populated
LOCATION: Hoover Wilderness and Yosemite National Park
MAPS: USGS 7.5-min. *Twin Lakes, Buckeye Ridge, Matterhorn Peak,* and *Piute Mtn.*
BEST SEASON: Late summer through early fall

PERMITS

Humboldt-Toiyabe National Forest administers the Hoover Wilderness, at the start of this trip. It is easier to get permits from them than from very busy Yosemite National Park. Trailhead quotas are in effect for the Robinson Creek Trail, beginning on the last Friday in June and running through September 15. Half of all permits are available on the first day of your trip from the Bridgeport Ranger

Photo: The Sawtooth Ridge and Mattherhorn Peak

TAKE THIS TRIP

This is Yosemite at its finest: sweeping subalpine vistas, soaring granite peaks, and delightful, trout-filled lakes. From the Robinson Creek Trail, this route leads quickly into breathtaking subalpine terrain around glittering Peeler Lake. After traversing Kerrick Canyon, it follows the Pacific Crest Trail (PCT) to Benson and Smedberg lakes, both of which have good fishing. Halfway through the trip, it arrives at Matterhorn Canyon, the jewel of northern Yosemite, with a dazzling array of smooth cliffs sculpted by glaciers that once passed through this 13-mile trough. The route ascends the entire canyon before passing right under spiky Sawtooth Ridge.

Station (located on U.S. Highway 395, just 0.5 mile south of Bridgeport). The other half can be reserved by mail.

Download a wilderness permit application from the Hoover Wilderness website: www.fs.fed.us/htnf/hoover.htm. You can make reservations beginning January 1, up to three weeks before your trip. A $3 per-person, nonrefundable processing fee is charged. Make checks payable to "USDA-USFS" and send the application and permit to: Bridgeport Ranger Station, HCR 1, Box 1000, Bridgeport, CA 95317. You can also call the ranger station at 760-932-7070.

CHALLENGES ·

Camping is not allowed within 100 feet of Barney Lake, which also has a one-day camping limit.

HOW TO GET THERE · · · · · · · · · · · · · ·

From Highway 395 near the west side of Bridgeport, take paved Twin Lakes Road south 13.6 miles to the Mono Village entrance at the western head of upper Twin Lake. Park within the village for a nominal fee.

TRIP DESCRIPTION · · · · · · · · · · · · · · · ·

Begin in Mono Village, a private resort at the head of upper Twin Lake, and follow signs to the Barney Lake Trail, branching right (west), away from a pretty meadow. Your level path strikes west, staying north of Robinson Creek under a canopy of white fir, Jeffrey pine, Fremont cottonwood, and aspen.

The trail winds gently uphill into more open terrain, and soon, the cobbled, dusty path approaches Robinson Creek, where the canyon—and the vista—open up. Your path continues westward, well above lodgepole pines in beaver-dammed Robinson Creek. Here, the dry surroundings support mule ears and patches of gooseberry. The route passes through an aspen grove and then through

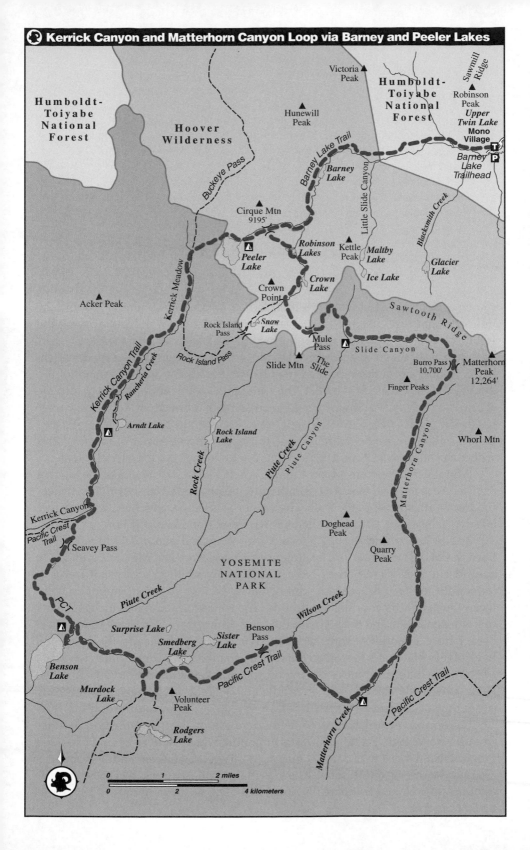

Humboldt-Toiyabe National Forest

Hoover Wilderness

▲ Victoria Peak

Humboldt-Toiyabe National Forest

Sawmill Ridge

▲ Robinson Peak

Upper Twin Lake

Mono Village

▲ Hunewill Peak

Barney Lake Trail

Barney Lake

Little Slide Canyon

🅣🅟 Barney Lake Trailhead

▲ Cirque Mtn 9195'

Robinson Lakes

▲ Kettle Peak

Maltby Lake

Blacksmith Creek

🏕 *Peeler Lake*

Crown Lake

Ice Lake

Glacier Lake

▲ Acker Peak

Crown Point

Kerrick Meadow

Sawtooth Ridge

Kerrick Canyon Trail

Rock Island Pass

Snow Lake

Mule Pass 🏕

Slide Canyon

Burro Pass 10,700'

▲ Matterhorn Peak 12,264'

Rock Island Pass

Rancheria Creek

Slide Mtn ▲

The Slide

▲ Finger Peaks

🏕 Arndt Lake

Rock Island Lake

Rock Creek

Piute Creek

Piute Canyon

Matterhorn Canyon

▲ Whorl Mtn

Kerrick Canyon

Pacific Crest Trail

Seavey Pass

▲ Doghead Peak

▲ Quarry Peak

PCT

Piute Creek

YOSEMITE NATIONAL PARK

Wilson Creek

🏕 *Surprise Lake*

Smedberg Lake

Sister Lake

Benson Pass

Pacific Crest Trail

Benson Lake

Murdock Lake

▲ Volunteer Peak

Pacific Crest Trail

Matterhorn Creek 🏕

Pacific Crest Trail

Rodgers Lake

0   1   2 miles

0   2   4 kilometers

TWIN LAKES

Twin Lakes lie behind curving recessional moraines left by the last ice age. The moraines form bouldery, sagebrush-dotted benches high above the lakes' shores, indicating that the last glacier filled the canyon here to a depth of about 1500 feet.

Summits to the north of Twin Lakes are composed of former volcanic rocks and limestone. They were metamorphosed by the later intrusion of magma from below, which solidified to form the canyon's white walls of Cathedral Peak granodiorite.

more sagebrush and boulders to the Hoover Wilderness boundary, about 2.5 miles from Mono Village. Minutes later, you can stop for a drink at tumbling Robinson Creek—a good rest spot for the climb ahead.

Now gear down to accommodate more than a dozen well-graded switchbacks leading north through head-high brush, but always within earshot of unseen Robinson Creek. Still higher, the trail bends south about halfway into the ascent, and it levels out to for a simple crossing of a branch of Robinson Creek. Just a few yards later, a level use trail branches south to campsites along Barney Lake's outlet stream. Soon after, come to the northwest corner of Barney Lake, where a sandy beach, good after a swim, makes a fine spot for a lunch break.

About 4.5 miles from Mono Village, reach 14-acre Barney Lake, nestled, at 8290 feet, in a narrow, glaciated trough, rimmed on the east by the broken, lichenmottled north spur of Kettle Peak. The western shoreline, which the trail follows, is a dry, talus slope. Cirque-girdled Crown Point dominates the horizon.

Follow the trail along the western shoreline, and about 0.75 mile beyond Barney Lake, come to a ford of Robinson Creek. Pan-size rainbow and brook trout occur here, as in Barney Lake. Climb easily south in a pleasant forest of lodgepole pine, red fir, western white pine, and a new addition: mountain hemlock, which reflects your higher altitude. The trail soon returns to the west bank of Robinson Creek and then crosses the cascading stream from Peeler Lake. Rest here, before ascending a long series of switchbacks just ahead—though you'll have plenty of excuses to stop on the way up to take in the impressive views east of stunted whitebark pines growing on rough, ice-fractured outcrops of Kettle Peak. Eventually come to a small saddle at 9195 feet, which has a trail heading south for Rock Island Pass and Slide Canyon—this is your return route.

Bound for Peeler Lake, continue moderately up, northwest. About 8 miles from Mono Village, Peeler Lake's startling blue waters appear behind car-sized granodiorite blocks that dam its outlet. Many good, conifer-shaded campsites are found along the north shore. The lake margin, mostly rock, has a few stretches of meadowed beach, where it's possible to fly-cast for rainbows and brookies up to 14 inches.

Leaving Peeler Lake near its northwest end, the path climbs slightly to a granitic bench dotted with bonsai-like lodgepole pines and then leads to the Yosemite National Park boundary. Beyond the festoon of signs, you soon reach a junction, from which the Buckeye Pass Trail goes north, and this route, Kerrick Canyon Trail, goes south. Now about 9.25 miles into your trek, head south through Kerrick Meadow, a frost-hummocked expanse of sedge, rice-grass, reed-grass, and dwarf bilberry—quite typical of Sierran subalpine meadows—that covers a vast ground moraine at the head of Rancheria Creek. Numerous young lodgepole pines encroach upon the grassland but die where the soil gets too boggy.

Head down-canyon (south) along the path, which is rutted up to 2 feet deep in the delicate turf, and soon cross the seasonal headwaters of Rancheria Creek. Now descend easily along the west margin of Kerrick Meadow.

About 1.5 miles from the junction with the Buckeye Pass Trail, you descend past at a junction with the Rock Island Pass Trail. Later, emerge at the northern end of an even larger meadow with long views south down upper Kerrick Canyon, topped by Piute Mountain. After another 1.5 miles of rolling, sandy trail, you approach an oxbow in 20-foot-wide Rancheria Creek, where the broad canyon pinches off above a low hill. Here you'll find the north-flowing outlet creek of Arndt Lake. This lake, 0.25 mile south, has good campsites.

STREAM SAFETY: BE A TRIPOD

Northern Yosemite has some of the most treacherous stream crossings in the Sierra. To improve your chances of a safe passage, do the following:

- Wear your shoes, for better footing (stow your socks!).
- Find a long, sturdy stick to use as your "third leg."
- Cross at the *widest* part of the stream. That's where the current will be weakest and the stream will be shallower.
- Face *upstream* and lean onto your stick.
- Proceed slowly, moving only one foot at a time.
- Unclip your pack's hip belt, so you can jettison it quickly should you fall in!

Rancheria Creek's banks become a broken gorge, as you drop down over broken slabs and then traverse shaded slopes to a junction with the PCT. Turn left (south) toward Seavey Pass, and climb sometimes steeply up the PCT into a ravine, over two false summits, and then down southwest to another gap, the real Seavey Pass, at 17.3 miles from the trailhead.

From this point, the path winds down to a large tarn, where vistas are had, over the confusing array of rust-stained cliffs surrounding Piute Creek, to Volunteer Peak on the horizon. The route switchbacks steeply down, and you get a glimpse of the next highlight of your trip, Benson Lake. Finally, reach the valley bottom, a sometimes swampy tangle of willows and bracken ferns, under lodge-pole pines and firs. At the floodplain's south end, some 2.75 miles from Seavey Pass, is the 0.4-mile Benson Lake spur trail, which heads south for a broad, sandy beach. Campsites lie just back from shore. Angling here is for large rainbow and brown trout.

Retracing your steps to the PCT, turn southeast across wide Piute Creek and climb up a brushy saddle. A short distance later, you reach the creek that drains Smedberg Lake, which poses a difficult ford in early summer. Beyond the ford, the path climbs steeply up a rocky slope before two more crossings in a tight canyon walled by tremendous bluffs. Once again south of the stream, tackle a steep hillside. Almost 700 feet higher, but still under the stony gaze of Volunteer Peak, find a trail branching southwest to shallow Murdock Lake, about 0.5 mile away, which has campsites. Continue 0.3 mile east on the PCT to a meadow and junction with a trail heading south to Rodgers Lake, which is even nicer and has campsites as well.

In the next mile to Smedberg Lake, the PCT switchbacks down, then up to a slabby, polished bench overlooking the lake's south shore, 24.8 miles from the trailhead. Named for an army cartographer who, with lieutenants Benson and McClure, mapped the Yosemite backcountry in the early 1900s, 30-acre Smed-berg Lake is dotted with low, grassy islets, and rimmed with strips of sedge-and-bilberry meadow and pockets of conifers. Pan-size rainbow trout are common in its shallow waters, which reflect the brooding vertical profile of Volunteer Peak. Most camps are found on the west and north shores.

Leave Smedberg Lake and begin a climb northeast that becomes steeper as you approach Benson Pass. At the pass (26.7 miles from the trailhead), which is sprinkled with a few whitebark pines and covered with coarse, granitic sand, you can catch your breath while enjoying views to the northeast over Doghead and Quarry peaks to Whorl Mountain.

A steep stretch rapidly leads down to the hop-across ford of Wilson Creek in a steep-walled trough—a classic, glaciated, hanging tributary canyon. Turn-ing down-canyon, the trail crosses Wilson Creek twice more, and soon you be-gin two dozen tight, rocky switchbacks, as Wilson Creek canyon debouches into deeper Matterhorn Canyon. Bottoming out a few minutes later, turn up Matter-horn Canyon and pass a large camping complex, 31.2 miles from the trailhead. It lies just before the wide, cobbled ford of Matterhorn Creek. On the east bank, your trail starts up the canyon, while the PCT continues south.

Leaving the PCT, head north for a 6-mile ascent to Burro Pass, and if you aren't camping near the ford of Matterhorn Canyon creek, do so higher up in the beautiful canyon. At first, the trail climbs imperceptibly. In about 1.5 miles, you enter an open, bouldery stretch, then cross Matterhorn Creek via boulders. You recross the creek at a horseshoe bend.

About 0.75 mile upstream, you ford again to the west side, then wind past rapidly thinning forest patches. Here are a few very nice, remote camps—your last desirable camping opportunities before the pass. Ahead, it's pretty much open going, with Burro Pass clearly in sight. Soon, the cobbled, riprapped trail dissolves into a chaos of eroded, miniature switchbacks leading to Burro Pass, 32.2 miles from the trailhead and at nearly 10,700 feet. From here, a 360-degree panorama unfolds. Aptly named Sawtooth Ridge, to the north, forms a picket line of fractured granite gendarmes, culminating in 12,264-foot Matterhorn Peak. To the east, massive Twin Peaks dwarfs Whorl Mountain, which spawns a text-book rock glacier. Vistas south down the trough of Matterhorn Canyon, stop at the exfoliating slopes of Quarry Peak. On a clear day, you may get a real treat—a view of Yosemite's Clouds Rest and Half Dome, over the east flank of Quarry Peak. Leaving Burro Pass, the trail drops steeply and is often obscured by long-lasting snowfields. Hop across infant Piute Creek, and then follow that raucous stream west on a sometimes steep descent into clustered whitebark pines, which soon become an open forest. Continue down, crossing the creek twice more, to the floor of Slide Canyon (40.1 miles from the trailhead). Truly remote, essentially pristine camping lies along the creek down this canyon—a worthy layover day.

Now the trail begins to head back uphill, and you can look down-canyon to the feature that gave this canyon its name: the Slide.

THE SLIDE

It was first noted by Lieutenant Nathaniel F. McClure, while mapping the Yosemite north country:

After traveling three-and-one-half miles down the canyon, I came to the most wonderful natural object that I ever beheld. A vast granite cliff, two thousand feet in height, had literally tumbled from the bluff on the right-hand side of the stream with such force that it not only made a mighty dam across the canyon, but many large stones had rolled far up the opposite side.

McClure somewhat overestimated Slide Mountain's 1600-foot wall, but he understated the magnitude of the rockfall. About 2.5 million cubic yards fell—some boulders the size of small houses—and the debris cut a swath across Piute Creek about a quarter mile wide and rolled almost 200 vertical feet up the far bank!

After a few switchbacks, you reach the top of Slide Canyon's rim. Here, step across the small stream you've been paralleling, and then ascend more steeply, eventually gaining the 10,460-foot saddle dividing the Piute and Robinson creek drainages. This windy col, about 4 miles beyond Burro Pass, gives views north-east over the head of Little Slide Canyon, guarded by a cliff named the Incredible Hulk.

Leaving Yosemite National Park, the trail first descends a half dozen switch-backs to a small tarn. Then it descends a rocky path of talus blocks through a maze of head-high whitebark pines along the tarn's outlet stream. Soon, the northward path plunges steeply, losing 500 feet of elevation via rocky switchbacks, to a pocket meadow, where you cross to the stream's west bank. Below, trace the sharp western lateral-moraine crest. It descends to upper Robinson Creek, as do you, where, in a sandy, willowed flat, you meet a junction, about 1.5 miles from the col, with the Rock Island Pass Trail.

This route continues down (northeast). Across the stream, 100 yards east, sits a large, pretty tarn—a secluded alternative to camping at sometimes crowded Crown Lake. Below it, descend via gentle switchbacks to the sodden west shore of Crown Lake. At the lake's north outlet (44.7 miles from the trailhead), use trails lead to campsites in grouped whitebarks and hemlocks above the lake's rocky east shore. Anglers will be pleased to find a self-sustaining fishery of rainbow trout.

The next leg of the descent leads steeply down to the two small Robinson Lakes, on a 9200-foot bench under towering Crown Point. Just above the larger, eastern lake, you get nice views north over its shallow waters to Hunewill and Victoria peaks.

Leaving the swampy, grassy western lakelet, climb through a chaos of mammoth talus blocks—the terminal moraine of the Crown Point cirque glacier—and soon reach a sunny gap to meet the Peeler Lake Trail (46.3 miles from the trailhead). From here, turn right (east) to retrace your first day's steps downhill all the way to Mono Village.

SNOW SAFETY: SCREW YOUR SHOES!

Early-summer snowfields are often hard and icy, especially in the morning. Lightweight hiking boots and running shoes don't "bite" into the snow as well as older, heavier vibram-soled boots or crampons. But who wants to carry all that extra weight just to cross a few snow patches? Instead, armor your thin-soled shoes with a few ½-inch sheet-metal screws. They're available at any hardware store and can be mounted with your Swiss Army knife. Two screws each, on the inner edge and outer edge of each shoe, and one in each heel, will give your shoes plenty of grip.

BUILD-UP AND WIND-DOWN TIPS ·

For gratuitous carbo-loading, there is no better place than the **Bridgeport Bakery**, right on Highway 395 in the heart of Mono Village. Get there early for heavenly gooseberry streudel, pecan danish, and their piece de résistance: the most elegant, melt-in-your-mouth cake donut ever to grace this earth.

The definitive cure for trail-pounded feet is a soak in **Buckeye Hot Springs**: From the Bridgeport Bakery, take Twin Lakes Road 7.3 miles back toward Mono Village, and turn right (north) on dirt Buckeye Creek Road. From the trailhead at Mono Village, Buckeye Creek Road is 6.3 miles out.

Once on Buckeye Creek Road, drive 2.75 miles to cross a bridge over Buckeye Creek. On the other side, bear right at a junction with a road that continues up-canyon to Buckeye Campground. Head down-canyon for about 0.2 mile. Stop for the hot springs at an unsigned parking area on the right. There are numerous smaller pools at the rim of the scarp, but be sure to sample the biggest and hottest spring down below, just beside a gravelly bend of Buckeye Creek.

59

COUNTY LINE TRAIL TO SWORD AND LOST LAKES

Jeffrey P. Schaffer

MILES: 6.0
RECOMMENDED DAYS: 2
ELEVATION GAIN/LOSS: 1510´/1510´
TYPE OF TRIP: Out-and-back
DIFFICULTY: Easy
SOLITUDE: Moderately populated
LOCATION: Carson-Iceberg Wilderness, Stanislaus National Forest
MAPS: USGS 7.5-min. *Spicer Meadow Res.*,
U.S. Forest Service *Carson-Iceberg Wilderness*
BEST SEASON: Summer

PERMITS

For overnight stays in Carson-Iceberg Wilderness via Highway 108, contact the Summit Ranger District (Stanislaus National Forest), Star Route 1295, Sonora, CA 95370, 209-965-3434. The office is immediately past the Pinecrest Lake turn-off, some 30 miles above Sonora and about 19 miles before the Clark Fork Road junction. During the summer season, it is open every day from 8 AM to 5 PM.

Photo: Sword Lake

CHALLENGES

Since there can be abundant hordes of mosquitoes before August, be sure to bring a tent and insect repellent.

HOW TO GET THERE

From the junction of Highway 49 and 108 in Sonora, drive about 30 miles northeast up 108 to the Summit Ranger Station, which is immediately past the Pinecrest Lake road. Get a wilderness permit here, and continue 19 miles northeast to the Clark Fork Road junction. Branch left and take it 0.7 mile down to a bridge over Middle Fork Stanislaus River and then 0.2 mile farther to a bridge over the cascading Clark Fork. Immediately past it, branch left onto Road 6N06. Just 0.3 mile up it is a spur road right, which leads into nearby, primitive Fence Creek Campground. Should you stay here, you can get water from the Clark Fork, but do so safely well above its cascades by the Clark Fork bridge. Continue ahead on the main road 6.0 miles to its end, with abundant trailhead parking.

TRIP DESCRIPTION

From the trailhead at 7170 feet, the lesser-used, lakeless McCormick Creek Trail goes right, while your trail goes more or less straight ahead, soon making your only significant ascent, which tops out at a lava outcrop at 0.5 mile and 7580 feet that offers a fair view south toward Donnell Reservoir. From here you could scramble some 1200-plus feet up to the 8796-foot southern summit of the Dardanelles. The oldest, lowest unit of this volcanic formation, rhyolite, erupted 20-plus million years ago, then andesites came next, and finally a huge latite flow, which capped the series 10 million years ago. Streams and glaciers removed most of the volcanic products, exhuming the buried canyons. From the summit you have excellent views of the Stanislaus River drainage, and can identify Sword

TAKE THIS TRIP

Lying barely an hour's walk from the trailhead, Sword and Lost lakes are popular destinations, so to avoid the crowds, visit them during the weekdays. Both lakes, among the warmest in the Sierra Nevada, offer slab benches, some of which are great for high-diving or jumping and all of which are great for sunbathing. From Monday through Thursday you have the lakes almost to yourself, but they can be quite popular from Friday afternoon through Sunday afternoon.

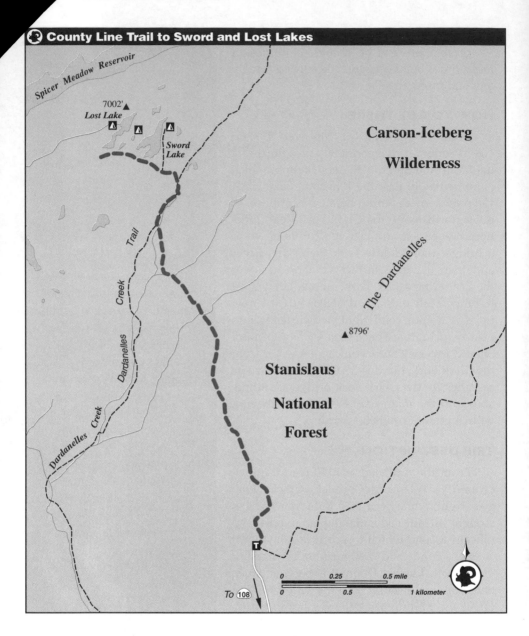

and Lost lakes, which some 20,000 years ago lay under about 1300 feet of glacier ice. Should you climb to this summit, retrace your steps; all other routes are more difficult and dangerous.

From where the trail tops out, it roller-coasters to a nearby broad, open saddle at 0.8 mile and 7420 feet, and your only "major" descent—your only significant ascent out. About midway along it, you cross a 1990s landslide that has exposed some rhyolite that had buried a granitic ridge upon which lies the Dardanelles. Not far beyond this slide and its creeklet you head north down a gully and parallel a low rhyolite cliff for some 200 yards, about 1000 feet below the buried ridge, which means that the eruptions that buried this drainage must have been absolutely stupendous, the kind that cause significant global cooling for a couple of years.

The trail turns west and your descent quickly ends with a crossing of the east branch of Dardanelles Creek at 1.6 miles and 6980 feet, which you parallel momentarily downstream and then cross a trivial gap. A moderate descent ensues, which ends with the crossing of two tributaries of the west branch at 2.0 miles and 6790 feet. You follow the second tributary briefly upstream to a junction with the Dardanelles Creek Trail at 2.2 miles and 6880 feet, and on it have an easy walk a little farther, skirting a seasonal linear pond midway to your final junction at 2.5 miles and 6880 feet and a similar pond. Ahead, a trail goes about 2 miles northeast down to Spicer Meadow Reservoir.

You veer left, make a short climb west up a minor gully, and then start an equally short descent to the south shore of Sword Lake at 2.7 miles and 6859 feet. While there is camping down here, some old sites are closed for rehabitation, so you should consider the lake's east-side campsites, reached from a trail that branches right a few paces along your descent to the lake. To reach Lost Lake,

The Dardanelles rise high above Sword Lake's high-dive rocks.

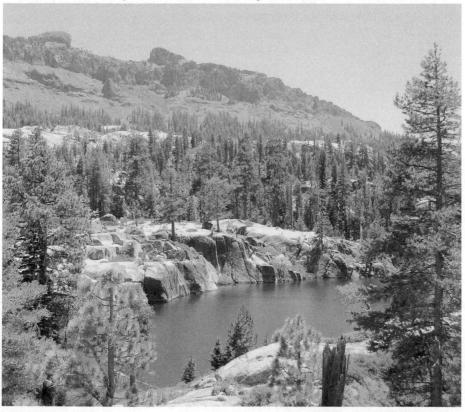

take the main trail to the southwest arm of Sword Lake, and then climb briefly up to a long, sloping granitic slab. Rather than take the trail down, contour across the slab to its end, just above Lost Lake's south shore at 3.0 miles and 6890 feet.

Of the two lakes, Sword Lake is larger and more popular and has more campsites. East-side cliffs offer high diving, up to 25-plus feet, but regardless where you dive or jump from, make sure the water is deep enough first. Linear Lost Lake is smaller and shallower, so it tends to be a few degrees warmer. Most backpackers camp above its east shore, but the west shore also has camping, although it is harder to reach. Above its southwest shore is a conspicuous cliff for jumping or diving some 15-plus feet into the lake. A conspicuous ridge above its west shore provides views of Spicer Meadow Reservoir, which for much of the summer is not full and has an unattractive "bathtub ring" along its shore.

BUILD-UP AND WIND-DOWN TIPS

Your last chance for supplies is a store in **Strawberry**, which is a combination store and inn. After a hot hike, you can bathe in potholes below the Clark Fork bridge, which you can access from the bridge's east side. Take a short trail down to them if the water isn't swift. Then, drive to Pinecrest Lake Road, and take it to the nearby, popular reservoir. For food and drinks, try Pinecrest Lake's **Steam Donkey** restaurant and bar. To avoid weekend crowds, try Highway 108's **Strawberry Inn Restaurant and Bar**, with deck seating above the South Fork Stanislaus River, about 1 mile north of Pinecrest Lake Road.

60

PACIFIC GRADE SUMMIT TO BULL RUN LAKE

Jeffrey P. Schaffer

MILES: 7.6
RECOMMENDED DAYS: 2
ELEVATION GAIN/LOSS: 1970´/1970´
TYPE OF TRIP: Out-and-back
DIFFICULTY: Easy
SOLITUDE: Moderately populated
LOCATION: Carson-Iceberg Wilderness, Stanislaus National Forest
MAPS: USGS 7.5-min. *Pacific Valley* and *Spicer Meadow Res.*,
U.S. Forest Service *Carson-Iceberg Wilderness*
BEST SEASON: Midsummer

PERMITS

For overnight stays in Carson-Iceberg Wilderness via Highway 4, contact the Calaveras Ranger District (Stanislaus National Forest), P.O. Box 500, Hathaway Pines, CA 95232, 209-795-1381. The office is on Highway 4 at Hathaway Pines. You can mail in or call in a permit request, but you have to pick up the permit in person during normal business hours or just outside the office after hours. You can also get a permit at the Alpine Ranger Station on Highway 4 between Bear

Photo: Near-shore island in Bull Run Lake

Valley and Lake Alpine, which is open Thursday through Monday, 8:30 AM to 5 PM, during the summer season.

CHALLENGES

There can be locally abundant hordes of mosquitoes before August so be sure to bring a tent that time of year.

HOW TO GET THERE

From the junction of Highways 49 and 4 in Angels Camp, drive about 56 miles northeast up 4 to the conspicuous Bear Valley entrance. About 1.5 miles farther is the Alpine Ranger Station, on the left. Get a wilderness permit here if you haven't gotten one below. You soon reach Lake Alpine Lodge, beside its namesake, and at the lake's end, at about mile 60, is its east-shore access road, which has three campgrounds. From this road, ascend 5.8 miles northeast up Highway 4 to a small parking area for a picnic ground. This parking area is about 70 yards west of Mosquito Lakes Campground, whose entrance, in turn, is 0.25 mile west of Pacific Grade Summit, which is 7.8 miles west of Ebbetts Pass. For most of the summer there is one Mosquito Lake, but as the water drops later in the season, the lake's two lobes become separate lakes.

TRIP DESCRIPTION

Mosquito Lake lives up to its name through mid-July in average years, and if the mosquitoes are active at the lake, then they will pester you along the trail and at both lakes. From the trailhead at 8050 feet in elevation you arc around the lake's end and start a moderate, diagonal ascent to a broad flat, 250 feet higher than your trailhead. A few paces east, barely above the trail, is a view that offers a sweeping panorama. From northeast to northwest you see Reynolds and Raymond peaks, Jeff Davis Peak and the Nipple, with Freel Peak, due north on the distant skyline

TAKE THIS TRIP

Trout-stocked Bull Run Lake is only a two-hour hike for the average backpacker, and with a mountain backdrop and bedrock island that's an easy swim away, it is a classic subalpine lake. A side trip to smaller Heiser Lake takes only about an hour roundtrip and so is a good destination for novices or those with children. Both lakes are popular destinations—to avoid the crowds, visit them on weekdays.

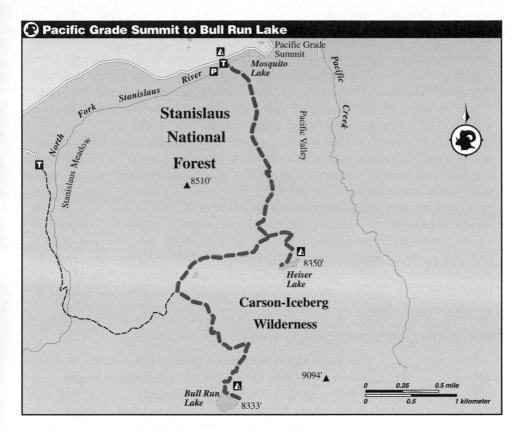

Pacific Grade Summit to Bull Run Lake

between them, and then Round Top. Onward, you make a minor, forested descent to a grassy pond, then after a short climb south you reach an open granitic crest. Next you descend about 200 feet in elevation to a snowmelt creeklet and then make a short ascent to a junction at 1.6 miles.

Your main route goes to Bull Run Lake, but should you wish to visit Heiser Lake, just 0.5 mile away, turn left and head about 0.2 mile up a gentle grade to a switchback, from which you diagonal up to a minor ridge crest, with views, and make a similar descent to nearby 8350-foot Heiser Lake. The best campsites are along its north shore, but others exist along its south shore. The lake is quite shallow at both ends, although its center is about 15 feet deep, good for both trout and swimmers. However, so many dayhikers come here to fish that you may not catch any. Glacial striations in this part of the Sierra indicate that the last glacier through here was just over 1000 feet thick, having flowed west across Pacific Valley and onward across other canyons without modifying them.

Bound for more-scenic Bull Run Lake, at the junction with the Heiser Lake turnoff turn right and traverse briefly southwest before making a plunge that eases after about 300 feet of elevation loss. You then have an easy, half-mile creekside stroll to a second junction at 2.5 miles and 7860 feet. An alternate, lakeless route, starting from Stanislaus Meadow, arrives here. Ahead, you quickly cross Heiser Lake's seasonal creek and then stroll southeast for one-third mile to face a 500-plus-foot, three-stage ascent south. The first stage diagonals south up across several creeklets, and then the second stage proceeds usually steeply from slab to granitic slab. Finally you reach a snowmelt pond and commence your final climb, also convoluted, but with a moderate grade. After another one-third mile of progress you crest a granitic slab and almost fall into Bull Run Lake at 3.8 miles and 8333 feet. After the taxing climb, that isn't a bad idea.

Bull Run Lake offers brisk swimming, usually in the mid-60s in midsummer, and you may find the lake's rock-slab island a tempting goal for a bit of sunbathing. Lying about 50 yards from the shore, this island is an easy swim. Anglers go after brook trout, planted since at least 1950 in this 30-foot-deep lake. The best campsites are along the lake's northeast shore, although isolated ones lie just beyond a large meadow bordering the lake's southeast shore—all of them provide a base camp for further exploration of the area. From the lake, you can climb a half mile south up granitic slopes to a saddle and then angle east up a gully to another saddle, this one separating Peak 9352 to the south from Peak 9413. The latter offers better, panoramic views, including dark, volcanic Bull Run Peak, almost due east of it.

BUILD-UP AND WIND-DOWN TIPS ·

For many people, the **Lake Alpine Recreation Area** is a destination in itself, with folks staying in its campgrounds or in cabins at **Lake Alpine Resort**. You may wish to stop there to buy food or drinks at its store or at its restaurant and bar, and sit on the deck just above Lake Alpine. This island-dotted reservoir is relatively warm, making it great for swimming and sunbathing. Be aware that it is so popular on weekends that you may have trouble finding a parking space.

Bull Run Lake

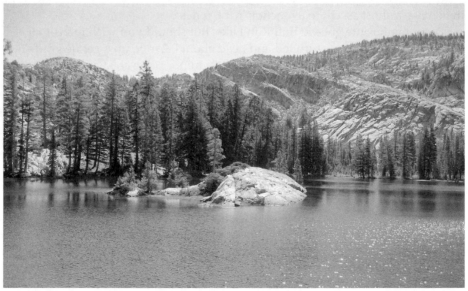

61

GLEN ALPINE TO HALF MOON LAKE

Mike White

MILES: 10.0
RECOMMENDED DAYS: 2
ELEVATION GAIN/LOSS: 1480´/1480´
TYPE OF TRIP: Point-to-point
DIFFICULTY: Easy
SOLITUDE: Moderately populated
LOCATION: Desolation Wilderness
MAPS: USGS 7.5-min. *Emerald Bay*, *Echo Lake*, and *Rockbound Valley*;
　　　　U.S. Forest Service *A Guide to the Desolation Wilderness*
BEST SEASON: Summer through early fall

PERMITS •

Both backpackers and dayhikers must obtain a wilderness permit for entry into Desolation Wilderness. Dayhiking permits are free and may be obtained at Taylor Creek Visitor Center, Pacific Ranger Station in Pollock Pines, or Lake Tahoe Basin Management Unit in South Lake, or by self-issue at the trailhead.

A zone quota system is in effect for overnight visitors, with half of the quota available by advanced reservation beginning the third Thursday in April, and half available on a first-come, first-served basis. Each reservation is subject to a

Photo: The Desolation crest from the trail to Half Moon Lake

TAKE THIS TRIP

As one of the most heavily used wildernesses in the West, Desolation Wilderness can be a difficult nut to crack when searching for some solitude and serenity. Since Half Moon Lake lies off the beaten track at the head of a dead-end cirque and the trailhead quota is a mere 5 backpackers per day, overnighters can expect at least a modicum of elbow room and some peace and quiet while enjoying the fine scenery. The lake is an excellent base camp for setting out on adventures to some of the surrounding points of interest, including 9735-foot Mt. Tallac and the incomparable view of the Tahoe basin from its 9735-foot summit.

$5 fee. Overnight wilderness permits cost $5 per person for one night and $10 per person for two or more nights. The cost of a single permit will not exceed $100. (Group size is limited to 12 individuals, and children under 12 are free).

Advanced reservations can be made with a credit card by calling 530-647-5415 or with a credit card, check, or money order by mail to Pacific Ranger Station, 7887 Highway 50, Pollock Pines, CA 95726. First-come, first-served permits may be obtained at the U.S. Forest Service facilities listed above. The quota for Half Moon Lake is 5 backpackers per day, resulting in fierce competition for permits, especially on weekends.

CHALLENGES

Campfires are not allowed in Desolation Wilderness. Bears are active throughout Desolation Wilderness, and so hikers must observe proper food storage guidelines at all times. While bear canisters are not required, they are highly recommended.

HOW TO GET THERE

On the west side of Lake Tahoe, follow Highway 89 to Fallen Leaf Road (3 miles northwest of the Y-junction with Highway 50) and drive south to the far end of Fallen Leaf Lake. Turn left at a junction for Glen Alpine and follow the narrow road 0.5 mile to the trailhead parking area just beyond a bridge over Glen Alpine Creek. The trailhead has vault toilets. Plan to arrive early on weekends, as the small parking lot fills up rather quickly.

TRIP DESCRIPTION

From the trailhead, follow a closed gravel road past unseen Lily Lake to your right, obscured by a floral barrier of tall willows, and then proceed past a number of summer cabins to pause near a scenic cascade on Glen Alpine Creek. Beyond the watery splendor,

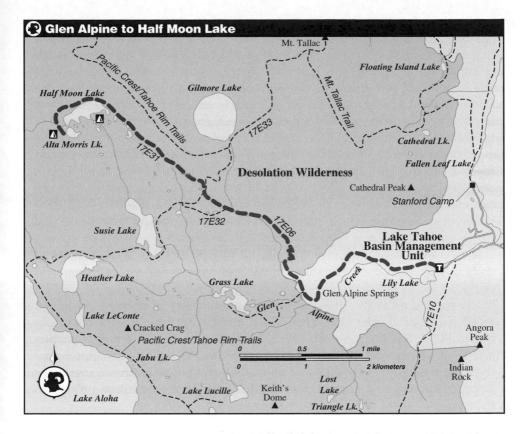

Glen Alpine to Half Moon Lake

Mt. Tallac

Floating Island Lake

Half Moon Lake

Gilmore Lake

Pacific Crest/Tahoe Rim Trails

Mt. Tallac Trail

Alta Morris Lk.

17E33

17E31

Cathedral Lk.

Fallen Leaf Lake

Desolation Wilderness

Cathedral Peak ▲

Stanford Camp

Susie Lake

17E32

17E06

Lake Tahoe Basin Management Unit

Heather Lake

Grass Lake

Creek

Lily Lake

Glen Alpine Springs

Lake LeConte

Glen

Alpine

17E10

▲ Cracked Crag

Angora Peak

Pacific Crest/Tahoe Rim Trails

0   0.5   1 mile

Jabu Lk.

0   1   2 kilometers

▲ Indian Rock

Lost Lake

Lake Aloha

Lake Lucille

Keith's Dome ▲

Triangle Lk.

you continue up the rocky road that is steep in places to Glen Alpine Springs, site of a former resort established by Nathan Gilmore in the late 1800s. The area has undergone some restoration recently, and docents provide informative tours on summer weekends. Beyond the springs, you proceed on single-track trail through mixed forest and open, shrub-covered slopes with fine views of the surrounding peaks and ridges. Pass into Desolation Wilderness and shortly reach a junction with the trail to Grass Lake.

Veer right at the Grass Lake junction and make an extended, switchbacking climb across open, granite slopes up the narrow canyon of the outlet from Gilmore Lake. Returning to forest cover, you hop over an alder-lined rivulet and continue climbing to ford the outlet and soon reach a junction with Trail 17E32, a shortcut to the combined Pacific Crest and Tahoe Rim trails (PCT/TRT), as well as the nearby destinations of Susie and Heather lakes.

Turn right and continue northwest through a scattered, mixed forest of lodgepole pines, western white pines, and firs, as lupine and paintbrush line the path through midseason. Emerge from the forest to cross an open, shrub-covered hillside and then pass a pond covered with lily pads on the way to a junction with the PCT/TRT. From this junction, the PCT/TRT heads southbound to Susie Lake and northbound to a junction with a short lateral to Gilmore Lake.

Leaving the PCT/TRT behind, you veer left at the junction and continue climbing, initially through shady forest with a lush understory but eventually back onto open, chaparral-covered slopes, where pinemat manzanita is the dominant shrub. Mildly rising trail leads back into the trees, which now includes a few mountain hemlocks. The forest becomes more scattered as you pass the first of several ponds and tarns on the way to Half Moon Lake. If you want to camp here, look for good sites between the tarns and the southeast shore of the lake. Approaching Half Moon Lake, the trail breaks out onto a wildflower- and willow-covered slope above the northeast shore and then wraps around the crescent-shaped lake to Alta Morris Lake. Located near Half Moon Lake's southeast tip, Alta Morris offers more secluded camping opportunities. The two lakes repose majestically within the largest and deepest cirque within Desolation Wilderness. Towered over by the dark summits of Dicks and Jacks peaks, the cirque wall tops out near 1300 feet. From early to midseason, snowmelt streams cascade down the cirque face and plunge into the placid lakes, creating quite an enjoyable display. Later in the summer, the chilly waters warm up just enough to provide a refreshing swim.

Layover days at the lake can be spent on a variety of pursuits. Susie and Heather lakes, and Lake Aloha are well within striking distance along the southbound PCT/TRT. To climb Mt. Tallac, retrace your steps back to the junction and head northbound on the PCT/TRT on a climb to a junction with the trail to Gilmore Lake. Pass the lake and then climb continuously up the southwest slopes of the peak to a junction with the Mt. Tallac Trail. From there, proceed to the top.

BUILD-UP AND WIND-DOWN TIPS ·

South Lake Tahoe offers a plethora of alternatives for food, drinks, lodging, and entertainment. **Camp Richardson**, on Highway 89 just south of the Fallen Leaf Road intersection, offers a number of ways to satisfy your palate after your trip. **The Ice Cream Parlor** is the place to enjoy "the best ice cream cones in Lake Tahoe." Across the street, you can grab a fresh, made-to-order deli sandwich from the **General Store**. On the scenic lakeshore, the **Beacon Bar & Grill** (530-541-0630) offers fine dining in a casual atmosphere. Be forewarned that, during the height of the summer tourist season, you may have to work as hard to get into these establishments on a weekend as you did obtaining a wilderness permit for your trip.

62

VELMA, FONTANILLIS, AND DICKS LAKES

Mike White

> **MILES:** 11.5
> **RECOMMENDED DAYS:** 2
> **ELEVATION GAIN/LOSS:** 2300´/2300´
> **TYPE OF TRIP:** Out-and-back
> **DIFFICULTY:** Moderate
> **SOLITUDE:** Moderately populated
> **LOCATION:** Desolation Wilderness
> **MAPS:** USGS 7.5-min. *Emerald Bay* and *Rockbound Valley*;
>   U.S. Forest Service *A Guide to the Desolation Wilderness*
> **BEST SEASON:** Summer through early fall

PERMITS •

Both dayhikers and backpackers must obtain a wilderness permit for entry into Desolation Wilderness. Dayhiking permits are free and may be obtained at Taylor Creek Visitor Center, Pacific Ranger Station in Pollock Pines, or Lake Tahoe Basin Management Unit in South Lake, or by self-issue at the trailhead.

A zone quota system is in effect for overnight visitors, with half of the quota available by advanced reservation beginning the third Thursday in April, and half available on a first-come, first-served basis. Each reservation is subject to a

Photo: A glorious view of Lake Tahoe and Emerald Bay from the trail to Velma Lakes

$5 fee. Overnight wilderness permits cost $5 per person for one night and $10 per person for two or more nights. The cost of a single permit will not exceed $100. (Group size is limited to 12 individuals, and children under 12 are free).

Advanced reservations can be made with a credit card by calling 530-647-5415 or with a credit card, check, or money order by mail to Pacific Ranger Station, 7887 Highway 50, Pollock Pines, CA 95726. First-come, first-served permits may be obtained at the U.S. Forest Service facilities listed above.

CHALLENGES

Campfires are not allowed in Desolation Wilderness. Bears are active throughout Desolation Wilderness, and so you must observe proper food storage guidelines at all times. While bear canisters are not required, they are highly recommended.

HOW TO GET THERE

Follow Highway 89 along the west side of Lake Tahoe to Emerald Bay to the road to the Bayview Trailhead, about 7.5 miles north of the Y-junction with Highway 50 and 19.5 miles south of Tahoe City. Proceed 0.2 mile to the parking area at the end of the road.

TRIP DESCRIPTION

Immediately beyond the trailhead, you turn right at a junction with the trail on the left to Cascade Falls and begin a stiff, breath-stealing ascent that switchbacks up the hillside through mixed forest. Beyond the wilderness boundary, the ascent continues along the crest of a ridge, where the forest parts just enough to allow fine views of Emerald Bay and deep blue Lake Tahoe. Leaving the ridge, the trail follows the alder-lined outlet of Granite Lake on a gentler ascent through ferns, wildflowers, and shrubs to the lake. The trail remains well above the lake, with use trails descending

TAKE THIS TRIP

The sparkling granite and lake-dotted terrain for which Desolation Wilderness is famous is represented well on this semiloop trip past four cirque-bound lakes below 9974-foot Dicks Peak. Although it makes for a fine weekend backpack, extra layover days give you plenty of time to explore the area or simply to languish along the lakeshore while enjoying the splendid scenery.

This trip can be done as a dayhike by hikers in reasonable condition. Past the cirque of Dicks Lake, you could follow the Eagle Lake Trail to the Eagle Falls Trailhead. However, such a route would necessitate arranging for the short shuttle between trailheads.

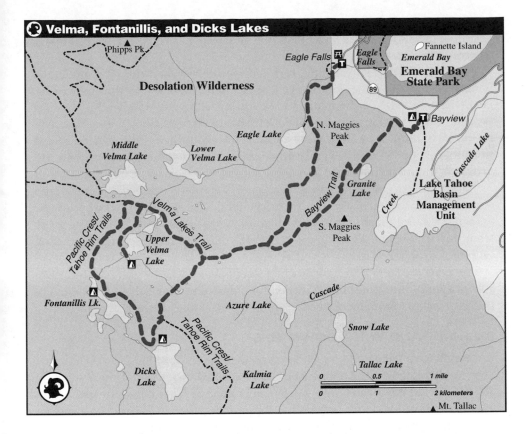

Velma, Fontanillis, and Dicks Lakes

steeply to the shoreline. Near the far end of the lake, the path switchbacks numerous times up the south-facing slope beneath the twin summits of Maggies Peaks, taking you out of the basin and around the backside of the south peak on more pleasantly graded trail. A gentle descent then leads to a saddle and a junction with the Eagle Lake Trail.

Veer right at the junction and follow sandy tread on a mildly undulating route through widely scattered, mixed forest and around granite boulders and slabs to a junction with the Velma Lakes Trail.

Bear right and proceed on a downhill course amid acres of granite slabs, boulders, and rocks, interspersed with widely scattered pines. The descent bottoms out along the north shore of the unnamed pond northeast of Upper Velma Lake known to some as Velma's Chum. Just after a ford of the outlet, you reach a junction with the lateral to Upper Velma Lake.

Turn left (south) and follow the lateral through forest and granite slabs to the west shore of picturesque Upper Velma Lake and good campsites at 4.6 miles near the cascading stream spilling down granite slopes below Fontanillis Lake.

Retrace your steps to the junction and proceed a short distance west to a junction of the combined Pacific Crest and Tahoe Rim trails (PCT/TRT). If you plan to visit or camp at Middle Velma Lake, head north from the junction on a short and easy cross-country ramble down to the south shore. Surrounded by granite slabs, this popular lake offers fine swimming, sunbathing, and camping opportunities.

From the PCT/TRT junction, turn left (southwest) and follow a moderate, winding climb across the slope above Upper Velma Lake. Where the grade eases, Dicks Pass and slender Fontanillis Lake spring into view, followed by a short descent to the crossing of the lake's outlet. The trail travels along the east shore of the lake's multihued basin in the shadow of towering Dicks Peak. Due to a location along a popular trail, several campsites are spread around the shore beneath groves of mountain hemlocks and lodgepole pines.

From the far end of Fontanillis Lake, a brief ascent across boulder-covered slopes leads to the top of a rise and a short lateral to Dicks Lake, where backpackers will find additional campsites with good views of Dicks Peak. Bending away from the cirque of Dicks Lake, the PCT/TRT makes a mild ascent to a junction with the Eagle Lake Trail.

Leaving the PCT/TRT, you descend steeply before gently graded tread leads across a pond-dotted basin to a junction with the Velma Lakes Trail at the close of the loop section. From there, retrace your steps 2.7 miles to the trailhead.

BUILD-UP AND WIND-DOWN TIPS· ·

South Lake Tahoe offers a plethora of alternatives for food, drinks, lodging, and entertainment. The **Cantina Bar & Grill**, located just north of the Y-junction at 765 Emerald Bay Road (Highway 89), opened in 1977 and has repeatedly won awards for best Mexican restaurant and best margaritas in Tahoe. For more details, visit www.cantinatahoe.com or call them at 530-544-1233.

Fontanillis Lake backdropped by Dicks Peak

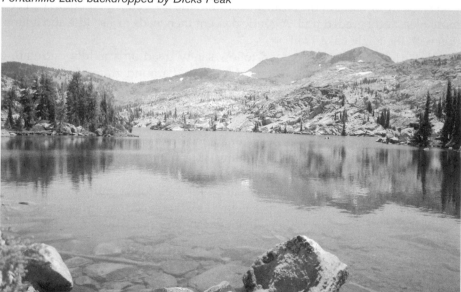

63

MEEKS BAY TO EMERALD BAY

Mike White

MILES: 17.8
RECOMMENDED DAYS: 2
ELEVATION GAIN/LOSS: 3690´/3350´
TYPE OF TRIP: Point-to-point
DIFFICULTY: Moderate
SOLITUDE: Moderately populated
LOCATION: Desolation Wilderness
MAPS: USGS 7.5-min. *Emerald Bay*, *Homewood*, and *Rockbound Valley*;
U.S. Forest Service *A Guide to the Desolation Wilderness*
BEST SEASON: Summer through early fall

PERMITS

Both backpackers and dayhikers must obtain a wilderness permit for entry into Desolation Wilderness. Dayhiking permits are free and may be obtained at Taylor Creek Visitor Center, Pacific Ranger Station in Pollock Pines, or Lake Tahoe Basin Management Unit in South Lake, or by self-issue at the trailhead.

A zone quota system is in effect for overnight visitors, with half of the quota available by advanced reservation beginning the third Thursday in April, and half available on a first-come, first-served basis. Each reservation is subject to a $5 fee. Overnight wilderness permits cost $5 per person for one night and $10

Photo: A fine view from the Tahoe-Yosemite Trail

per person for two or more nights. The cost of a single permit will not exceed $100. (Group size is limited to 12 individuals, and children under 12 are free).

Advanced reservations can be made with a credit card by calling 530-647-5415 or with a credit card, check, or money order by mail to Pacific Ranger Station, 7887 Highway 50, Pollock Pines, CA 95726. First-come, first-served permits may be obtained at the U.S. Forest Service facilities listed above.

CHALLENGES ·

Campfires are not allowed in Desolation Wilderness. Bears are active throughout Desolation Wilderness, and so you must observe proper food storage guidelines at all times. While bear canisters are not required, they are highly recommended.

HOW TO GET THERE · · · · · · · · · · · · · · ·

Parking is at a premium at the Eagle Falls Picnic Area and Trailhead all summer long, so plan to arrive early if you want to leave a vehicle there. The U.S. Forest Service charges a $3 per day parking fee. By riding the free Emerald Bay Shuttle between the Eagle Falls and Meeks Bay trailheads you can avoid paying the fee and drive only one vehicle. (For information about the shuttle, visit www.laketahoetransit.com or call 775-323-3727.)

Meeks Bay Trailhead: Follow Highway 89 along the west side of Lake Tahoe to a closed road 0.1 mile north of Meeks Bay Campground, about 16.5 miles north of the Y-junction with Highway 50 and 11 miles south of Tahoe City. Park your vehicle on the west shoulder of the highway.

Trailhead at Eagle Falls Picnic Area: Follow Highway 89 to the Eagle Falls Picnic Area near Emerald Bay, about 9 miles north of the Y-junction with Highway 50 and 19 miles south of Tahoe City. A limited amount of free parking is available along the highway near the entrance to the picnic area and trailhead.

TAKE THIS TRIP

Beginning near Meeks Bay, this trip into Desolation Wilderness follows 13-plus miles of the northernmost section of the 186-mile Tahoe-Yosemite Trail, visiting the string of lakes known as the Tallant Lakes and then the Velma Lakes before passing by ever-popular Eagle Lake on the way to an exit at the Eagle Falls Trailhead near Emerald Bay. Swimmers, sunbathers, and anglers will find plenty of diversions along the way.

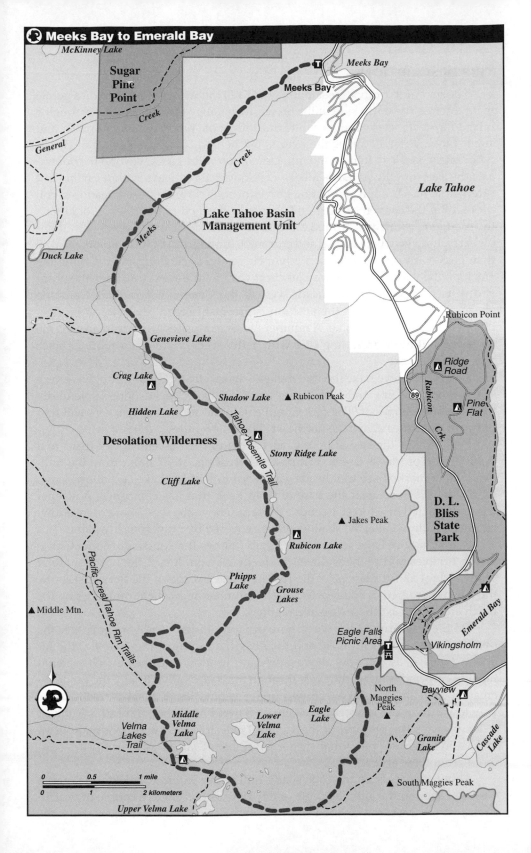

McKinney Lake

Sugar Pine Point

Meeks Bay

Meeks Bay

Creek

Lake Tahoe

General

Creek

Duck Lake

Meeks

Lake Tahoe Basin Management Unit

Rubicon Point

Genevieve Lake

Crag Lake

Shadow Lake ▲ Rubicon Peak

Hidden Lake

Desolation Wilderness

Tahoe-Yosemite Trail

Stony Ridge Lake

Ridge Road

89

Rubicon Crk.

Pine Flat

Cliff Lake

▲ Jakes Peak

D. L. Bliss State Park

Rubicon Lake

Pacific Crest/Tahoe Rim Trails

Phipps Lake

Grouse Lakes

▲ Middle Mtn.

Emerald Bay

Eagle Falls Picnic Area

Vikingsholm

North Maggies Peak ▲

Bayview

Middle Velma Lake

Lower Velma Lake

Eagle Lake

Velma Lakes Trail

Granite Lake

Cascade Lake

0   0.5   1 mile

0   1   2 kilometers

▲ South Maggies Peak

Upper Velma Lake

TRIP DESCRIPTION

The start of the Tahoe-Yosemite Trail (TYT) follows a closed road on a gentle incline across the north side of the broad, lush valley of Meeks Creek through a mixed forest of incense cedars, white firs, lodgepole pines, ponderosa pines, and sugar pines. After 1.5 miles the road is left behind, as single-track trail climbs moderately past lush foliage and into Desolation Wilderness. Beyond the boundary, the trail roughly parallels Meeks Creek, which is always within earshot but rarely in sight. Through alternating groves of conifers and pocket meadows, you proceed up the canyon to a log-and-timber bridge across the creek. From there, the moderate climb arcs around a red-fir-forested side canyon filled with thimbleberry, fireweed, vine maple, and currant. Climbing out of this canyon, the trail then passes around the nose of a minor ridge and back alongside the tumbling creek on the way to a three-way junction with a little-used trail near the north end of Genevieve Lake that heads west to the General Creek Trail. Continue ahead, where just beyond the junction is greenish-tinged, shallow, and lodgepole-fringed Genevieve Lake. A number of fair campsites are spread around the far shore, but more appealing sites with better scenery are just a short distance away at Crag Lake.

After Genevieve Lake the trail makes a short, steady climb through western white pines, red firs, and Jeffrey pines to Crag Lake, backdropped splendidly by the granite slopes of 9054-foot Crag Peak to the south. Backpackers will find pleasant campsites above the northeast shore at 4.9 miles.

Pass around the east side of Crag Lake and then ascend rocky tread to a boulder hop of Meeks Creek. Just past the crossing, at 5.7 miles from the trailhead, an unmarked use trail heads southwest to Hidden Lake, a shallow, irregularly-shaped pond near the base of Crag Peak that has campsites. A steeper climb through dense forest ascends a moraine above the west shore of meadow-rimmed Shadow Lake, the shallow waters covered by numerous lily pads.

From Shadow Lake, a moderate climb follows the course of Meeks Creek, which tumbles and plunges down the rocky canyon. Reach the north shore of Stony Ridge Lake, the largest of the Tallant Lakes. Except for the steep east shore, the lake is bordered by lodgepole pines. A number of excellent campsites on the north and northeast shore lure overnighters.

On the way around the west shore of Stony Ridge Lake, you hop over the outlet from isolated Cliff Lake and then begin a mildly rising ascent at the far end of the lake, as you pass above a verdant meadow and then a well-watered hillside carpeted with wildflowers through midseason. Eventually the grade increases, switchbacking between two upper tributaries of Meeks Creek on the way toward the last lakes in the chain. At 8 miles from the trailhead is Rubicon Lake, perhaps the prettiest of the Tallant Lakes, rimmed with mountain hemlocks and lodgepole pines that shelter a number of fair-to-good campsites scattered around the shore.

About 100 yards up the cool, shady trail above Rubicon Lake is a lateral to Grouse Lakes on the left. The route of the TYT veers right to a couple of switchbacks, where the snow-covered slope of Mt. Tallac springs into view above the gray-green valley of Eagle Creek. You ascend moderately on a rocky trail until the grade eases on a traverse of the far side of a ridge overlooking Grouse Lakes and the Eagle Creek drainage, along which Cascade and Fallen Leaf lakes are visible to the southwest. Pass a junction with a lateral to Phipps Lake and continue the south-southwest traverse to where the route unexplainably contours around the south side of Phipps Peak until it heads almost due north, where hikers may begin to wonder if they're on the right trail, knowing that they should be heading south toward the Velma Lakes.

Veering west onto the dry and exposed west flank of Phipps Peak, the TYT offers excellent views of the northern Crystal Range, including Rockbound Pass—the deepest notch visible from this point—and the basins of Lois and Schmidell, landmarks that remain in sight for the next mile or so as the trail arcs around Phipps Peak. Finally, on a hairpin turn, the trail heads in a southerly direction toward Velma Lakes on a steady, sandy descent that incorporates three long-legged switchbacks. In dense forest, you reach a junction with the shared course of the Pacific Crest and Tahoe Rim trails (PCT/TRT).

You head southbound on the TYT/PCT/TRT on a moderate, forested descent, eventually crossing the sluggish outlet of Middle Velma Lake before ascending to a junction with the Velma Lakes Trail. Just before the junction, the trees part enough to allow a fine view of Middle Velma Lake. A short, off-trail descent will take you to the shoreline, where fine camping (at 13.4 miles) and swimming opportunities await.

Bathers at one of the Tallant Lakes

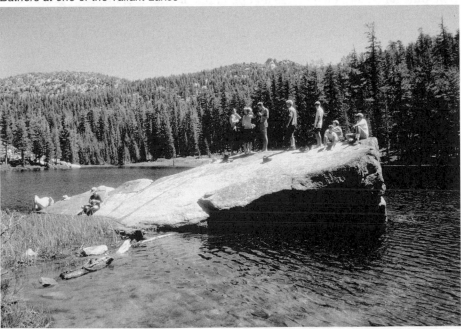

Turn left at the junction and follow the shared route of the trail to Velma Lakes and the TYT/PCT/TRT west a short way to another junction. Here the TYT/PCT/TRT turns south toward Fontanillis Lake, but your route continues west on the Velma Lakes Trail, soon reaching a junction with the lateral to Upper Velma Lake. To visit this scenic body of water, turn right (south) and follow the lateral through forest and granite slabs to the west shore and good campsites near the cascading stream spilling down granite slopes below Fontanillis Lake.

From the Upper Velma Lake junction, follow the Velma Lakes Trail to a ford of the outlet from the unnamed pond northeast of Upper Velma Lake and continue along the north shore. Proceed on an uphill course amid acres of granite slabs, boulders, and rocks, interspersed with widely scattered pines for 0.9 mile to a junction.

Veer right at the junction and follow sandy tread on a mildly undulating route through widely scattered, mixed forest and around granite boulders and slabs for 0.6 mile to a saddle and a junction with the Eagle Lakes Trail.

For the next 1.5 miles, the trail makes a moderate descent across the west slope below Maggies Peaks to a junction with a lateral to Eagle Lake. To visit the lake, turn sharply left and climb shortly to the northwest shore. The scenic lake reposes serenely in an impressive cirque composed of steep cliffs. The steep, shrub-covered slopes surrounding the lake offer limited access to the abrupt shoreline, providing a bit of a challenge to swimmers interested in a chilly dip and anglers plying the waters for trout. Located a mere mile from the trailhead, Eagle Lake is a very popular destination for both hikers and tourists—be prepared to meet a wide variety of people at the lake and on the way to the trailhead.

From the Eagle Lake junction, the descent continues, initially through lodgepole pine forest and then across an open area of granite slabs, with good views of Lake Tahoe and the towering cliffs of the canyon. Pass through an area of lush trailside flora and dense shrubs on the way to a junction with the Eagle Loop Nature Trail just prior to a bridge over Eagle Creek. After the bridge, descend 0.2 mile to the Eagle Falls Trailhead, passing the lower junction of the nature trail along the way.

BUILD-UP AND WIND-DOWN TIPS

In the heart of Homewood, the **Old Tahoe Café** dishes up ample portions of hearty meals at a reasonable price for breakfast and lunch from 7 AM to 2 PM. If you haven't been able to locate a "real" milkshake lately, look no farther than the Old Tahoe Café.

64

TAHOE RIM TRAIL: SHOWERS LAKE

Tim Hauserman

MILES: 15.3
RECOMMENDED DAYS: 2
ELEVATION GAIN/LOSS: 1485´
TYPE OF TRIP: Point-to-point
DIFFICULTY: Moderate
SOLITUDE: Moderately populated Big Meadow to Showers Lake, Moderate solitude Showers to Echo Summit
LOCATION: Lake Tahoe Basin Management Unit
MAPS: Tom Harrison's *Lake Tahoe Recreation Map*, *The Tahoe Rim Trail Elevation-Profile Trail Map* by Take it Outdoors!
BEST SEASON: Summer through fall

PERMITS ·

No permits are required for this trip on the Tahoe Rim Trail.

CHALLENGES ·

Water is limited but available. Sources include Round Lake, Showers Lake, Upper Truckee River, and numerous small streams in the bowl to the northwest of Showers Lake. Be careful on the northern half of the trail as water is much

Photo: Wildflowers between Meiss Meadows and Showers Lake

less prevalent. Bears in the area look forward to enjoying your food—carry your food in a bear canister to deter them.

HOW TO GET THERE · · · · · · · · · · · · · ·

From the intersection of Highways 50 and 89 in South Lake Tahoe take the combined route 8 miles south and then turn left onto Highway 89 as Highway 50 heads over Echo Summit. Proceed 5.5 miles on Highway 89 to the TRT Big Meadow Trailhead on your left. From the trailhead parking lot, the trail begins across the street.

TAKE THIS TRIP

This trip has something for everyone: several mountain lakes perfect for swimming, spectacular volcanic rock formations, and incredible wildflower displays in Meiss Meadows and in a bowl just north of Showers Lake (mid-July is your best bet). In fact, that bowl may be the most magical mile of the Tahoe Rim Trail (TRT)—it has cascading streams, leftover snowfields, castlelike rock formations, and wildflowers galore.

TRIP DESCRIPTION · · · · · · · · · · · · · · ·

Get ready for some of the best miles you will find on the TRT. Your journey begins at the edge of the parking area, where a short stroll brings you to a crossing of Highway 89. Across the street you hike uphill through boulders and Jeffrey pines, western white pines, and firs. Soon you pass aspen groves and a stream and in about 0.7 mile reach aptly named Big Meadow.

A pleasant walk across the meadow brings you to another mile of uphill trekking, through a thinning forest, providing more room for wildflowers and bushes. You reach a saddle and begin seeing beautiful mountain views on a steep descent to a junction. Here a right turn takes you to Dardanelles Lake, at just 1.4 miles each way, a very worthwhile goal or side trip. The TRT continues straight ahead past intriguing volcanic mudflow formations to Round Lake, a fairly large mountain lake good for camping and swimming but with a green to blue hue caused by the volcanic sediment. The Dardanelles, a spectacular volcanic cliff, reaches skyward to your left. Fortunately, you will have many more glimpses of this interesting feature as the hike progresses.

For the next 2 miles you pass through several meadows loaded with wildflowers in season as well as lots of aspen trees. Your views are enhanced by the high ridges on both sides

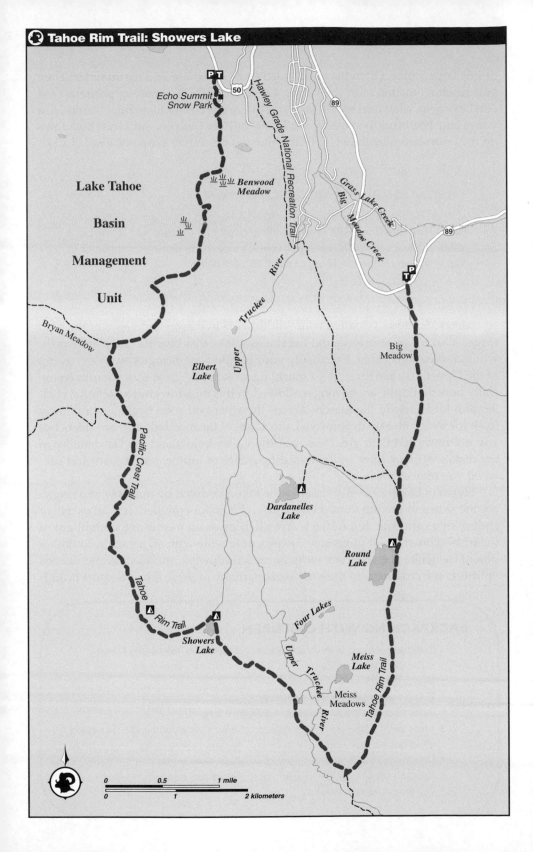

Echo Summit
Snow Park

50

Hawley Grade National Recreation Trail

89

Grass Lake Creek

Big Meadow Creek

89

Benwood Meadow

Lake Tahoe

Basin

Management

Unit

Bryan Meadow

Upper Truckee River

Big Meadow

Elbert Lake

Pacific Crest Trail

Dardanelles Lake

Round Lake

Tahoe Rim Trail

Four Lakes

Showers Lake

Upper Truckee River

Meiss Lake

Tahoe Rim Trail

Meiss Meadows

0   0.5   1 mile

0   1   2 kilometers

of this large valley. Often they hold patches of snow late into the summer. Then you reach a junction with the Pacific Crest Trail (PCT), where opposite an old cowboy cabin, a left turn would take you to Carson Pass in just under 3 miles, but your route heads north in the Upper Truckee River Canyon and Meiss Meadows on the path shared by the PCT, TRT, and even the Tahoe Yosemite Trail (TYT).

THE TAHOE RIM TRAIL ASSOCIATION

The Tahoe Rim Trail Association (TRTA) helped build and maintains the Tahoe Rim Trail. The TRTA provides information to the public and conducts a series of hikes over the summer and winter months. For more information or to help, visit www.tahoerimtrail.org or call 775-298-0012.

Meiss Meadows is loaded with wildflowers in season and views of the high ridges above. The meadows and the shallow lake that bear its name are worthwhile destinations alone. Eventually your gentle walk brings you to a crossing of the Upper Truckee River. It's a sparkling stream and great water source (especially now that cattle are no longer allowed in this meadow) but a potential challenging ford early in the season. Across the river you soon begin a climb away from the valley and up to Showers Lake. Parts of the next half mile are steep, but you are rewarded with great views of the valley below and the Dardanelles in the distance. Enjoy some of the thickest patches of lupine, paintbrush, and fireweed you may ever see.

Showers Lake is a very pleasant little lake, bordered by meadow and marsh on one side and granite slabs on the other. If it is not crowded, it is an excellent choice for a campsite. If the lake is crowded, press on past it to the highlight of the trip—a bowl about three-quarters of a mile wide with an amazing combination of castlelike volcanic rock formations, wildflowers, snowfields, and dozens of little creek crossings. In the early season, many of those streams sport beauti-

BACKPACKING WITH CHILDREN

When backpacking with your children, remember a few simple things:
* Have them bring a friend.
* Don't go too far the first time.
* Camp near a lake for some great fun.
* Relax and forget trying to teach—just have fun.
* Arrange for a layover day so everyone can wander around without carrying a big pack.
* Don't scare them.
* Spend a lot of quiet time looking at the stars and sunsets.
* Tell them you love them.

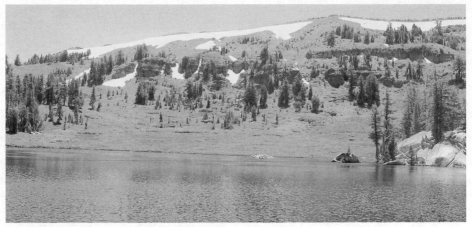

Showers Lake from its granite-bordered northern edge

ful cascades from the lofty slopes above. A gentle climb across the bowl leads you out of the lushness and into a more sandy saddle.

Now at close to 9000 feet you pass scattered western white pine, lodgepole, and hemlock as you gently ascend. Then you find a mostly viewless up-and-down hike along the top of a broad ridge, passing several junctions. At 4.4 miles from Showers Lake you reach Bryan Meadow, with about 4 miles to go to Echo Summit. From the meadow your trail heads uphill fairly steeply for a half mile before a steep descent. A rock outcropping to your right provides views over the South Lake Tahoe airport to Lake Tahoe in the distance. Your trail levels off and you pass perhaps the last good campsite next to a creek before beginning a steep descent along the edge of a granite canyon. An ancient juniper provides a last view of the Dardanelles, as well as Round Top peak which can hold snow well into late summer. After a grueling 2-mile drop you reach a bridge crossing and more level terrain. A pleasant section with tiger lilies and assorted other wildflowers and Benwood Meadow through the trees to your right now awaits you. Just 0.75 from the end you reach a junction. Turn left and head through tall Jeffrey pines to the finish at a large parking lot.

BUILD-UP AND WIND-DOWN TIPS ·

Lower Echo Lake is just another 2.3 miles of hiking or a short drive from your finishing trailhead. Here summer cabins perch above a beautiful mountain lake surrounded by granite. The lake provides a water taxi across to **Upper Echo Lake**, as well as fishing and a small store. I still remember fondly a sandwich and ice cream from the store on Day 11 of a thru-hike of the TRT. Here on the PCT/TRT you are just a few miles from Desolation Wilderness. From Echo Summit, **South Lake Tahoe** is just a few miles away and loaded with restaurants and everything else you could need, perhaps more than you need. Just north of South Lake Tahoe on Highway 89 you can go to **Taylor Creek**. Here a stream profile chamber, which provides a view of the creek through a glass pane, is prime territory in the early fall to watch the spawning of the kokanee salmon.

65

TAHOE RIM TRAIL: STAR LAKE AND FREEL PEAK

Tim Hauserman

MILES: 13.6 to Star Lake, with trip up Freel Peak
RECOMMENDED DAYS: 2–3
ELEVATION GAIN/LOSS: 1000´/1000´ to Freel Saddle;
2100´/2100´ to Freel Peak
TYPE OF TRIP: Out-and-back
DIFFICULTY: Moderate to Star Lake,
Moderately strenuous to Freel Peak
SOLITUDE: Moderately populated on weekends and prime season,
Moderate solitude off-season and weekdays
LOCATION: Lake Tahoe Basin Management Unit
MAPS: Tom Harrison's *Lake Tahoe Recreation Map*,
Tahoe Rim Trail Elevation-Profile Trail Map by Take It Outdoors!
BEST SEASON: Summer through fall

PERMITS ·

No permit is required for this trip on the Tahoe Rim Trail.

Photo: Freel Peak

CHALLENGES

Water is limited but available. Several creeks cascade down from Freel Peak to cross the trail on the way to the Freel Saddle, as well as swiftly moving Cold Creek and Star Lake. Bears, while not as prevalent here as on the west shore of Lake Tahoe, are still an issue and are too smart for their own good. To keep your food safe, bring and use a bear canister. Do not leave any food or valuables in your car. Higher-clearance vehicles are recommended for the last few miles of dirt road to the Armstrong Pass Trailhead.

HOW TO GET THERE

From South Lake Tahoe take Highway 50 8 miles south to Meyers. Then head south on Highway 89 to Luther Pass, just past Grass Lake on your right. Continue downhill on Highway 89 toward Hope Valley 0.8 mile to Forest Service Road 051 on your left (1.8 miles north of the Highway 89/88 junction in Hope Valley). Take the Forest Service road steeply uphill. At 1.1 miles, veer left. At 1.6 miles bear left again. You reach your first bridge at 2.4 miles as you follow a stream. At 2.7 miles, go straight ahead at a fork in the road. At 3.4 miles cross a second bridge and then immediately your road makes a 180-degree turn into a small parking area. Park here and begin your walk on a trail bridge across a small stream.

TRIP DESCRIPTION

From the bridge go 0.5 mile uphill on the now-abandoned road to the former Armstrong Pass parking area. Here the single-track trail begins, and you walk steeply uphill 0.4 mile to a saddle and your junction with the Tahoe Rim Trail (TRT). From the junction a left turn takes you first uphill and later downhill to the Big Meadow Trailhead in 9.5 miles. You turn right and head toward Star Lake. The good news is that you are already at 8700 feet in elevation and thus have only another 1000 feet

TAKE THIS TRIP

Journey past Lake Tahoe basin's highest peak (10,881 feet) to the Tahoe areas highest lake (Star Lake at 9100 feet) while enjoying a well-graded, beautiful trail that is not too difficult. Enjoy views of Desolation Wilderness, Lake Tahoe, ancient juniper trees, and a favorite section of the lightly forested Carson Range. For a real treat, head up to Freel Peak and then over to Jobs Peak and Jobs Sister, bagging three of the four highest peaks in the Tahoe basin. Star Lake is a great destination for families with older children. To top it all off, it is almost always less crowded than nearby Desolation Wilderness.

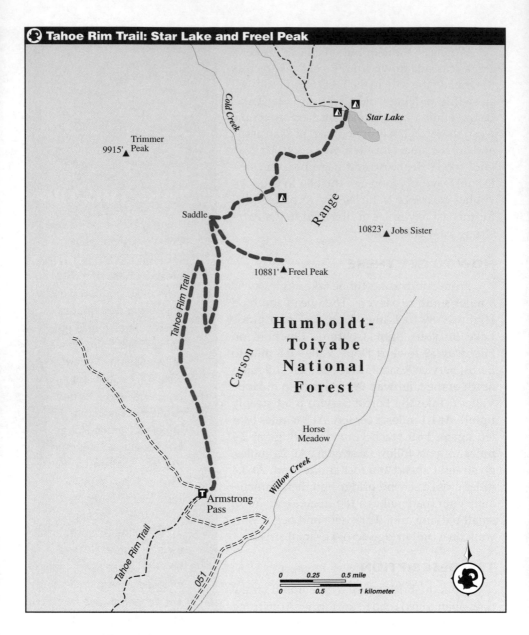

Tahoe Rim Trail: Star Lake and Freel Peak

Cold Creek

Star Lake

Trimmer
9915' ▲ Peak

Range

Saddle

10823' ▲ Jobs Sister

Tahoe Rim Trail

10881' ▲ Freel Peak

Humboldt-Toiyabe National Forest

Carson

Horse
Meadow

Willow Creek

Tahoe Rim Trail

Armstrong
Pass

051

0   0.25   0.5 mile
0   0.5   1 kilometer

to climb to reach the Freel Peak saddle. The trek begins with gentle rolling terrain past some lovely junipers in a scattered forest. Views open up as you begin a big traverse around a ridge, pass Fountain Face, a large granite face just off the trail, and begin climbing north. It's a steady but only moderately difficult climb, well suited to most backpackers. You pass three streamlets along the way, each lined with late season wildflowers and serving as a water source well into the fall. Two long switchbacks lead you through the lightly scattered forest, with plenty of views into Desolation Wilderness and its rampart, the Crystal Range.

TAKE THE TYKES

One of the best things you can do with your children is take them backpacking in the wilderness. Aside from being a great opportunity for your kids to learn about nature, once you're both away from cell phones, TV, and computers, you might actually get a chance to have a conversation with your offspring and perhaps even find out what is really going on in their life.

In the foreground is evidence of the Angora Fire of 2007 which destroyed more than 200 homes in South Lake Tahoe. Eventually, you reach a saddle at the head of the canyon.

Here, a right turn onto the signed Freel Peak trail leads you in a mile and about 1100 feet of climbing, to the highest peak in the Tahoe basin, Freel Peak at 10,881 feet in elevation. From the top of Freel you get panoramic views of Lake Tahoe in the distance with Jobs Peak and Jobs Sister nearby, both of which can be accessed via a use trail from the top of Freel.

If you want to save Freel for a layover day, continue downhill from the saddle toward Star Lake. This next mile is a real treat. Scattered and wind-beaten white-bark pines, western white pines, and hemlock frame the desolate high peaks above. You cross a tiny patch of green at easily jumpable, swift-moving Cold Creek. Follow this creek upstream a few hundred yards for spectacular camping just below a lush meadow. Past the creek your trail continues a descent to the edge of Star Lake. Find a campsite in the ridge above the lake and then take a dip in the usually chilly water; if you catch it after a warm spell, it's better. Near Star Lake's outlet are dramatic views of Jobs Sister above. Once you are settled in, take a lovely walk above the northern and eastern shores of the lake. The views are great and you will spot a little mountain of shiny white quartz.

To return, retrace your steps to the trailhead. If you're looking for a longer trip, hike a 23-mile section of the TRT by starting near Kingsbury Grade and hiking to Big Meadow.

BUILD-UP AND WIND-DOWN TIPS ·

Just a few miles downhill from the Armstrong Pass turnoff on Highway 89, you reach **Hope Valley**. This large, lovely valley is filled with aspens and surrounded by high peaks that hold patches of snow into midsummer. Beautiful views can be found year-round but are particularly special in the fall when the aspens turn into a blaze of gold. Situated in the aspens is **Sorenson's Resort**, a rustic retreat popular with tree gazers and cross-country skiers. A few miles farther to the south near Markleeville lies **Grover Hot Springs State Park** with spring-fed hot pools, a campground, and hiking trails.

66

LITTLE JAMISON CANYON TO GRASS, ROCK, JAMISON, AND WADES LAKES

Mike White

MILES: 7.5
RECOMMENDED DAYS: 2
ELEVATION GAIN/LOSS: 2090´/2050´
TYPE OF TRIP: Semiloop
DIFFICULTY: Easy
SOLITUDE: Moderately populated
LOCATION: Plumas-Eureka State Park, Lakes Basin Recreation Area
MAPS: USGS 7.5-min. *Gold Lake*; U.S. Forest Service *Lakes Basin, Sierra Buttes, and Plumas-Eureka State Park Recreation Guide*
BEST SEASON: Summer through early fall

PERMITS •

In a throwback to the pre-1960s Sierra, permits are not required in Plumas-Eureka State Park or Lakes Basin Recreation Area.

Photo: Scenic Jamison Lake

CHALLENGES · · · · · · · · · · · · · · · · · · ·

The short distances to these lakes makes for relatively easy backpacking, which leads to stiff competition for campsites on weekends. To fully enjoy the area, visit midweek.

HOW TO GET THERE · · · · · · · · · · · · · ·

In the quaint town of Graeagle, leave Highway 89 and follow County Road 506 west toward Plumas-Eureka State Park. Cross the park boundary and continue to a left-hand turn onto a dirt road, 4.6 miles from Highway 89, signed JAMISON MINE, GRASS LAKE TRAIL. Proceed to the end of the dirt road and park in the gravel area near the trailhead.

TRIP DESCRIPTION· · · · · · · · · · · · · · · ·

Walk around a closed steel gate and follow the old, rocky road on a moderate climb past some of the historic buildings of the Jamison Mine. Beyond the structures, you follow single-track trail beneath the cover of a mixed forest above tumbling Jamison Creek. After 0.6 mile pass a signed junction with a 1.3-mile lateral to Smith Lake, and continue another 0.2 mile to a junction with an unmarked path that leads shortly to a view of Jamison Falls, a 60-foot waterfall on Jamison Creek that puts on quite a display when the creek is flowing near full capacity. A half mile of gentle ascent then leads to Grass Lake, providing good views from the east shore of Mt. Washington rising sharply into the sky above the far side of the lake. A use trail at the north end of the lake leads across the outlet to fair campsites on the west shore at 1.3 miles, before the path dies out in a tangle of thick brush.

Beyond Grass Lake, you follow gently graded tread through lush groundcover and light forest, across a small meadow, and then over to a crossing of Jamison Creek, which may be difficult in early season. A slightly climbing trail continues past the crossing to a

TAKE THIS TRIP

Short hikes to a quartet of delightful lakes lures backpackers on this semi-loop trip. Grass, Rock, Jamison, and Wades lakes are among the few lakes in the area where camping is allowed, which partially explains their popularity. However, camping is not the only appeal, as the scenery is superb, fishing is fair, and swimming can be quite refreshing on a typically hot summer afternoon.

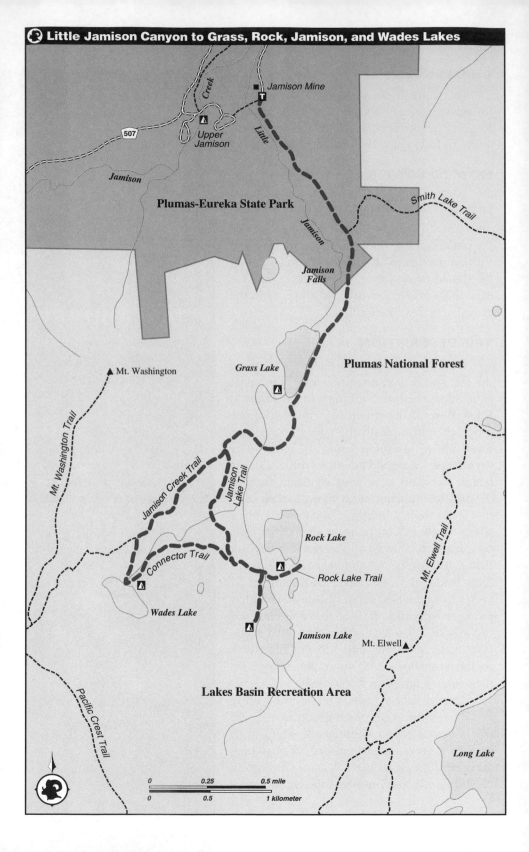

T-junction of the Jamison Creek Trail on the right and the Jamison Lake Trail on the left.

Head left (south) from the junction and climb mildly for a brief spell until the grade increases at the beginning of some switchbacks. Shortly after crossing the outlet from Wades Lake you reach a junction with the Wades Lake and Jamison Lake Connector. Remaining on the Jamison Lake Trail on the left, you soon come to a Y-junction, where the path splits to access Rock Lake on the left-hand path and Jamsion Lake on the right-hand path. The short walk to Jamison Lake (at 3.1 miles) brings you to the old rock dam, where lush foliage covering the structure gives the appearance of an ornamental garden. To visit the shoreline, you'll have to backtrack a few steps to where a much more obscure path follows an open, bedrock ridge above the west shore to the far end. Other than a few dead stumps left over from when the dam was built, Jamison Lake is a pleasing sight at the base of 7818-foot Mt. Elwell. Small islands on the north side of the lake offer fine swimming destinations and sunbathing spots. Campsites are very limited.

To visit aptly named Rock Lake, retrace your steps to the Y-junction and proceed to a ford of Jamison Creek. Beyond the ford, a short climb leads to the south shore of the windswept, rockbound lake. A few campsites on the south and southeast shores at 3.2 miles seem to get plenty of use.

After a visit to Jamison and Rock lakes, backtrack to the junction with the Wades Lake and Jamison Lake Connector and begin a moderately steep, zigzagging climb across an open, brushy slope toward Wades Lake—try to get an early start to beat the heat. Tight switchbacks lead to the top of a rock outcrop with

The restored buildings of the Jamison Mine near the trailhead

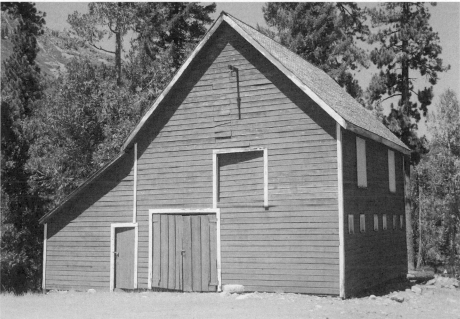

good views of Grass Lake and Jamison Creek canyon. From there, more gently graded trail heads through scattered conifers, past a small pond, and around the head of a small canyon before a stiffer climb resumes. The trees thicken a bit where you enter the drainage of Wade Lake's outlet and follow the stream to a crossing just before reaching the south shore and a large and shady camping area at 4.5 miles. Grasses and willows border the near side of the lake, but the far side has a dramatic backdrop from steep and rocky cliffs.

The trail connecting to the Jamison Creek Trail may be difficult for first-time users to locate, but you should be able to find the path on the west side of the outlet near the ford (which was marked only by a four-by-four post when I last scouted it). Head downstream through a lodgepole pine forest on gently descending tread. Very soon, western white pines, Jeffrey pines, and an assortment of shrubs begin to intermix with the lodgepoles. About a quarter mile from Wades Lake, you reach a junction with the Jamison Creek Trail.

The descent increases beyond the junction, as you follow a rocky trail through shrubs and scattered conifers to a rock promontory with good views of Grass Lake, Jamison Creek canyon, and the surrounding mountains. The stiff, rocky descent continues to a junction with the Jamison Lake Trail at the close of the loop. From there, retrace your steps 2.2 miles to the trailhead.

BUILD-UP AND WIND-DOWN TIPS ·

The mill town of Graeagle was founded in the 1800s to support a vigorous logging operation that continued until 1957. A decade or so later, the quaint town, with its row of red company houses, became the centerpiece for what is now a thriving resort community complete with upscale homes and golf courses. The Graeagle area has several eateries, spanning the spectrum from casual to fine dining. The **Graeagle Fros-Tee** is the place to grab an old-fashioned burger, fries, and shake. In the nearby community of Blairsden, **Gumba's Pizzeria and Grill** serves up a pretty good pie. **Café Mohawk** offers decent breakfasts or lunches every day except Tuesday.

For more urbane fare, the **Iron Door**, located in the historic mining town of Johnsville within Plumas-Eureka State Park, has been serving hearty meals in the rustic setting of the old general store and post office since 1961. The restaurant is open Wednesday through Monday from April to November, and reservations are required (530-836-2376).

The **Mt. Tomba Inn Dinner House**, located off Highway 70 in Cromberg, offers perhaps the most unique dining experience in the area, as the restaurant is a virtual shrine to John Wayne, with every meal bearing the name of one of the Duke's movie titles (except for the vegetarian choice, of course). Call 530-836-2359 for reservations.

67

BUCKS LAKE WILDERNESS LOOP

Mike White

> **MILES:** 21.4
> **RECOMMENDED DAYS:** 3–4
> **ELEVATION GAIN/LOSS:** 4500´ / 4500´
> **TYPE OF TRIP:** Loop
> **DIFFICULTY:** Moderate
> **SOLITUDE:** Solitude
> **LOCATION:** Bucks Lake Wilderness, Plumas National Forest
> **MAPS:** USGS 7.5-min. *Bucks Lake*;
> U.S. Forest Service *A Guide to the Bucks Lake Wilderness*
> **BEST SEASON:** Summer through early fall

PERMITS ·

Wilderness permits are not required in Bucks Lake Wilderness.

CHALLENGES ·

The first leg of this loop is definitely the least enjoyable stretch of trail, as very steep climbing combines with a route near and sometimes on a dirt road before better conditions prevail beyond the Mill Creek Trailhead. A portion of Bucks Lake Wilderness is used for cattle grazing, a practice that dates back to the

Photo: The Bucks Lake Loop offers backpackers several far-ranging views.

TAKE THIS TRIP

While Bucks Lake is an extremely popular summer hangout for Northern Californians, the trails within the neighboring Bucks Lake Wilderness offer plenty of solitude and serenity. This scenic loop, which incorporates a short section of the famed Pacific Crest Trail, offers visitors picturesque lakes, cascading streams, wildflower-filled meadows, shady forests, and wide-ranging views. The general lack of use has resulted in few developed campsites, so backpackers will have to plan their route carefully and may have to branch off the loop in order to find the best spots. During the month of July, the area puts on a surprising display of wildflowers.

early 1900s. For a bovine-free experience, plan to visit the area prior to August 1, or after September 30.

HOW TO GET THERE········

From Highway 70 in Quincy, follow Bucks Lake Road to Forest Road 33, just west of Haskins Bay and Bucklin Dam, and proceed northbound for 4.4 miles to a Y-junction. Veer right onto Forest Road 24N69X, as Road 33 on the left turns to dirt, and follow the paved road a half mile to Mill Creek Campground, which has running water and vault toilets.

TRIP DESCRIPTION ···············

From Mill Creek Campground, follow the single-track trail on a rising climb for a quarter mile to a junction with the Mill Creek Trail above the ford of Mill Creek just before the stream pours into the northern arm of Bucks Lake. Beyond this junction the grade increases substantially on a climb toward Chucks Rock. Fortunately, a mixed forest of conifers shades most of the brutally steep route. Just below Chucks Rock, the trail crosses over Forest Road 33 and continues a short distance to cross the road again farther up the slope. Despite what is shown on the U.S. Forest Service map, there seems to be no discernible trail from here to the Mill Creek Trailhead, requiring you to walk a section of road. Fortunately, the grade of the road is much more pleasant than that of the previous stretch of trail.

Single-track resumes past the Mill Creek Trailhead, immediately crossing Mill Creek to follow gently graded tread through a light forest of lodgepole pines and white firs to a boulder hop back over the creek. The tread briefly disappears in a small, grassy meadow on the far side but is easily found again just past a snow survey marker, where the trail reenters forest cover. Leaving Mill Creek behind, the lupine-lined trail begins a moderate climb through shady forest with occasional pockets of meadow carpeted with grasses, sedges,

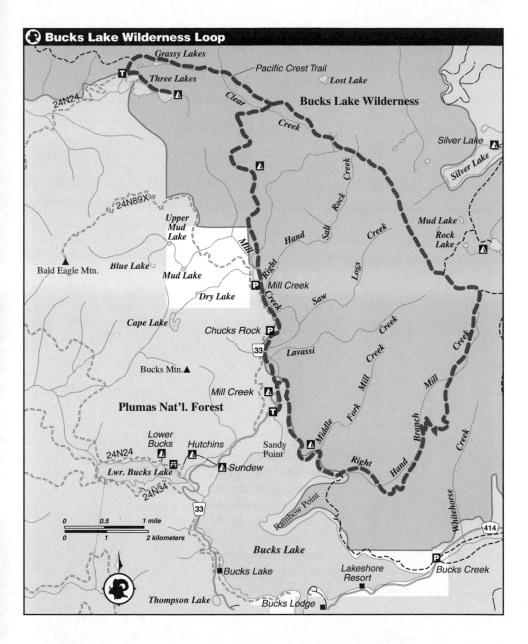

Bucks Lake Wilderness Loop

Grassy Lakes

Pacific Crest Trail

Three Lakes

Lost Lake

24N24

Clear

Bucks Lake Wilderness

Creek

Silver Lake

Silver Lake

24N89X

Upper
Mud
Lake

Hand

Salt

Rock

Creek

Mud Lake

Rock
Lake

Bald Eagle Mtn.   Blue Lake

Mud Lake

Mill

Right

Logs

Cape Lake

Dry Lake

P Mill Creek

Creek

Saw

Creek

Chucks Rock P

Creek

33

Lavassi

Creek

Mill

Bucks Mtn.▲

Plumas Nat'l. Forest

Mill Creek

T

Fork

Branch

Creek

Lower
Bucks

Hutchins

Sandy
Point

Middle

Mill

24N24

Right

Hand

Lwr. Bucks Lake

Sundew

24N34

Whitehorse

33

414

0   0.5   1 mile

0   1   2 kilometers

Rainbow Point

Bucks Lake

P Bucks Creek

Bucks Lake

Lakeshore
Resort

Thompson Lake

Bucks Lodge

shrubs, and wildflowers in early to midseason. Around the 1.5-mile mark, the trail draws alongside an alder-lined tributary of Mill Creek and then continues climbing to a high point, south-southeast of Point 6738. Nearby, at an unmarked junction, a use trail drops down to a horse camp, from where the faint path continucs to a water source at a nascent stream.

From the high point, the trail descends toward the Three Lakes area, passing through a pair of meadows, the tread temporarily disappearing in the verdant vegetation of the second one. Continue the descent, hopping across a trio of thin, lushly lined rivulets and passing by a shallow pond bordered by tall grasses and covered with lily pads. Just past the pond, you reach a three-way junction with the Pacific Crest Trail (PCT).

Turn left (west) and follow the gently graded PCT past the pond and alongside an alder-lined seasonal stream draining into the pond from Grassy Lakes.

A splendid view from the PCT across Bucks Lake Wilderness

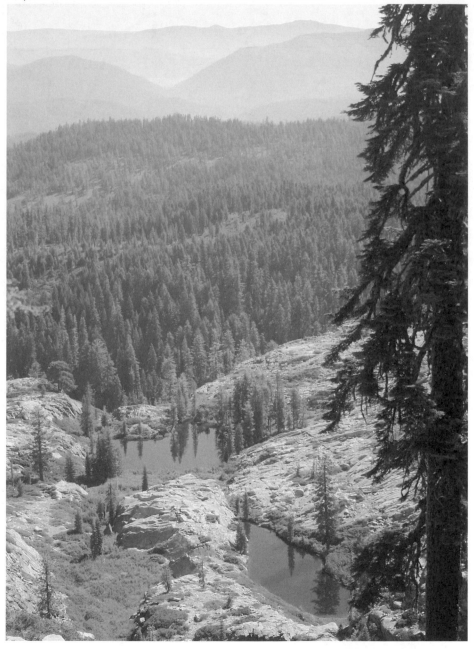

A fern-lined section of trail leads through open forest with evidence of a previous fire on the right-hand hillside. Continue past the larger Grassy Lake, which, except in early season, will appear to be more like a grassy meadow with a small pond near the end than a bona fide lake. Reach a junction with the unmaintained trail to Kellogg Lake, a second-rate body of water made even more unappealing by the recent fire, and then proceed a short distance to a junction with the lateral to Three Lakes.

Leaving the PCT, the lateral drops moderately through open forest past a Bucks Lake Wilderness sign to another junction. The path ahead leads to the Three Lakes Road, a little used four-wheel-drive road, but you turn left and soon catch a glimpse of the lower lake and the dam at the far end. After crossing an old wood bridge over a narrow creek, the path continues through dense forest to the middle lake, a natural body of water rimmed by grey cliffs—a much more scenic locale than the artificial lake below. Past a couple of campsites at 5.1 miles, the encroaching water at the far end of the middle lake inundates the trail, where thick brush makes circumventing this obstacle a bit difficult, at least not without getting your feet wet. Once you are beyond this minor inconvenience, the trail makes a short climb to the upper lake, clearly the most attractive of the Three Lakes. Unfortunately, the upper lake offers only small, marginal campsites above the northwest shore. Deteriorating tread continues above the lakeshore but disappears entirely before reaching the far end of the lake. After a night at Three Lakes, retrace your steps 1.8 miles to the junction of the PCT and Mill Creek Trail.

From the junction, head southeast on the flower-lined PCT through open to light forest, crossing a seasonal swale and passing a small, flower-filled meadow on the way to a crossing of Clear Creek, where a small campsite is just above the stream. After a while the trail draws alongside the creek near some cascades and a small pool before quickly moving away again. Climbing moderately through light forest, the path approaches and crosses a number of lushly lined rivulets below the southwest slope of Mt. Pleasant, directly south of the broad-topped peak.

A short, mild descent leads to the start of a gently undulating traverse along the northeastern escarpment between Mt. Pleasant and Spanish Peak. Beginning in thick forest, the traverse eventually leads out of the trees to impressive views of the lakes below in their granite basins and the terrain beyond, including the deep gash of North Fork Feather River, a slice of Sierra Valley, nearby Meadow Valley, and the more distant Quincy area. The traverse lasts for 2.5 miles, stands of forest intermittently interrupting the stunning views. At Granite Gap, in one such stand of forest, you reach a junction with the trail descending toward Silver Lake.

Since decent campsites are few and far between Right Hand Branch Mill Creek and the shore of Bucks Lake, you may want to consider spending the night at Rock Lake (or even Gold Lake). To visit Rock Lake, drop down from Granite Gap on a series of switchbacks through a rocky gully for three-quarters of a mile to a junction with the lateral to Rock Lake. Turn right and head through brush and boulders to the lip of the lake's basin, where large rocks line a shoreline backdropped by rocky bluffs and outcrops. If you're staying at Rock Lake, locate campsites in groves of conifers at 13 miles. Otherwise, you can always enjoy the lake and return to the main trail. When you're ready to continue the loop, retrace your steps to the junction at Granite Gap.

Heading southeast on the PCT, a section of open forest allows more views before being obscured by thickening forest on the way to a saddle and a junction with the Right Hand Branch Mill Creek Trail. Before heading down Right Hand Branch Mill Creek, you should consider a short extension to the marvelous view from the old lookout site on Spanish Peak: Head southeast on the PCT through a stand of conifers prior to open slopes carpeted with pinemat manzanita and continue to a junction of the lateral to Spanish Peak. Turn left (east) and proceed toward the peak on mildly rising tread through more pinemat manzanita before entering a red fir forest. Pass the old, dilapidated shack that formerly served as the outhouse for the ranger who staffed the lookout and immediately break out of the trees for the final, short climb to the top. The sweeping view includes such noteworthy landmarks as Lassen Peak and Lake Almanor to the north and Sierra Buttes to the southeast. Once you've thoroughly enjoyed the view, retrace your steps back to the Right Hand Branch junction.

At the junction, leave the PCT and follow Right Hand Branch Mill Creek Trail over a low rise before embarking on a nearly continuous, 5-mile descent to the east shore of Bucks Lake. Beyond the low rise, the trail enters a small meadow, where the tread is momentarily lost in the lush vegetation—cairns should help you to stay on course. Step across the usually dry streambed in the uppermost part of the canyon and continue to a second, larger meadow, where, once again, the trail disappears for a while in the thick grasses and cairns should be an aid. Follow the creek, which by now should be flowing with water, to an easy stream crossing.

After the crossing, the trail moves away from the creek for a while, more or less traversing the east side of the canyon. The traverse ends at the beginning of an extended switchbacking descent leading steeply down the forested hillside. After a couple of miles and countless switchbacks, the trail drops to a boulder hop of the main branch of the creek. A level spot just above the creek bears the closest resemblance to a campsite so far.

Beyond the creek, a couple more short-legged switchbacks lead to the crossing of a tiny rivulet that is easily negotiated. Soon afterward, you get your first glimpse through the trees of the blue waters of Bucks Lake. Hop across a second rivulet just before a junction with the Mill Creek Trail.

Turn right (north-northwest) at the junction and proceed along the forested lakeshore path. A sandy beach near the junction offers a passable campsite, albeit with the intermittent noise from passing pleasure craft slicing across the lake's surface. Veer into the next side canyon and a usually ankle-deep ford of Middle Fork Mill Creek. Follow the trail as it wraps around Point 5450 at 18 miles, where overnighters may find better campsites on the bluff overlooking the lake, and then crosses a seasonal, alder-lined stream. Reach a stretch of open forest, where the white beach from Sandy Point glistens in the sun across the north arm of the lake. Back into forest, the trail follows the shore across more seasonal streams surrounded by lush vegetation toward the end of the north arm, where a moderate ascent leads across an open slope covered with tobacco brush. Briefly enter the wilderness on the way to the top of the climb, head back into forest, and then drop steeply to a ford of Mill Creek, which may be difficult in early season.

From the west bank of Mill Creek, climb the hillside to a junction with the Mill Creek Trail. Turn left (south) and retrace your steps 0.4 mile to the end of the trail and proceed to Mill Creek Campground.

BUILD-UP AND WIND-DOWN TIPS

Bucks Lake has a couple of all-year resorts scattered around the south side of the lake. Both **Lakeshore Resort** (530-283-6900) and **Bucks Lake Lodge** (www. buckslakelodge.com, 530-283-2262) have housekeeping cabins, small general stores, cafes, boat rentals, and gas pumps. Bucks Lake Lodge also operates Timberline Inn, a separate structure with motel rooms. The **Haskins Valley Inn** (www. haskinsvalleyinn.com, 530-283-9667) is a bed-and-breakfast with a general store next door. **Bucks Lake Marina** (530-283-4243) has boat and kayak rentals, a campground, and cabins during summer.

Plumas National Forest manages several campgrounds in the area, including **Mill Creek**, **Lower Bucks**, **Hutchins**, **Sundew**, **Grizzly Creek**, **Whitehorse**, and **Silver Lake**. **Haskins Valley Campground** is managed by Pacific Gas & Electric.

Between Bucks Lake and Quincy, in the community of Meadow Valley, the **Ten-Two Dinner House** offers great food with all-natural ingredients from a changing menu. Summertime diners can sit outside and enjoy the sounds of the nearby creek. The town of Quincy, 17 miles from Bucks Lake, has many lodging and dining options. **Morning Thunder Café** at 557 Lawrence St. is the spot for breakfast, while **Moon's** at 487 Lawrence St. is arguably the best restaurant for dinner. If you just want to grab a sandwich for lunch, check out the **Courthouse Café** at 525 Main St.

CASCADE RANGE

Geographic tradition defines the Cascade Range as extending from southernmost British Columbia to the volcanic terrain south of the Mt. Lassen area. That puts about 130 miles of Cascadia within California. Outdoors enthusiasts can find lots of good fishing, hunting, and water sports in the state's share of this great range, but most of this is hilly country with more timber harvesting than hiking. The Pacific Crest Trail is as well-located as a trail can be to take advantage of the scenic terrain in this stretch, but for the average backpacker California's Cascades offer two very notable areas of attraction: Mt. Lassen and Mt. Shasta.

LASSEN VOLCANIC NATIONAL PARK

Situated about 75 miles southeast of Mt. Shasta, the centerpiece of Lassen Volcanic National Park is the 10,457-foot Cascade Range volcano Lassen Peak. Prior to the 1980 eruption of Washington's Mt. St. Helens, Lassen Peak was the most recent volcano to blow in the continental U.S., erupting numerous times from 1914 to 1917. These eruptions, along with several active hydrothermal areas, and plenty of evidence of previous volcanic activity, compelled the federal government to give the area national park status in 1916.

Lassen is more than just a place for a geology lesson, however. The scenery—the flower-covered meadows, crystal lakes, rushing streams, serene forests, and rich red summit of Lassen Peak itself—is stunning. The 150 miles of maintained trails in the 106,000-acre park tempt hikers to enjoy its wonders, and a fine network of connecting trails provides many loop options. Best of all, the park is well away from California's major urban areas, so backpackers won't have to contend with crowds on most trails.

CARIBOU WILDERNESS

On the eastern border of Lassen Volcanic National Park is the 20,625-acre Caribou Wilderness, a land of rolling, forested terrain and numerous lakes. While you won't find any caribou in this misnamed wilderness, you will have the opportunity to backpack to a number of peaceful lakes on the trip described in this section. The gentle terrain characteristic of Caribou Wilderness makes the area well suited for short backpacks for outdoor enthusiasts of all ages and physical condition. Despite the short and easy trails, the remote location insures that you won't have to share the area with too many others.

MOUNT SHASTA

Mt. Shasta stands in solitary dominance as the most striking mountain in northern California. Its volume—estimated by various geologists at between 80 and 120 cubic miles—makes it, arguably, the largest volcanic peak in the continental U.S., and its base-to-summit relief compares with many of the world's greatest peaks. Indeed, if Shastina, Mt. Shasta's secondary cone, stood alone, it would be the third highest mountain in the Cascade Range after Mts. Rainier and Shasta. And yet, ironically, Mt. Shasta was the last major mountain of the Pacific Northwest to be discovered by Euro-American explorers. Mts. Rainier, Hood, St. Helens, Baker, and St. Elias were all named and mapped before 1800. Shasta, midway between the British settlements at Fort Vancouver and the mouth of the Columbia River and the Spanish enclaves in San Francisco and Monterey, was not seen by explorers until they had journeyed overland nearly 300 miles from these settlements into unknown territory.

Mt. Shasta's slopes are continuous and vast, and so it is justifiably known as a climber's and backcountry skier's mountain. Thousands of people dayhike on and climb Shasta every year, and most of the summit-bound backpack in for at least one night, but few people go backpacking per se on Shasta. However, a timber line circumnavigation of the peak is one of California's least appreciated wonder-tours, a multiday adventure that John Muir described glowingly.

68

SUMMIT LAKE TO CLUSTER, TWIN, RAINBOW, SNAG, HORSESHOE, AND SWAN LAKES LOOP

Mike White

MILES: 22.0
RECOMMENDED DAYS: 2–4
ELEVATION GAIN/LOSS: 2500´/2500´
TYPE OF TRIP: Loop
DIFFICULTY: Easy
SOLITUDE: Moderate solitude
LOCATION: Lassen Volcanic National Park
MAPS: USGS 7.5-min. *Reading Peak*, *West Prospect Peak*,
        Prospect Peak, and *Mt. Harkness*
BEST SEASON: Summer through early fall

PERMITS

A free wilderness permit, required for overnight stays in Lassen Volcanic National Park, can be obtained in person from any ranger or information station during regular business hours. Applications may be downloaded from the park's website (www.nps.gov/lavo/planyourvisit/wilderness-permit-information.htm) and returned to the park via email or fax (530-595-3262). Allow two

Photo: Snag Lake, one of the larger lakes in Lassen Volcanic National Park weeks for processing. After business hours, backpackers may self-register at the Kohm Yah-mah-nee visitor center near the southwest entrance.

CHALLENGES

Campfires and pets are not permitted within Lassen Volcanic National Park. Mosquitoes can be problematic through midsummer—bring a tent and repellent.

HOW TO GET THERE

From either the Manzanita Lake or the southwest entrances, follow the main park road to the access road to the Summit Lake ranger station, 0.3 mile north of the turnoff for the North Summit Lake Campground. Head east, past the ranger station, and park in the overnight parking area.

TRIP DESCRIPTION

From the overnight parking area, follow a boardwalk east across a spongy clearing—a finger of Dersch Meadows—into a mixed forest of red firs, lodgepole pines, and western white pines. After crossing a lush swale, make a brief ascent over a low hill to the northeast shore of Summit Lake, passing a junction with a lateral from North Summit Lake Campground. Continue a short distance to a well-signed Y-junction with a trail to Corral Meadow.

Turn left (east), following signs toward Echo Lake, and make a moderate climb up a gully and a ridge to a switchback, where you have an excellent view of Lassen Peak to the west and Crescent Crater on the peak's north flank. Continue climbing through open forest, across a slope carpeted with pinemat manzanita and some greenleaf manzanita. Reach a plateau, where you find a junction with the trail continuing west toward Echo Lake (this is your return route).

TAKE THIS TRIP

Numerous lakes, easy terrain, and a lack of crowds make this trip a backpacker's paradise. This loop takes you to several of the best lakes in the park, and since these lakes are never too far apart, you have plenty of opportunities for camping and swimming. (However, fishing is limited.) The gentle terrain makes getting around fairly easy, a particular bonus for families with young children. And with a remote location in northeastern California, far from any of the state's urban centers, there are no quotas and few people to share the backcountry with too many others. Other options are also possible with this trip: It's easily reversible, and thanks to a number of connecting trails, you could extend your trip, or use layover days to dayhike to a variety of destinations.

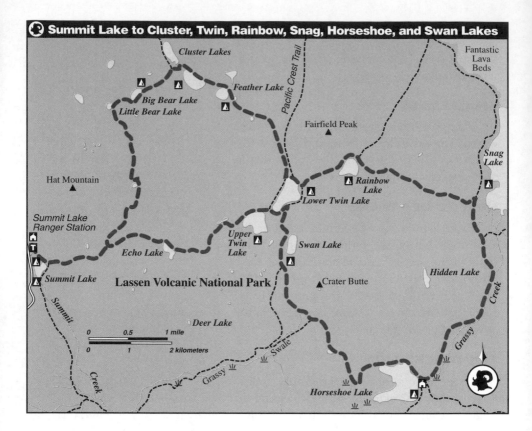

Turn left (north) at the junction, and make a gradual then moderate climb to a high point atop a rumpled plateau of old lava flows. From there, follow a northward descent to a shallow unnamed lake, a pleasant swimming hole by midsummer. A half mile of gently graded trail leads across the plateau, past a tiny pond, before a moderate-to-steep descent takes you down a ridge that separates a pair of small, glaciated canyons. The grade eases and the forest thickens on the approach to shallow, lodgepole-lined Little Bear Lake, which has good swimming but hordes of mosquitoes through midsummer. It also lacks campsites due to the sloping topography around the lake. A short but steep descent brings you to Big Bear Lake, also ringed by lodgepole pines but not quite as shallow as its counterpart. Passable campsites near the northeast and south shores lure tired backpackers.

Away from Big Bear Lake, a gentle, half-mile descent leads to a junction with a trail to Badger Flat. The northernmost Cluster Lake, which has good campsites near its north end, is just 200 yards down this trail. This lake becomes less attractive by mid-July, when the surface level drops about a foot and the western arm disappears entirely, reducing the lake size by about a third. Unfortunately, prior to mid-July, this and the other Cluster Lakes suffer from a healthy population of mosquitoes.

Continuing ahead (east) from the junction, reach the north shore of Silver Lake after an easy stroll. Follow the trail around the lake's northeast side, through a mixed forest of western white pines, lodgepole pines, and red firs—the trademark forest of Lassen's backcountry. Shallow Silver Lake, the largest of the Cluster Lakes, has several campsites, but make sure you select a site at least 100 feet from the water. In early morning, sunlit Lassen Peak reflects brightly in the dark, placid surface.

Continue ahead (southeast) over a low drainage that separates Silver and Feather lakes, the latter of which is perhaps the best of all the Cluster Lakes. The unnamed triangular lake 200 yards north of Feather Lake is also quite pleasant, for, despite its shallowness, the lake doesn't attract many mosquitoes—an important consideration for campers prior to late July. By early August, all of the Cluster Lakes, as well as the Twin Lakes, drop a foot or so, and a narrow ring of tiny, yellow, primrose monkeyflowers bloom around the lakes.

Leaving Cluster Lakes behind the trail proceeds southeast through mixed forest, past a chest-deep pond to a low point at the usually dry, rocky swale that serves as the seasonal outlet for Twin Lakes. A short climb from there brings you to a junction, where your trail merges with the wide path of an old roadbed that now serves as a section of the famed Mexico-to-Canada Pacific Crest Trail.

On a not-too-scenic section of this usually scenic trail, you pass a small, seasonal pond on the right, and the backcountry cabin that serves as the Twin Lake ranger station on your left. Proceed a short distance to the north shore of Lower Twin Lake and a junction. Remaining on the PCT, head around the east side of the large, but relatively shallow lake past several lodgepole-shaded campsites. The water temperature is usually warm enough by mid- to late July to provide refreshing swimming. Expect voracious mosquitoes before late July and vociferous Stellar jays throughout the season. Proceed shortly to another junction, where the southbound PCT continues ahead.

Leaving the PCT, turn left and travel east and then northeast on a gentle climb to crescent-shaped Rainbow Lake. Peakbaggers can leave the trail just before the lake and head north cross-country 0.5 mile to the top of 7160-foot Fairfield Peak. Steep terrain surrounding Rainbow Lake limits the number of available campsites. However, at the south end, a use trail heads around the lake to a few small campsites with filtered views of Lassen Peak. Above the northeast shore is a junction with a trail heading northeast toward Cinder Cone.

From the junction, follow the right-hand trail on a brief climb southeast to the crest of a low ridge, and then drop to a nearby gully. A protracted traverse leads across rolling terrain on tread so deep and loose, it feels like you're walking on a sandy beach. A profusion of Bloomer's goldenbush—a late-blooming sunflower that thrives in dry, gravelly flats—binds the loose soils somewhat, offering some stability. Midway between Rainbow and Snag lakes, the trail begins a steep descent that may be accompanied by more gravel-loving wildflowers, including cycladenia, with tubular rose flowers and broad, smooth-edged leaves; and Lobb's nama, with tubular magenta flowers and narrower, shallow-toothed leaves. Less attractive is the increasing evidence of a fire that has devastated acres of lodgepole pine forest. About a quarter mile before Snag Lake, you cross a rivulet and proceed to a junction a good distance away from the southwest shore.

Due to the fire, campsites along Snag Lake's northwest shore have lost much of their appeal. However, the peninsula just north of the junction has an intact grove of trees that shades several good campsites. The water around the peninsula is fairly shallow—5 to 10 feet in most places—and therefore quite warm, luring weary backpackers with the prospect of a refreshing swim. Anglers can ply the waters in search of good-size rainbow trout.

If you're not camping at Snag Lake, turn south at the junction, and soon pass a junction with a trail heading around the south and east sides of the lake. Continue ahead, and follow the Grassy Creek Trail on a gentle-to-moderate ascent a little more than 2 miles to Horseshoe Lake. Initially, the trail crosses moist-to-dry soils characterized by spreading phlox, coyote mint, dwarf lousewort, California stickseed, and California butterweed. After a half mile, the trail draws alongside the creek, where July visitors will be presented with a lush, wildflower extravaganza that includes several dozen species, including corn lily, marsh marigold, alpine shooting star, Nuttall's larkspur, crimson columbine, wandering daisy, common dandelion, and yarrow. Fortunate botanists may find all three of the park's stickseeds, all six violets, and many representatives of the figwort and buttercup families.

Follow the charming creek through a forest of western white pines and firs and an understory of thick shrubs that threaten to overgrow the trail. About halfway to Horseshoe Lake, the narrowing canyon forces you to make a couple creek crossings over a set of log rounds. Beyond the crossings, it becomes evident why the stream is named Grassy Creek: Lush grasses line the banks all the way to a verdant swale near the Horseshoe Lake ranger station, where you reach a junction with a trail to Juniper Lake.

Turn right (northwest) and travel briefly upstream along the bank of Grassy Creek to the outlet of Horseshoe Lake, which, with a view of Lassen Peak across the water, is a fine setting for lunch or a rest stop. A sign and map indicates that camping along the north shore of the lake is not allowed (backpackers wishing to camp nearby should backtrack to the junction and head south to the camping area near the east shore). Proceed along the north shore, past a small peninsula that affords a good, if rather plain, view across the lake. The north half of the lake offers a very attractive, oversized swimming hole; the lake's pebbly bottom quickly drops away from the shore to level off at about 10 to 15 feet, without rocks, snags, and other submerged obstacles for swimmers to fret about. Since the middle of the lake is relatively shallow—less than 5 feet deep in places—colder water from the deeper, southern half is effectively kept out of the north end, where water temperatures become relatively warm by midsummer.

Away from Horseshoe Lake, the trail follows a nearly level course for nearly 1.5 miles through the forest and past a handful of seasonal ponds on the way to a junction with a lateral to the trail down Grassy Swale.

Proceed ahead (northwest) on the right-hand trail, dipping across a verdant swale lined with vibrant wildflowers and lush plants at the head of Grassy Swale, and then begin a moderately steep climb up a side canyon that is nearly as verdant. A mosaic of flowers includes Applegate's paintbrush, Christine's lupine, California stickseed, coyote mint, and mountain violet. Where the grade eventually eases, on the way around the western base of Crater Butte to a junction with the Pacific Crest Trail, you may notice silver-leaved lupine and pumice paintbrush monopolizing the gravelly forest floor. A 0.6-mile, 500-foot ascent southeast to the summit of Crater Butte is a straightforward enterprise from the vicinity of the junction; it takes about an hour round trip. Like nearby Fairfield Peak, the butte is composed mainly of lava flows instead of cinders, although both peaks are technically referred to as cinder cones.

Proceed north on the PCT for about 250 yards to the crest of a low divide, and then drop into the Butte Creek drainage on the way to forest-rimmed Swan Lake. Backpackers who plan to overnight at this typical, forest-rimmed Lassen lake can find passable campsites above the south shore, or along an east-shore bench. The trail draws near to the lake at the northeast corner, then immediately crosses the barely discernible outlet before leaving Swan Lake.

Rainbow Lake

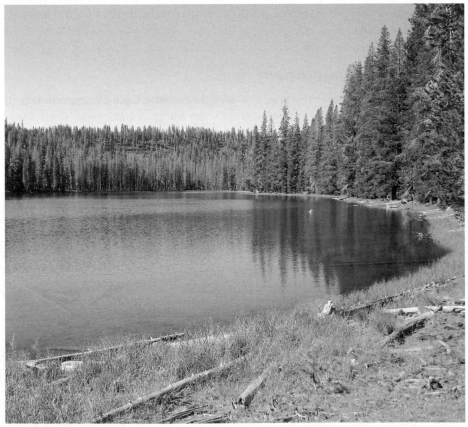

After surmounting a low rise north of Swan Lake, you make a mild descent on the lupine-lined PCT to a junction near the southeast shore of lodgepole-fringed Lower Twin Lake. Turn left at the junction, and pass around the south shore of Lower Twin Lake to a junction on the far side.

At that junction, turn left again to follow the usually dry outlet a short distance to Upper Twin Lake. From there, the trail skirts the north shore along the base of a steep slope that limits potential campsites to the west, south, and east shores. Beyond Upper Twin Lake, a moderately steep climb incorporating a few switchbacks takes you past a fair-size pond. A long stretch of gentle ascent, followed by a short, stiff climb leads to another pond, this one backdropped by a talus slope. More climbing precedes a short drop to Echo Lake, which displays a fine, forest-lake ecotone—a transition zone between forest plants and lakeshore plants. Pinemat manzanita, characteristic of well-drained forest slopes, gives way to red mountain heathers only a few feet from shore. In turn, heathers give way to a thin band of shoreline species, most notably western blueberry, primrose monkey flower, and moss. Sedges flourish along the shoreline and advance into the shallow water near the lake's edge. Due to its proximity to the trailhead, camping is not allowed at Echo Lake.

A mild climb across the floor of Echo Lake's basin is followed by a steeper ascent of a shrub-covered slope, where tobacco brush, chinquapin, and manzanita flourish. Where the grade eases, you stroll across the top of a lightly forested bench to the trail junction at the close of the loop. Turn southwest to retrace your steps to the trailhead.

BUILD-UP AND WIND-DOWN TIPS ·

Before your trip, reserve a spot at one of the **Summit Lake campgrounds** (call 877-444-6777), and get a jump on acclimatizing for your backpack. The restaurant at the **Kohm Yah-mah-nee visitor center** (opening fall of 2008) and the snack bar at the **Manzanita Lake Camper Service Store** are the only two places within the park to grab a bite to eat or get something to drink.

Although reservations at the **Drakesbad Guest Ranch** (530-529-1512, www. drakesbad.com) are difficult to come by—it has a 99 percent occupancy rate during July and August—you could experience a grand end to your backpack with a stay at this historic resort. On the National Registry of Historic Places, the ranch is operated in much the same way it was when it was established in 1900—without phones or electricity. The 17 guest rooms, with either a half or full bath, are lit by kerosene lamps and heated by propane. Perhaps the most notable feature of the ranch is the swimming pool heated by natural hot springs. Excellent meals are served for breakfast, lunch, and dinner, and the restaurant has a good selection of beers and wines.

69

CENTRAL CARIBOU LAKES LOOP

Mike White

MILES: 12.0
RECOMMENDED DAYS: 2
ELEVATION GAIN/LOSS: 900´/900´
TYPE OF TRIP: Loop
DIFFICULTY: Easy
SOLITUDE: Moderately populated
LOCATION: Caribou Wilderness
MAPS: USGS 7.5-min. *Bogard Buttes* and *Red Cinder*;
U.S. Forest Service *A Guide to Ishi, Thousand Lakes, and Caribou Wildernesses*
BEST SEASON: Summer through early fall

PERMITS

Wilderness permits are not required for trips in Caribou Wilderness.

CHALLENGES

Mosquitoes are problematic through midsummer—bring a tent and plenty of repellent.

Photo: Jewel Lake in Caribou Wilderness

TAKE THIS TRIP

Lakes, lakes, and more lakes await you in the Caribou Wilderness—and the good news is that most of them are well suited for camping, swimming, and angling. The terrain here is relatively flat, making this trip a good choice for backpackers of all ages and conditions. (Although, with few significant landmarks, getting lost away from the trail is quite possible.) Dramatic peaks are lacking here, but the part of the route that climbs to Rim and Cypress lakes provides scenic views from the edge of a prominent escarpment.

HOW TO GET THERE

County Road A21 provides a shortcut between Highway 36 in the town of Westwood to Highway 44. From A21, about 14 miles north of Westwood and 4.5 miles south of the Highway 44 junction, turn west onto Silver Lake Road (County Road 110) and proceed 5 miles to a junction with Forest Service Road 10. Following signed directions for Caribou Wilderness, turn right and travel on Road 10 for 0.4 mile to another junction. Remaining on Road 10, continue another 0.2 mile and then turn left at a road marked CARIBOU WILDERNESS EAST TRAILHEAD, CARIBOU LAKE. Proceed on single-lane road for 0.1 mile to a fork, and then follow the left-hand road a short way to the large overnight parking area.

TRIP DESCRIPTION

From the overnight parking lot, make a short climb northwest up a hillside to the trailhead above heavily fished Caribou Lake. From there, proceed west through a forest of lodgepole pines, Jeffrey pines, and firs, passing a feeder trail from the private homes around Silver Lake just before the signed wilderness boundary. The trail skirts a fair-size pond covered with lily pads and then passes a smaller pond before reaching a junction, where the loop portion of the trip begins.

Follow the right-hand trail west, and very shortly arrive at the east shore of Cowboy Lake, which is mostly too shallow for decent swimming. However, the shoreline does provide a scenic spot from which to enjoy a view of the lake, picturesquely backdropped by low cliffs on the west side. Proceed around the north shore of the lake to the west end, where the trail turns sharply north-northwest on a moderate, switchbacking climb up an escarpment into a dry, open forest, where pinemat and greenleaf manzanita flourish and a few juniper take root. Soon, the trail heads back into deeper forest cover, reaching Jewel Lake

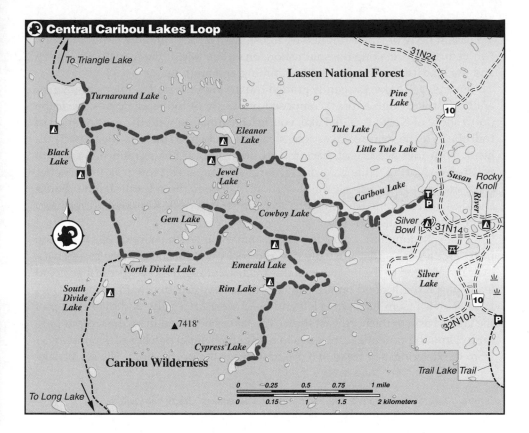

Central Caribou Lakes Loop

To Triangle Lake

Turnaround Lake

Lassen National Forest

Pine Lake

10

Eleanor Lake

Tule Lake

Little Tule Lake

Black Lake

Jewel Lake

Caribou Lake

Susan Rocky Knoll

River

T P

Gem Lake

Cowboy Lake

Silver Bowl

31N14

North Divide Lake

Emerald Lake

South Divide Lake

Rim Lake

Silver Lake

10

▲7418'

32N10A

P

Cypress Lake

Caribou Wilderness

Trail Lake Trail

To Long Lake

| 0 | 0.25 | 0.5 | 0.75 | 1 mile |
| 0 | 0.15 | 1 | 1.5 | 2 kilometers |

at the top of the climb, where good campsites may be found above the north shore, as well as near the southwest shore of nearby Eleanor Lake, which is accessible from the main trail via a pair of use trails heading north. Both of these shallow lakes possess their own unique charm—Jewel has a scenic setting and greater depth, and Eleanor offers a peaceful, secluded environment. Despite its appearance on USGS and USFS maps, the connecting trail from the east end of Jewel Lake heading south to the trail from Gem Lake no longer exists.

From Jewel Lake, the trail winds through an open forest past some small ponds before climbing moderately along the base of a brushy escarpment. Where the grade eases again, you pass more ponds, some seasonal in nature, before gently descending trail leads to a three-way junction between a trail north to Turnaround Lake and south to Black Lake.

To visit Turnaround Lake, follow nearly level path 0.15 mile to the south shore. In early season, a very shallow finger extends south of the lake's main body. Spacious campsites can be found near the south shore, west of this finger. More campsites are located along the east side of the lake, but the ones offering the most solitude are on the less-traveled west side. After a visit to Turnaround Lake, retrace your steps south to the junction north of Black Lake.

Turn left (south) and walk about 200 yards to the north shore of Black Lake, a pleasant body of water rimmed by forest, with a rock cliff above the far shore. Fair campsites are along the south shore on either side of the usually dry outlet, and the lake itself offers passable swimming and angling.

From Black Lake, the gently graded trail follows the outlet downstream generally south through a forest composed primarily of lodgepole pines. Near the north shore of North Divide Lake, you reach a junction with the continuation of trail ahead to the string of lakes accessible primarily from the Hay Meadow Trailhead. Your trail heads east, back toward the Caribou Lake Trailhead. Knee- to waist-deep North Divide Lake offers marginal campsites. However, much better campsites may be had above the west shore of deeper, though still shallow, South Divide Lake, 0.3 mile to the south, across a stretch of flower-covered meadow and through a stand of forest.

From the junction, the route passes above the north shore of North Divide Lake, crosses the outlet's usually dry and rocky channel, and then crosses back over the channel to the north bank. Gently descending tread veers northeast and leads past a small pond on the way to a three-way junction with a trail to Gem Lake. To visit Gem Lake, turn left and head west up a gully and over the lip of the lake's basin to the northeast shore. The lake is hemmed in by the steep topography, limiting potential campsites to a few small, level patches of ground away from the deteriorating tread of a use trail above the north shore. The scenic lake

Emerald Lake offers anglers fine fishing and backpackers shady campsites.

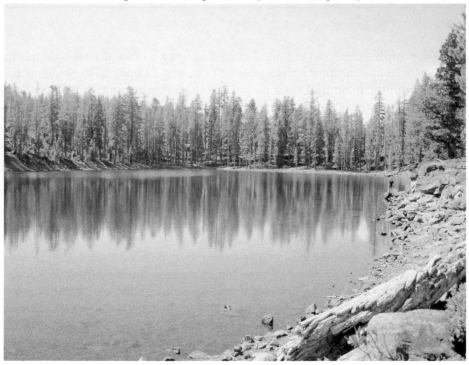

offers refreshing swimming and fair fishing. After visiting Gem Lake, retrace your steps to the junction. From there, head southeast and stroll past a seasonal pond/meadow to a junction with the trail to Emerald, Rim, and Cypress lakes.

Turn right (south) and make a very brief climb through open forest, across pinemat manzanita-covered slopes, to the northeast shore of Emerald Lake, one of the deepest lakes in Caribou Wilderness. The low, rocky bench on the lake's north side has several good campsites. Anglers should find the fishing to be fair to good, and swimmers will enjoy a refreshing dip throughout the summer season.

Beyond the steep-sided bowl of Emerald Lake, the trail follows a winding course through mostly open terrain past a seasonal pond/meadow to the edge of an escarpment with a good view of Caribou and Silver lakes and the surrounding terrain. The trail then winds among sparse forest and bedrock slabs toward Rim Lake. The route over these slabs may be difficult to discern at times, but a preponderance of ducks should help keep you on track. If you happen to lose the route, simply walk upslope toward the west for about a half mile, and you're almost certain to run into Rim Lake, which is located on the very edge of a steep escarpment. On a hot day, Rim Lake can be a welcome sight, despite the shallow waters at the east end; swimmers will find the depth adequate and diving rocks midway along the south shore to be much more inviting. Spartan campsites are scattered between rock slabs around the well-named lake; what they lack in shade, they make up for in sweeping views from the edge of the escarpment. A persistent breeze helps keep the mosquitoes at bay, at least until their numbers diminish after midseason.

A winding, rocky trail continues the climb away from Rim Lake for a half mile to an unnamed lake backdropped by a prominent cliff. The trail swings around the lake's south arm, which is also at the brink of a cliff, and then rolls over a low divide to Cypress Lake. Rockbound and scenic, Cypress Lake was mistakenly named for the few western junipers nearby; true cypress trees are nonexistent in these parts. Secluded campsites may be found among the small slabs and gravel flats tucked around the lakeshore. From the low divide near the lake, cross-country enthusiasts can follow a straightforward route north and then northeast to the summit of North Caribou Peak in about an hour. After fully enjoying Cypress, Rim, and Emerald lakes, retrace your steps to the junction north of Emerald Lake.

Turn right and proceed east-southeast through mixed forest on a moderate descent that is interrupted briefly by a gently graded stretch of trail. Where the descent resumes, switchbacks lead down the steep wall of a prominent escarpment until the trail bottoms out near the base of talus slope. Soon, the trail turns north and passes to the right of an unnamed pond before intersecting the main trail from Caribou Lake at the close of the loop. Turn right (east) and retrace your steps 0.7 mile to the trailhead.

BUILD-UP AND WIND-DOWN TIPS••••••••••••••••••••••••••••

Except for two **Forest Service campgrounds**, Rocky Knoll and Silver Bowl, there are no amenities near the Caribou Wilderness. If you happen to be traveling back home by way of Chester, you'll have some options for grabbing a post-trip meal. The **Pine Shack Frosty** (321 Main St., 530-258-2593) offers old-fashioned hamburgers, fries, and shakes, while the **Pizza Factory** (197 Main St., 530-258-3155) serves up a decent pie. A caffeine fix for the long drive home can be satisfied at **Three Beans Coffee House & Bakery** (150 Main St., 530-258-3312). **Cynthia's** (278 Main Street; 530-258-1966), where indoor and outdoor seating is available during the summer months (reservations recommended), is the best spot for upscale fare. The restaurant serves lunch (Monday and Tuesday, and Thursday through Saturday) and dinner (Monday and Tuesday, Thursday through Sunday).

70

TREELINE CIRCUMNAVIGATION OF MOUNT SHASTA

Michael Zanger and Andy Selters

MILES: 25.0–30.0, depending on specific route
RECOMMENDED DAYS: 5–7
ELEVATION GAIN/LOSS: 2500´/2500´
TYPE OF TRIP: Loop
DIFFICULTY: Moderately strenuous
SOLITUDE: Solitude
LOCATION: Mount Shasta Wilderness, Shasta-Trinity National Forest
MAPS: *Mt. Shasta Wilderness Recreation Map* from Wilderness Press;
USGS 7.5-min. *Mt. Shasta* and *Hotlum*
BEST SEASON: Summer through early fall

PERMITS ·

While there is currently no quota limiting backpacking, the Forest Service requires a permit for overnight stays in Mt. Shasta Wilderness. You can get one at the Ranger District office: 204 W. Alma Street, Mt. Shasta, CA 96067, 530-926-4511. Otherwise, you can get a self-issue permit from the bulletin board outside the office or at the trailhead. There is no fee for the permit.

Photo: Mt. Shasta from the north

CHALLENGES

In route finding, strenuousness, and terrain, this trip should be considered a moderate but long mountaineering endeavor. Very fit hikers can complete the route in four days, and five should be comfortable for most backpackers. Plan your route carefully to camp at water sources, and find passages across some of the canyons. Shasta's relatively open slopes help make route finding fairly easy, but the soft, ashy ground occasionally gets tedious. It's necessary to know how to self-arrest and to carry an ice ax in early season on the high snowfields.

HOW TO GET THERE

There are two trails to Horse Camp, your starting point, off Everitt Highway, one from Bunny Flat Trailhead and another from Sand Flat Trailhead. More people take the trail from Bunny Flat because it climbs more gradually and starts 100 feet higher. From the town of Mt. Shasta, Bunny Flat is 10.9 miles up Everitt Highway, and the trailhead is right beside the road. A large parking area, an outhouse, and a bulletin board with information and self-issuing wilderness permits are located here.

TAKE THIS TRIP

When John Muir, America's most eloquent and far-traveled naturalist, first caught sight of Shasta from the Sacramento River canyon in 1875, he exclaimed, ". . . I was fifty miles away and afoot, alone and weary. Yet all my blood turned to wine, and I have not been weary since." Muir, the quintessential mountaineer, who circled the mountain in segments over more than a decade, found Shasta's circumnavigation to be perhaps more appealing than the ascent:

> Arctic beauty and desolation, with their blessings and dangers, all may be found here, to test the endurance and skill of adventurous climbers; but far better than climbing the mountain is going around its warm, fertile base, enjoying its bounties like a bee circling a bank of flowers . . . . As you sweep around so grand a center the mountain itself seems to turn . . . . One glacier after another comes into view, and the outlines of the mountain are ever changing.

Relatively few people take this ultimate Shasta backpack, partly because it's a fairly committing endeavor, with no trail to follow. But in these days of abundant trails on most mountains and in nearly every wilderness area, this kind of trip poses a welcome, off-trail adventure. Indeed, you can easily imagine that you're following John Muir's footsteps. Crossing the toes of several Shasta glaciers offers superb views, and the short side trips to view waterfalls—in particular Whitney and Ash Creek falls—are well worth the extra time. Experienced backpackers who are comfortable with occasional scrambling should not be deterred from taking this trip, one of California's finest and least-traveled backcountry hikes.

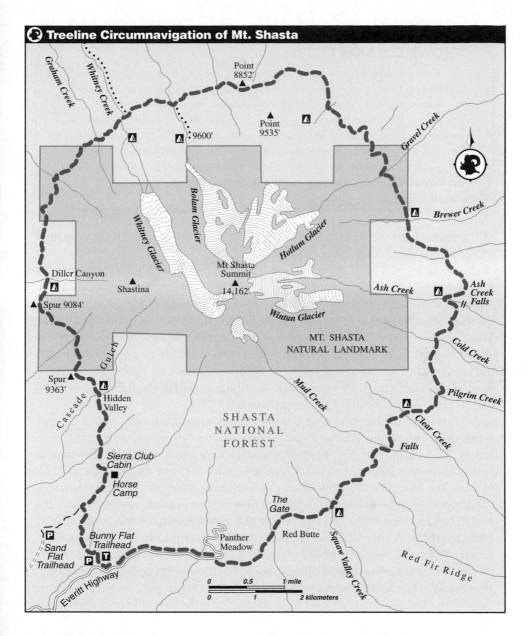

Treeline Circumnavigation of Mt. Shasta

Graham Creek
Whitney Creek
Point 8852'
Point 9535'
9600'
Gravel Creek
Brewer Creek
Bolam Glacier
Whitney Glacier
Hotlum Glacier
Diller Canyon
Shastina
Mt Shasta Summit 14,162'
Ash Creek
Ash Creek Falls
Spur 9084'
Wintun Glacier
MT. SHASTA NATURAL LANDMARK
Cold Creek
Spur 9363'
Cascade Gulch
Hidden Valley
Mud Creek
Pilgrim Creek
Clear Creek
Falls
SHASTA NATIONAL FOREST
Sierra Club Cabin
Horse Camp
The Gate
Red Butte
Squaw Valley Creek
Sand Flat Trailhead
Bunny Flat Trailhead
Panther Meadow
Red Fir Ridge
Everitt Highway

0   0.5   1 mile
0   1   2 kilometers

TRIP DESCRIPTION

While backpackers can choose to circle Mt. Shasta at different elevations, a clockwise direction, usually beginning and ending at the Sierra Club's cabin at Horse Camp, is preferred: water sources, campsites, and scenery continually improve in this direction, and most of the tiresome scree is dealt with initially. Though many route variations are possible—especially on the mountain's west flanks—most hikers will stay near the 8000-foot level (approximately at tree line). Since there is no beaten trail to follow, here is a very general description

SNOWFIELD SAFETY

Early summer in the mountains is a magical time: long days, early wildflowers, overflowing lakes, and . . . large snowfields. Consolidated summer snowfields can pose a hazard to ill-equipped hikers, especially during morning hours when the snow is still frozen. Consider carrying a lightweight set of crampons and an ice axe (and know how to use them) to safely traverse these snowfields; the alternative can be a dangerous slip or slide . . . or a lengthy detour. Light four-point instep crampons are usually adequate. You might also consider a basic mountaineering course in snow safety—it is time and money well spent.

of the route, with mention of key canyon crossings, important landmarks, and campsites.

Starting from Horse Camp, you can stay low, perhaps planning to spend the first night in Cascade Gulch or Diller Canyon. In dry years these canyons might not offer water although you can always count on finding snow to melt in Diller Canyon. An alternative route is to go high and spend the first night in Hidden Valley, where water is always available. This enables a slightly higher traverse around Shastina, over spurs 9363 and 9084. Staying high gives you a wonderfully scenic and somewhat shorter route, but it takes you across some trying scree slopes, and you have to negotiate some short cliff bands, 0.25 mile south of Diller Canyon and about 0.75 mile north of it.

To traverse the Graham Creek-Bolam Creek area, it's best to avoid the morainal hills below the Whitney and Bolam glaciers by going somewhat high across the terminus of the Whitney glacier. There are small grassy areas and springs for camping west of the Whitney Glacier toe, but they can be difficult to find. The beautiful Whitney Glacier is California's longest. Famous geologist Clarence King, who is credited with discovering the glaciers on Mt. Shasta, the first to be identified in the U.S., made one of the first ascents of this route in 1870. From the toe of Whitney Glacier enjoy a worthy side trip to scenic Whitney Falls. Follow Whitney Creek downhill for almost a mile, staying on the east side of the canyon for easier going and excellent views. For those who go high, good campsites await in the basin below the Bolam Glacier, at about 9600 feet. To continue clockwise from this area, it's best to descend along the east side of Bolam Creek to tree line.

In the North Gate vicinity, most hikers contour south of Point 8852 and gradually lose elevation as they continue east. Another option is to climb over the morainal benches near Point 9535, where there's excellent camping on flat, sandy ground, and almost always snowmelt for water. To continue east off these benches, descend sandy gullies through some cliff bands east-southeast of Point 9535 and contour toward Gravel Creek. Those who are relatively high will likely have some difficulty crossing Gravel Creek's canyon. The canyon walls consist of steep, unstable ash with large, precariously perched boulders. Members of a party must take special care to avoid knocking rocks onto one another, and not climb directly below or above one another. Below 7500 feet the canyon walls are safer and not as high. Here are excellent views of the Hotlum Glacier and its steep icefalls. Excellent campsites in a beautiful hemlock forest are found at Brewer Creek (reliable and clear).

The next key point is Ash Creek near the falls. To get there, hike through whitebark pine parklands near the 8000-foot level across Brewer Creek. Contour left around the ridge just north of the falls at 7800 feet and then cut back west to descend into the canyon above the falls. An 8-foot cliff on this descent requires some scrambling. Solid snow—avalanche debris—usually offers a convenient

Ash Creek Falls

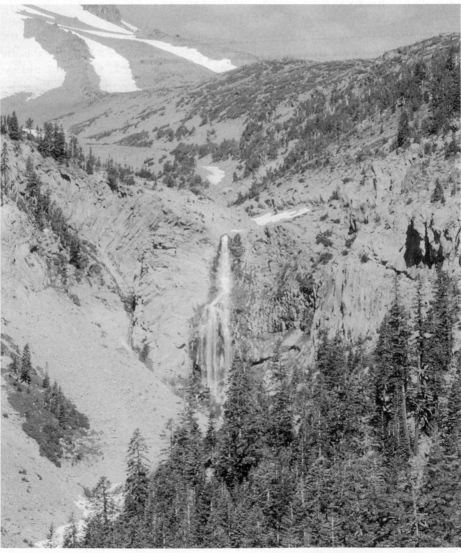

bridge across Ash Creek until late in summer. A short walk east offers spectacular views of the almost 300-foot Ash Creek Falls, one of John Muir's favorite sights on Mt. Shasta. On the south side of the canyon, climb directly upslope through a band of whitebark pines.

Cold Creek, Pilgrim Creek, and Clear Creek are all reliable and silt-free. Contour around Clear Creek's canyon at about 7800 feet to set up for the crucial crossing of intimidating Mud Creek canyon. From around 7700 feet on the canyon rim, drop straight into the canyon on a loose, sandy rib, at the uppermost grove of full-size Shasta red firs, just up-canyon from a bare, obvious landslide area. Near the canyon bottom, again take special care to avoid sending rocks onto partners. Cross Mud Creek a couple hundred yards above the falls, and climb directly up a steep, faint drainage to get back out of the canyon. This exit is important; large rocks offer reliable stepping stones to the rim. From the southwest rim of the canyon, a course that contours near 7800 feet takes you around Red Fir Ridge to Squaw Valley Creek. The lush meadows here offer one of the nicest campsites on the mountain. From here you can traverse north of Red Butte on an excellent use trail through the Gate to Panther Meadow (or the old ski bowl) and return to Everitt Highway. About 2 miles down this road (or 3 miles from the old ski bowl) is the Bunny Flat Trailhead.

BUILD-UP AND WIND-DOWN TIPS

Two establishments in the town of Mount Shasta should not be missed in preparing for this circumnavigation. The **Fifth Season** outdoor store (300 North Mt. Shasta Boulevard, 530-926-3606) has a complete range of outdoor equipment, including rental gear. Guidebooks, maps, and the latest information on mountain conditions are also available. **Berryvale Market** (305 South Mt. Shasta Boulevard, 530-926-1576) has an excellent selection of organic, natural, and hard-to-find foods, including lots of "goodies" for a backpack trip. **Castle Lake** and the many excellent swimming holes on the **South Fork Sacramento River** above Lake Siskiyou are fine places to wash off the trail dust and soak aching muscles after a long backpack.

WARNER MOUNTAINS

T he remote Warner Mountains are California's northeasternmost range, separating the Modoc Plateau to the west from the Great Basin to the east. Bearing affinities to both geologic provinces, the range is composed of multiple thick lava flows similar to the Modoc Plateau, and is a dipping fault-block range similar to those of the Great Basin. The Surprise Valley fault system trailing the Warner's eastern escarpment is the principal site of the area's ongoing faulting, stretching the land and causing Surprise Valley to sink over time. Today the valley is filled with deep sediments capped by three large, muddy, and extremely shallow alkali lakes. Thinning of the crust has allowed magma to work toward the surface, heating the groundwater and giving rise to a string of hot springs.

The tiny hamlet of Alturas is the nearest jumping-off point for trips into the Warner Mountains, located at the junctions of U.S. Highway 395 and State Highway 299. Alturas is the county seat of Modoc County, a vast volcanic region where cattle far outnumber people. Highway 299 bisects the Warner Mountains, the lower northern half traversed by four-wheel-drive roads and the higher southern half traversed by trails. This roadless area is home to the 70,385-acre South Warner Wilderness, a west-dipping range reminiscent of a miniature Sierra Nevada. The principal trail in the wilderness is the Summit Trail, a 22.5-mile route that traverses the north-south trending crest of the range. The lone entry from the South Warner Wilderness in this book follows the northern section of this scenic trail to lovely Patterson Lake, nestled below the rugged cliffs of 9710-foot Warren Peak.

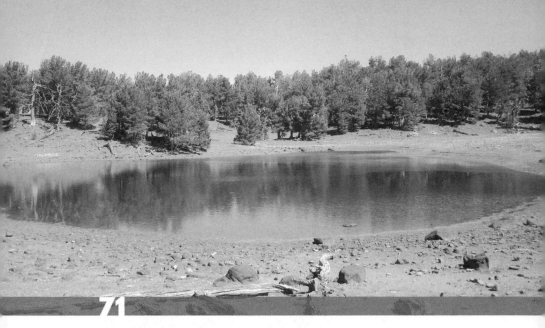

71

THE SUMMIT TRAIL: PEPPERDINE TRAILHEAD TO PATTERSON LAKE

Mike White

MILES: 12.0
RECOMMENDED DAYS: 2
ELEVATION GAIN/LOSS: 2400´/2400´
TYPE OF TRIP: Out-and-back
DIFFICULTY: Moderate
SOLITUDE: Moderate solitude
LOCATION: South Warner Wilderness, Modoc National Forest
MAPS: USGS 7.5-min. *Warren Peak*,
U.S. Forest Service *South Warner Wilderness*
BEST SEASON: Summer through fall

PERMITS ·

Permits are not required in the South Warner Wilderness.

Photo: Shallow Cottonwood Lake lies just to the north of the more prized Patterson Lake.

CHALLENGES

Cattle are allowed to graze within the South Warner Wilderness and may be encountered at any time between July and September. The remote location in extreme northeastern California makes for a long drive to the trailhead from any major urban area. Although there are a few stores in Alturas, backpacking gear is hard to come by in the area.

HOW TO GET THERE

From the south part of Alturas, about 1 mile south of the Highway 299 junction, leave U.S. Highway 395 and head east on County Road 56, passing Dorris Reservoir and remaining on Road 56 at a junction with County Road 58 on the left. Proceed 12.6 miles from 395 to the Modoc Forest boundary, where the surface turns to gravel and the road becomes Forest Road 5. Continue another 1.1 miles from the boundary to a junction, where Road 5 curves southwest, but you take the left-hand branch onto Forest Road 31. Drive 6.6 miles on 31 to a well-signed junction with the short road to the Pepperdine Trailhead on the right. Follow this road past the equestrian trailhead to the hiker trailhead near the entrance to Pepperdine Campground.

TRIP DESCRIPTION

Amid shady white firs, the trail immediately passes the path from the equestrian trailhead on the right and climbs moderately to moderately steeply up the forested slope. Break out of the trees near the signed wilderness boundary and climb more mildly across open volcanic slopes, where you will experience the first of the many impressive vistas to come. Westward views include Alturas and the upper Pit River valley, along with snowcapped Mt. Shasta and, farther up the trail, Lassen Peak. Eastward is the classic basin and range topography of the Great Basin, vividly displayed by Surprise Valley and the alkali

TAKE THIS TRIP

A narrow, linear range trending north-south, the South Warner Mountains are more similar in nature to mountain ranges in the Great Basin to the east than to those in the Golden State. Another dissimilarity to many other California mountain ranges is a lack of people—thanks to its remote setting in the extreme northeastern part of the state, you may not see another soul during this trip. On clear days, 100-mile vistas from this crest-hugging trail are quite common, stretching from the high desert of southern Oregon and northwestern Nevada to the Cascade summits of Mt. Shasta, Lassen Peak, and beyond. Patterson Lake is a cirque-bound, scenic body of water providing a destination worthy of the most discriminating backpacker.

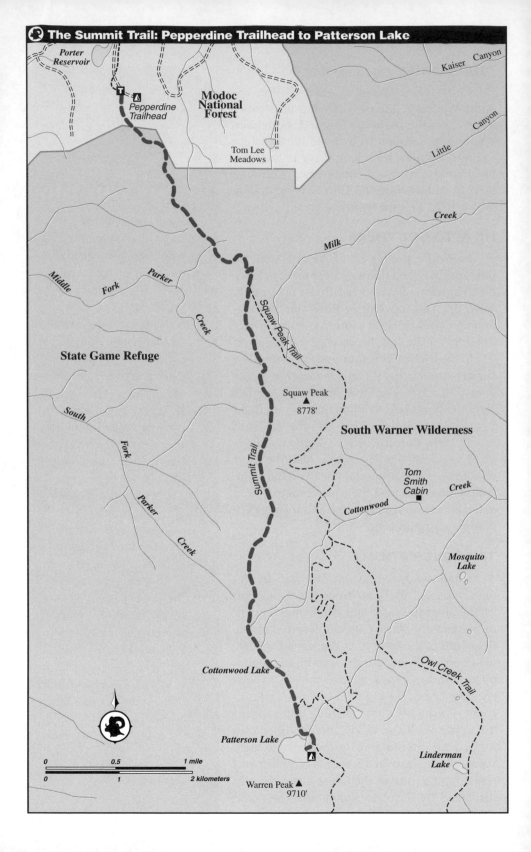

Porter
Reservoir

Kaiser Canyon

T

Pepperdine
Trailhead

**Modoc
National
Forest**

Little Canyon

Tom Lee
Meadows

Creek

Milk

Middle Fork Parker

Creek

Squaw Peak Trail

State Game Refuge

Squaw Peak
▲
8778'

South

Fork

South Warner Wilderness

Parker

Summit Trail

Tom
Smith
Cabin ■

Creek

Creek

Cottonwood

Mosquito
Lake

Cottonwood Lake

Owl Creek Trail

Patterson Lake

△

Linderman
Lake

0   0.5   1 mile
0   1   2 kilometers

Warren Peak ▲
9710'

lakes and the peaks of the Hays Canyon Range beyond. Gently rising tread, bordered by yellow-flowered mule ears in early season, takes you across mostly open terrain with a smattering of white fir and mountain mahogany before a stiffer climb leads to a view-packed, ridge-crest saddle and a junction shortly afterward with the Squaw Peak Trail, 2 miles from the trailhead.

Remaining on the Summit Trail, you climb moderately along the east side of the ridge, cross the crest to the other side, and then traverse the west face of Squaw Peak through very widely scattered whitebark pines. An ascent to the top of the 8778-foot summit is easily done via a half-mile, 400-foot ascent along the southwest ridge, where the top offers a nearly complete 360-degree panorama, with only the southernmost part of the range obscured behind Warren Peak and Devils Knob. From the end of the southwest ridge, you drop shortly into a saddle with fine eastward views down Cottonwood Creek canyon to the playa of Surprise Valley and then resume climbing along the spine of the narrow crest through wind-battered and prostrate mountain mahogany trees.

Just after the 4.5-mile mark, the trail veers away from the crest of the ridge and climbs toward Cottonwood Lake, passing above the fringe of some spring-fed meadows through light lodgepole pine forest. Despite a small and shallow stature, 8700-foot Cottonwood Lake offers the possibility of a less chilly swim

Scenic Patterson Lake lies below Warren Peak's rugged cliffs.

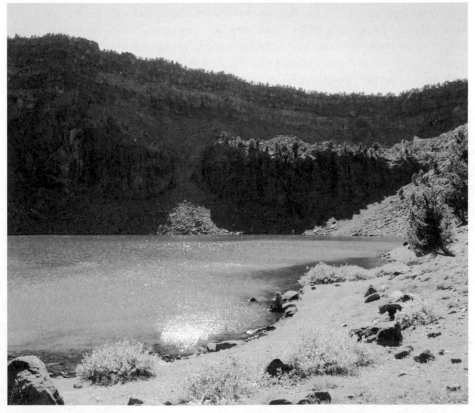

than the much deeper and colder lake ahead does, but campers will certainly want to push on to much more scenic campsites around Patterson Lake, especially if cows are present around Cottonwood Lake.

From Cottonwood Lake, climb steeply southeast for 0.3 mile to the southernmost junction of the Squaw Peak Trail, and then continue south a similar distance on a less steep grade to the northeast shore of Patterson Lake. The lake, 6 miles from the trailhead, sits in a deep, cirque rimmed with dark cliffs rising up to the summit of 9710-foot Warren Peak. Snow clings to crevices in the northeast-facing wall well into summer, intensifying the lake's rather chilly ambiance. A number of open campsites can be found on either side of the lake's outlet. Fishing is reported to be quite good. While camped at Patterson Lake, you may want to attempt the straightforward climb of Warren Peak by heading southbound on the Summit Trail for a short while to the east ridge and then following the ridge on an arcing route to the top.

When you're ready to head out the next day, retrace your steps to the trailhead. Although few backpackers are willing to accept the challenge, you could alter your return to the Pepperdine Trailhead by way of the Squaw Peak Trail; doing so requires a significant loss (2175 feet) and subsequent gain (1035 feet) in elevation over an extra 2.5 miles of hiking.

BUILD-UP AND WIND-DOWN TIPS ·

There are places to eat in Alturas, just not places to eat well. Fortunately, this small slice of Americana lacks the otherwise ubiquitous chains that make larger towns across the state into homogeneous and undistinguished replicas of themselves, but Alturas refuses to make up for this lack of franchise restaurants with any unique or memorable eateries or watering holes. A good option might be to stay overnight at the **Pepperdine Campground** before or after your backpack, where you could cook your own meals.

APPENDIX: TRIPS AT-A-GLANCE

TRIP NUMBER AND NAME	MILEAGE	DAYS	ELEVATION GAIN/LOSS
1 Noble Canyon Trail	10.0	2	650'/2400'
2 Horsethief Canyon	2.8	2	500'/500'
3 San Mateo Canyon	7.4	2	1300'/1300'
4 San Jacinto Peak	11.0	2	2600'/2600'
5 San Jacinto Loop	17.6	2–3	4500'/4500'
6 Art Smith Trail	16.0	2	3300'/3300'
7 San Gorgonio Mountain	15.6	2	5700'/5700'
8 San Bernardino Mountain Traverse	21.6	2–3	5500'/4500'
9 Holcomb Crossing Trail Camp Loop	5.6	2	900'/900'
10 Big Santa Anita Loop	9.4	2	2100'/2100'
11 Devils Canyon	5.4	2	2100'/2100'
12 East Fork San Gabriel River	14.5	2	200'/4800'
13 Point Mugu State Park Loop	23.2	2–3	5050'/5050'
14 Sykes Hot Springs	23.8	2–3	2380'/1490'
15 Black Cone Trail	30.2	3	2900'/2900'
16 Cone Peak Trail	10.2	2	3110'/3110'
17 Poverty Flat and Los Cruzeros Loop	13.9	2–3	2160'/2160'
18 Redfern Pond Loop	11.0	2	1352'/1352'
19 The Ohlone Wilderness Trail	19.5	3	6500'/6150'
20 Pescadero Creek Loop	28.0	3	5750'/5750'
21 Skyline to Big Basin	26.5	4	3550'/5150'

TYPE OF TRIP	DIFFICULTY	SOLITUDE	BEST SEASON
Point-to-point	Moderate	Moderately populated	Fall, winter, and spring
Out-and-back	Moderate	Moderate solitude	Winter and spring
Out-and-back	Moderate	Moderate solitude	Winter and spring
Out-and-back	Moderate	Moderately populated	Late spring, summer, and fall
Point-to-point or Loop	Moderate	Crowded	Summer through fall
Out-and-back	Moderate	Moderate solitude	Fall through early winter
Out-and-back	Moderately strenuous	Moderately populated	Late spring, summer, and fall
Point-to-point	Moderately strenuous	Moderately populated	Late spring, summer, and fall
Loop	Easy	Crowded	Spring and fall
Loop	Moderately strenuous	Moderately populated	Fall, winter, and spring
Out-and-back	Moderately strenuous	Moderate solitude	Fall, winter, and spring
Point-to-point	Moderately strenuous	Moderate solitude	Late spring, summer, and fall
Loop	Moderate	Crowded	Winter through spring
Out-and-back	Moderately strenuous	Crowded	Late spring through early fall
Out-and-back	Moderately strenuous	Solitude	Spring and fall
Out-and-back	Moderate	Moderate solitude	Spring and fall
Loop	Moderate	Moderate solitude to moderately populated	Spring and fall (depending on water)
Loop	Moderate	Moderate solitude to solitude	Spring and fall
Point-to-point	Moderately strenuous	Moderate solitude	Spring and fall
Loop	Moderate	Solitude	Year-round
Point-to-point	Moderate	Solitude	Year-round

TRIP NUMBER AND NAME	MILEAGE	DAYS	ELEVATION GAIN/LOSS
22 Skyline-to-the-Sea Trail	29.3	3	2500'/5100'
23 Coast Trail	14.6	2	2150'/1900'
24 Bear Valley Loop	15.8	2–3	2000'/2000'
25 Lost Coast Trail: Orchard Camp to Usal Camp	16.7	3	3800'/3800'
26 Lost Coast Trail: King Range Wilderness Loop	30.6	3–4	5800'/5800'
27 Canyon Creek Lakes and L Lake	16.5	2	4260'/4260'
28 North Fork Trinity River to Grizzly Lake	35.0	4–7	6925'/1775'
29 New River and Slide Creek to Historic Mining District and Eagle Creek	24.0	3–6	6875'/6875'
30 Deadfall Lakes, Mount Eddy, and the Sacramento Headwaters	12.2	2–3	1166'/4490'
31 Marble Rim via Sky High Lakes Basin	17.0	2	2800'/2800'
32 Shackleford to Campbell, Cliff, Summit, Little Elk, Deep, and Wrights Lakes Loop	32.0	4–6	8125'/8125'
33 Butler and Coyote Canyon Loop	18.0	2	2160'/2160'
34 Rockhouse Valley Loop	24.7	2–3	3650'/3650'
35 Marble Canyon to Cottonwood Canyon Loop	26.5	3	3750'/3750'
36 Surprise Canyon	24.0	4	9600'/8350'
37 Ubehebe Country Loop	23.0	3	4900'/4900'
38 Black Canyon	10.6	2	2300'/2300'
39 Cottonwood Basin Loop	9.4	2	1600'/1600'

TYPE OF TRIP	DIFFICULTY	SOLITUDE	BEST SEASON
Point-to-point	Moderate	Moderately populated	Spring and fall
Point-to-point	Moderate	Crowded	Spring and fall
Loop	Moderate	Crowded	Spring and fall
Point-to-point	Moderately strenuous	Moderate solitude	Spring and fall
Loop	Strenuous	Moderate solitude	Spring and fall
Out-and-back	Moderately strenuous	Moderately populated	Summer through early fall
Out-and-back	Moderately strenuous	Moderate solitude	Summer through early fall
Semiloop	Moderate	Solitude	Late spring and throughout fall
Point-to-point	Moderately strenuous	Moderately populated	Summer and early fall
Out-and-back	Moderate	Moderate solitude	Summer
Loop	Moderately strenuous	Solitude	Summer through fall
Loop	Moderately strenuous	Moderate solitude	Winter through spring
Loop	Strenuous	Solitude	Winter through spring
Loop	Moderately strenuous	Solitude	Spring and fall
Point-to-point or Out-and-back	Moderately strenuous	Solitude	Spring and fall
Loop	Moderately strenuous	Solitude	Spring and fall
Out-and-back	Moderately strenuous	Solitude	Spring and fall
Loop	Moderate	Moderate solitude	Summer

TRIP NUMBER AND NAME	MILEAGE	DAYS	ELEVATION GAIN/LOSS
40 Mineral King and Little Five Lakes Loop	40.5	5–7	10,710'/10,710'
41 Crescent Meadow to Whitney Portal via the High Sierra Trail	68.5	8–14	13,350'/11,850'
42 Lodgepole Campground to Deadman Canyon Loop	52.0	6–12	14,000'/14,000'
43 Rae Lakes Loop	39.0	4–7	3880'/3880'
44 Cottonwood Lakes to Upper Rock Creek Loop	27.0	4–7	4550'/4550'
45 Horseshoe Meadow to Whitney Portal	36.0	5–7	7405'/8885'
46 South Lake to North Lake	56.5	5–7	9240'/9790'
47 North Lake to Humphreys Basin Loop	27.0	4–6	5150'/5150'
48 North Fork Big Pine Creek Loop	16.0	3	3600'/3600'
49 Agnew Meadows to Devils Postpile	24.0	4–6	4360'/5120'
50 Lillian Lake Loop	12.6	2–3	2440'/2440'
51 Happy Isles to Half Dome	15.7	2	5400'/5400'
52 Happy Isles to Merced Lake	27.3	3	4670'/4670'
53 Glen Aulin and Waterwheel Falls	18.6	3	5210'/5210'
54 High Sierra Camps Loop, Northwest Part	17.6	3	2620'/3000'
55 High Sierra Camps Loop, Southeast Part	32.5	4	5930'/5550'
56 Tuolumne Meadows to Emeric Lake	21.0	2–3	2860'/2860'
57 Virginia Lakes Basin to Green Creek	11.9	2	1720'/3550'

TYPE OF TRIP	DIFFICULTY	SOLITUDE	BEST SEASON
Loop	Strenuous	Moderately populated	Late summer through early fall
Point-to-point	Strenuous	Moderately populated	Late summer through early fall
Loop	Strenuous	Moderate solitude	Late summer through early fall
Loop	Moderately strenuous	Moderately populated	Late summer through early fall
Loop or Point-to-point	Moderate	Moderate solitude	Late summer through early fall
Point-to-point	Moderately strenuous	Moderately populated	Late summer through early fall
Point-to-point	Strenuous	Moderately populated	Late summer through early fall
Loop	Strenuous	Moderately populated	Late summer through early fall
Loop	Moderately strenuous	Crowded	Summer
Point-to-point	Strenuous	Crowded	Late summer through early fall
Semiloop	Easy	Moderately populated	Midsummer
Semiloop	Strenuous	Crowded	Summer
Semiloop	Moderate	Moderately populated	Midsummer
Out-and-back	Moderate	Moderately populated	Early to midsummer
Point-to-point	Moderate	Moderately populated	Early to midsummer
Point-to-point	Moderately strenuous	Moderately populated	Midsummer
Out-and-back	Moderate	Moderate solitude	Midsummer
Point-to-point	Moderate	Moderate solitude	Midsummer

	TRIP NUMBER AND NAME	MILEAGE	DAYS	ELEVATION GAIN/LOSS
58	Kerrick Canyon and Matterhorn Canyon Loop via Barney and Peeler Lakes	53.6	5–7	9300'/9300'
59	County Line Trail to Sword and Lost Lakes	6.0	2	1510'/1510'
60	Pacific Grade Summit to Bull Run Lake	7.6	2	1970'/1970'
61	Glen Alpine to Half Moon Lake	10.0	2	1480'/1480'
62	Velma, Fontanillis, and Dicks Lakes	11.5	2	2300'/2300'
63	Meeks Bay to Emerald Bay	17.8	2	3690'/3350'
64	Tahoe Rim Trail: Showers Lake	15.3	2	1485'
65	Tahoe Rim Trail: Star Lake and Freel Peak	13.6	2–3	2100'/2100'
66	Little Jamison Canyon to Grass, Rock, Jamison, and Wades Lake	7.5	2	2090'/2050'
67	Bucks Lake Wilderness Loop	21.4	3–4	4500'/4500'
68	Summit Lake to Cluster, Twin, Rainbow, Snag, Horseshoe, and Swan Lakes Loop	22.0	2–4	2500'/2500'
69	Central Caribou Lakes Loop	12.0	2	900'/900'
70	Treeline Circumnavigation of Mount Shasta	25.0–30.0	5–7	2500'/2500'
71	The Summit Trail: Pepperdine Trailhead to Patterson Lake	12.0	2	2400'/2400'

TYPE OF TRIP	DIFFICULTY	SOLITUDE	BEST SEASON
Semiloop	Moderately strenuous	Moderately populated	Late summer through early fall
Out-and-back	Easy	Moderately populated	Summer
Out-and-back	Easy	Moderately populated	Midsummer
Point-to-point	Easy	Moderately populated	Summer through early fall
Out-and-back	Moderate	Moderately populated	Summer through early fall
Point-to-point	Moderate	Moderately populated	Summer through early fall
Point-to-point	Moderate	Moderately populated to moderate solitude	Summer through fall
Out-and-back	Moderate to moderately strenuous	Moderately populated to moderate solitude	Summer through fall
Semiloop	Easy	Moderately populated	Summer through early fall
Loop	Moderate	Solitude	Summer through early fall
Loop	Easy	Moderate solitude	Summer through early fall
Loop	Easy	Moderately populated	Summer through early fall
Loop	Moderately strenuous	Solitude	Summer through early fall
Out-and-back	Moderate	Moderate solitude	Summer through fall

INDEX

ABOUT THE CONTRIBUTORS

DOUG CHRISTIANSEN grew up in Arcadia, California, near the base of the San Gabriel Mountains, and has been an avid hiker for most of his life. Co-author, with John Robinson, of *Trail of the Angeles*, Doug makes his home near the mountains in Sierra Madre. When he is not hiking or spending time with his family, Doug travels throughout North America as a pilot for a major airline.

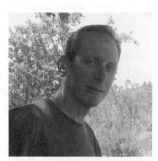

MICHEL DIGONNET is a physicist at Stanford University, where he teaches and carries out research on various aspects of light. Born and raised in Paris, France, he has explored many of the world's deserts, from eastern Africa to the Sahara and Baja California. He has hiked and backpacked extensively throughout the American West for nearly 30 years, especially on the Colorado Plateau and in the Mojave Desert. He is the author of *Hiking Death Valley*.

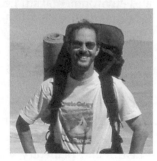

DAVID MONEY HARRIS began backpacking the Desolation Wilderness as a toddler in his father's pack. His books include the 6th edition of *San Bernardino Mountain Trails* and four textbooks on integrated circuit design. He is a professor of engineering at Harvey Mudd College. David can usually be found roaming the mountains of Southern California with his own toddler on weekends, scouting trails for a new guidebook.

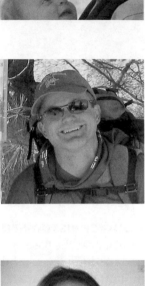

TIM HAUSERMAN leads hiking trips at Lake Tahoe, Yosemite, Death Valley, and the California Coast for Tahoe Trips and Trails. He is the author of *The Tahoe Rim Trail: A Complete Guide for Hikers, Mountain Bikers, and Equestrians* published by Wilderness Press; *Monsters in the Woods: Backpacking with Children;* and *Cross-Country Skiing in the Sierra Nevada.* In the winter he teaches cross-country skiing. His home base for backpacking adventures with his two daughters is the west shore of Lake Tahoe.

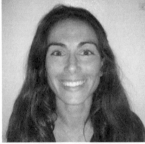

ANALISE ELLIOT HEID is an avid hiker, surfer, bird-watcher, and backpacker. She holds a bachelor's degree in forestry from the University of California, Berkeley and has worked as a naturalist, environmental educator, and outdoor education program director along the California coast and in the Sierra Nevada. She currently directs a nature and environmental studies program at Greenwood School in Mill Valley, California. Analise is the author of *Hiking and Backpacking Big Sur* and a contributor to *Sierra South*.

MATT HEID is the author of *101 Hikes in Northern California* and *Camping & Backpacking the San Francisco Bay Area.* He holds a bachelor's degree in earth and planetary science from Harvard University and currently resides in Anchorage, Alaska, where he is pursuing a passion for remote wilderness adventure.

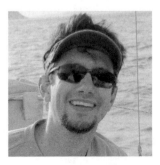

LOWELL and **DIANA LINDSAY** began backpacking together in the early 1960s as members of the UCLA Bruin Mountaineers. Anza-Borrego Desert State Park became their focus when Lowell was assigned to San Diego as a Navy helicopter pilot in 1966. He became aware of the Anza-Borrego area while on training flights over the area. The park then became part of Diana's study at San Diego State University as the subject of her master's thesis. In 1978 Wilderness Press published the first edition of *Anza-Borrego Desert Region*, now in its fifth edition. Other award-winning books on this desert area authored, coauthored, or edited by the Lindsays followed, including *Our Historic Desert*; *Geology of Anza-Borrego: Edge of Creation*; *Anza-Borrego A to Z: People, Places, and Things*; *Marshal South and the Ghost Mountain Chronicles*; and *Fossil Treasures of the Anza-Borrego Desert* (2007 winner of the PMA Ben Franklin Award in Science and Environment).

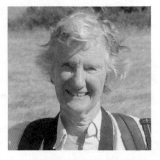

JEAN RUSMORE took her first backpacking trip at age 16 on Mt. Wilson in the San Gabriel Mountains with some food and a jacket rolled up in a blanket. Her outdoor experience was enlarged through her husband, Ted, whom she met at the University of California, Berkeley. They skied and backpacked with their six children, and all looked forward to their annual Sierra backpacking trip. She has long lived in the San Francisco Bay Area and written about its green spaces. She is the author of *Peninsula Trails*, *South Bay Trails*, and *Bay Area Ridge Trail*.

JERRY SCHAD is the author of 11 books on outdoor recreation in Southern California, and is a recognized expert on its trails. A fifth-generation Californian born in the Bay Area, Schad moved to San Diego County in 1972, and has remained there ever since. He is a professor of physical science and astronomy at San Diego Mesa College, and writes newspaper columns on topics of local interest for the *San Diego Reader*. Schad is an accomplished stock photographer with over 1500 photo credits in publications throughout the world. For Wilderness Press, he is the author of *Afoot & Afield San Diego County, Afoot & Afield Orange County, Afoot & Afield in Los Angeles County, 101 Hikes in Southern California, Trail Runner's Guide: San Diego*, and *Top Trails Los Angeles*.

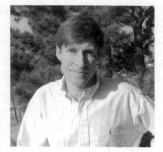

After 10 years of hiking, **JEFFREY P. SCHAFFER** began work in 1972 on his first Wilderness Press guidebook. Between then and the late 1980s, he wrote 12 guidebooks, mapped about 4000 miles of trail for them, and updated several U.S. Geological Survey 15-minute topographic maps. From 1990 onward he has engaged in serious fieldwork on Sierran uplift and glaciations. He started rock climbing in 1963 and still climbs today. He lives in Napa and teaches at three community colleges.

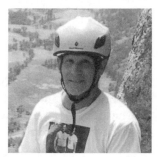

For Wilderness Press, he has written many books over the years: *Hiker's Guide to the High Sierra: Tuolumne Meadows, Hiker's Guide to the High Sierra: Sonora Pass, Carson-Iceberg Wilderness*, and *Crater Lake National Park and Vicinity*, all of which are out of print. He is also the author or coauthor of *Desolation Wilderness and the South Lake Tahoe Basin; The Geomorphic Evolution of the Yosemite Valley and Sierra Nevada Landscapes; Hiker's Guide to the High Sierra: Yosemite; Pacific Crest Trail: Northern California; Pacific Crest Trail: Oregon and Washington; Pacific Crest Trail: Southern California; The Tahoe Sierra;* and *Yosemite National Park*.

BEN SCHIFRIN began backpacking, sans parents, in Emigrant Wilderness and Yosemite National Park at age 12. He thru-hiked the Pacific Crest Trail in 1973. Mountaineering trips have taken him to most of the world's major mountain ranges. He is the author of *Emigrant Wilderness and Northwestern Yosemite* and coauthor of *Pacific Crest Trail: Southern California*.

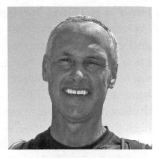

ANDY SELTERS started backpacking from his hometown of Los Angeles when he was in high school. He spent a summer as the custodian of the Sierra Club hut on Mt. Shasta, and at 19 he took up climbing. Andy worked for many years as a climbing guide and instructor, leading climbs from Alaska to Nepal, for the American Alpine Institute. Gradually he developed other mountain interests, including photography and studying the cultures of the Himalayas. He is the author or coauthor of *The Mt. Shasta Book: A Guide to Hiking, Climbing, Skiing, and Exploring the Mountain and Surrounding Area* and *Pacific Crest Trail: Oregon and Washington* and has gathered data for numerous maps.

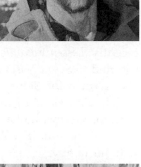

From childhood, **ELIZABETH WENK** has hiked and climbed with her family. Since 1995 Lizzy has spent most summers living in Bishop, a gateway to the Sierra Nevada and the White and Inyo Mountains. There, she has worked as a research assistant and completed her Ph.D. thesis research on the effects of rock type on alpine plant distribution and physiology. But much of the time, she hikes simply for leisure, continually exploring the backcountry. Since 2005 she, her husband, Douglas, and daughter, Eleanor, have been year-round Bishop residents, where she teaches biology at Cerro Coso Community College.

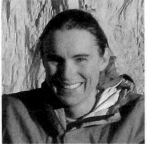

MIKE WHITE was born and raised in Portland, Oregon in the shadow of Mt. Hood. He learned to hike and climb in the nearby Cascade Range, honing his outdoor skills while earning a B.A. in political science at Seattle Pacific University. After college, Mike and his wife, Robin, were drawn to the beautiful and sunny Sierra and so they relocated to the high desert near Reno, Nevada.

In the early 1990s Mike began writing about the outdoors full time, expanding *The Trinity Alps* for Wilderness Press and then authoring his first solo guide, *Nevada Wilderness Areas and Great Basin National Park*. His subsequent books for Wilderness Press include *Snowshoe Trails of Yosemite, Snowshoe Trails Tahoe, Best Snowshoe Trails of California, Sequoia National Park, Kings Canyon National Park, Backpacking Nevada, Afoot & Afield Reno-Tahoe, 50 Classic Hikes in Nevada, Top Trails Lake Tahoe*, which won a Benjamin Franklin award in 2005, and, most recently, *Lassen Volcanic National Park*. He has contributed to *Sierra North* and *Sierra South*. Mike has also written for *Sunset* and *Backpacker* magazines and the *Reno Gazette Journal*. A featured speaker for outdoor groups, he has taught outdoor classes at his local community college. Mike resides in Reno with his family.

California native **MICHAEL ZANGER** has been hooked on the mountains ever since a family trip to Yosemite when he was five. He founded Shasta Mountain Guides in the mid-1970s, and has lived at the foot of Mt. Shasta for nearly 40 years. Beyond Mt. Shasta, Michael has participated in climbs and expeditions in North and South America, Europe, Africa, and Asia. He is the author of *Mt. Shasta: History, Legend, and Lore* and coauthor of *The Mt. Shasta Book: A Guide to Hiking, Climbing, Skiing, and Exploring the Mountain and Surrounding Area*.

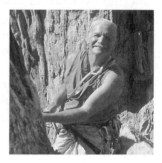